MW00882986

Over 350 Barbara O'Neill Inspired Herbal Healing Home Remedies & Natural Medicine.

Volume 1 & 2

Over 350 Barbara O'Neill Inspired Herbal Healing Home Remedies & Natural Medicine.

Volume 1

A Better You Everyday Publications
Email: info@abetteryoueveryday.com

Disclaimer
The information provided in this book is for educational and informational purposes only and is not affiliated with, authorized, endorsed by, or in any way officially connected with Barbara O'Neill or her affiliates or subsidiaries. The use of Barbara O'Neill's name in this book is for explanatory, educational, and reference purposes only, to discuss and provide insight into the theories and practices she has publicized through her teachings and public appearances. The views and interpretations presented in this book solely reflect those of the author and have not been reviewed or approved by Barbara O'Neill or her representatives.

The content within this book is not intended as medical advice and should not be taken as such. The author, Margaret Willowbrook, is not a medical professional. This book should not replace consultation with a qualified healthcare professional. It is essential that before beginning any new health practice, you consult with your physician, especially if you have any pre-existing health conditions.

While every effort has been made to verify the information provided in this book, the field of natural health is dynamic, and as such, the content may not reflect the most recent research or medical consensus. The author and publisher assume no responsibility for errors, omissions, or contrary interpretations of the subject matter herein.

Readers are encouraged to confirm the information contained within this publication through independent research and professional advice. Any perceived slights of specific people or organizations are unintentional. By reading this book, you agree that the author and publisher are not responsible for the success or failure of your health decisions related to any information presented.

A Better You Everyday Publications
email address info@abetteryoueveryday.com

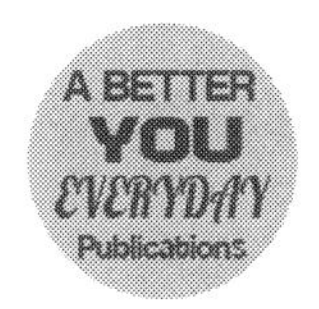

www.abetteryoueveryday.com

Printed or published to the highest ethical standard.

Over 350 Barbara O 'Neill Inspired Herbal Healing Home Remedies & Natural Medicine

Holistic Approach to Organic Health, Natural Cures and Nutrition for Sustaining Body and Mind Healing

Volume 1

By Margaret Willowbrook

USA
2024

CONTENTS

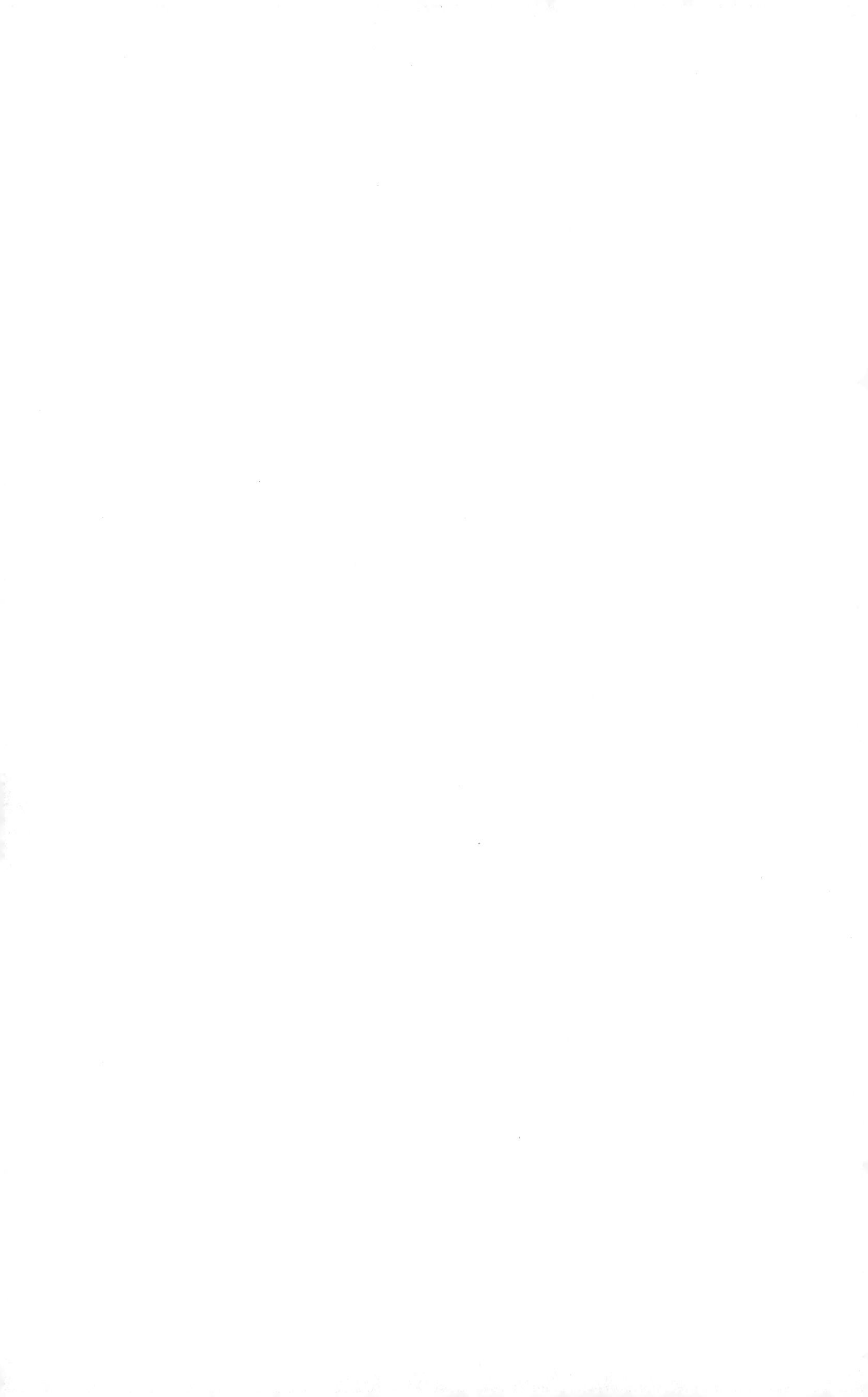

Glimpse into the Chapters Ahead

Embark on a transformative journey with Margaret Willowbrook as she delves into the holistic practices of herbal medicine, inspired by the teachings of Barbara O'Neill. This book goes beyond mere recipes and remedies—it reconnects us with the profound healing powers of nature, echoing the principles advocated by O'Neill. Margaret's tale begins with a personal anecdote about how a simple herbal remedy profoundly alleviated a chronic condition, setting the stage for a deep exploration into the art and science of herbal healing.

Chapter 1: Foundations of Herbal Medicine
Explore the core principles of herbal medicine as taught by Barbara O'Neill. Margaret introduces the subject with an engaging real-life story that highlights the power of herbs. This chapter covers the identification, benefits, and preparation methods of various herbs, offering a comprehensive entry into the ancient wisdom of natural healing.

Chapter 2: Herbal Safety and Contraindications
Understanding the safety and potential interactions of herbs is crucial. This chapter outlines O'Neill's safety protocols, discusses the potential side effects and interactions of various herbs, and details special precautions for different conditions and medications, ensuring readers are well-informed about the risks and benefits.

Chapter 3: Basic Herbal Preparations & Dosages
Dive into practical guidance on preparing and dosing herbal remedies. Margaret shares insights into the preparation techniques, dosage recommendations, and frequency of use as advised by O'Neill, emphasizing the application of these remedies in everyday life.

Chapter 4: Specialized Herbal Plans and Formulations
This chapter focuses on creating tailored herbal treatments for specific conditions. It includes interactive elements that encourage readers to personalize these treatments, enhancing the therapeutic effects of the herbs.

Chapter 5: Herbal Detoxification and Cleansing
Learn about the methods and routines for effective herbal detoxification. Margaret explains the significance of detox processes in holistic practices and provides actionable steps for safely implementing these routines.

Chapter 6: Women's and Men's Health
Address gender-specific health concerns using herbal remedies. This chapter explores herbal solutions for hormonal balance and reproductive health, supported by real-life success stories that illustrate the effectiveness of these treatments.

Chapter 7: Children's Herbal Remedies
Margaret offers guidance on formulating safe and effective herbal remedies for children. This chapter discusses how to adjust dosages for young ones and tackles common misconceptions about pediatric herbal care.

Chapter 8: Mental and Emotional Well-being
Focusing on mental health, this chapter presents herbs and lifestyle strategies for stress relief and overall mental well-being. It includes reflective exercises to help readers apply these strategies to their personal health scenarios.

Chapter 9: Seasonal Herbal Remedies
Adapt your herbal practices to the changing seasons. This chapter provides tips on modifying herbal treatments to align with seasonal needs, enhancing the natural rhythm of wellness.

Chapter 10: Incorporating Herbs into Daily Life
Discover practical ways to integrate herbs into your daily routine for enhanced wellness. Margaret provides a plan for readers to begin using herbs daily, emphasizing the lifestyle recommendations of O'Neill.

Chapter 11: Sustainable and Ethical Sourcing of Herbs
Focus on the sustainability and ethical considerations of sourcing herbs. This chapter includes discussions on the environmental impacts of herbal practice and the importance of supporting local communities.

Chapter 12: Herbal Preparation, Sourcing, Preservation, and Storage
Learn techniques for preserving and storing herbs to maintain their potency and effectiveness. This chapter provides practical tips and exercises for implementing these techniques effectively.

Chapter 13: Herbal First Aid Kit
Construct a basic herbal first aid kit for immediate needs. This chapter serves as a quick reference guide for emergency herbal treatments, coupled with a compelling narrative on the importance of being prepared.

Chapter 14: Empowering Yourself through Herbal Knowledge

Equip yourself with tools and resources for lifelong learning in herbal medicine. This chapter encourages further exploration and application of herbal knowledge, reflecting O'Neill's dedication to education.

Conclusion of the Book

Margaret Willowbrook concludes with a summation of Barbara O'Neill's teachings, inspiring readers to embrace the healing power of nature. Her final reflections draw on the wisdom gleaned from O'Neill, leaving readers empowered on their journey to natural health.

Last Words

The book concludes with a robust chapter offering over 300 detailed recipes for treating common conditions, inspired by O'Neill's remedies, making it an essential resource for anyone interested in herbal medicine.

References

Attetion!

Before you dive into this captivating book, we have an exclusive offer just for you! A fantastic FREE Bonus:

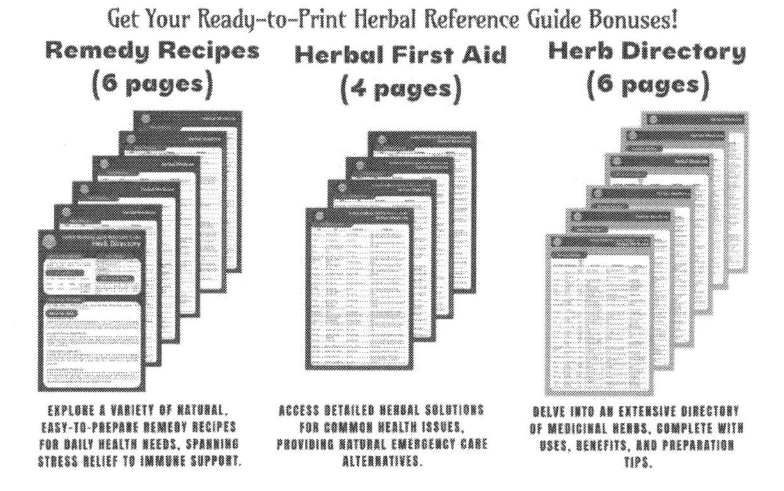

These printable guides, crafted after extensive research and dedication, offer quick, easy access to a wealth of herbal remedies, recipes, and first aid information. Designed for fast reference, they cover everything from specific herbs in our 'Herb Directory', to swift recipes in 'Remedy Recipes', and practical emergency care in 'Herbal First Aid'. Though we plan to sell them separately in the future, we're currently offering these guides for free as our appreciation for your book purchase, as a way of saying thank you and adding extra value to your reading experience.

For instant delivery, simply chat with our Facebook bot via the link below or scan the accompanying QR code.

http://tinyurl.com/Herbalbonuses

Alternatively, you can request the guides by emailing us at: info@abetteryoueveryday.com.
Enjoy your reading and these additional resources!

FOREWORD

My dear readers,

As you gently open the pages of "Over 350 Barbara O'Neill Inspired Herbal Healing Home Remedies & Natural Medicine," please know that you are not just launching into a book, but embarking on a journey very dear to my heart. This book, lovingly assembled, is not merely a compendium of herbal remedies; it is a vessel carrying the profound essence of nature's healing wisdom, a wisdom that has graced my life and which I now share with you.

My journey into the world of natural remedies began many years ago, under the quiet, watchful eyes of the towering trees and whispering herbs in my garden. Like many of you, I was once reliant on the quick fixes and promises of modern medicine, seeking relief but finding only temporary solace. It was in nature's embrace that I found true healing, not just for the body, but for the soul as well.

Barbara O'Neill's teachings were a revelation to me. Her approach to health and wellness, deeply rooted in the natural world, resonated with my own beliefs and experiences. She taught not just about herbs and their uses, but about a way of life; a life where one is in sync with the rhythms of nature, respectful of the body's innate wisdom, and mindful of the holistic nature of wellbeing. This book is my humble attempt to bring her teachings to a wider audience, woven together with my personal narrative and understanding.

Brought to light by these teachings, this book is my humble offering to you. I do not proclaim myself a specialist; rather, I see myself as a fellow traveler on the path to understanding the bounty of nature. It is my deepest hope that the wisdom shared here, a blend of Barbara's teachings and my own learning, will guide and comfort you as it has meAs we journey together through these pages, I invite you to join me with an open heart and mind. Embrace the possibilities nature unfolds, and let each piece of advice be a step towards better health and a deeper harmony with the world around us.

Learn the Role of Nature in Healing

In our fast-paced, technology-driven world, we often find ourselves disconnected from the natural environment. This disconnection can manifest in various forms of physical and mental health issues. By reconnecting with nature, not only do we find solace and peace, but we also tap into a powerful source of healing.

This book encourages you to view nature not just as a resource for ingredients but as a partner in healing. The plants, herbs, and natural elements around us are not mere commodities; they are part of a larger ecosystem to which we belong and with which we can interact to promote health and harmony.

The Importance of a Personalized Approach

Just as each plant has its unique properties and uses, each individual has unique health needs and conditions. This book aims to provide you with the knowledge and tools to understand how to select and use herbal remedies in a way that is most beneficial for your personal health.

In addition, the book addresses the importance of considering various factors such as lifestyle, diet, and emotional well-being when using herbal remedies. It's not just about treating symptoms; it's about addressing the root causes of health issues and fostering an overall state of well-being.

Finally, I must ask for your kindness and understanding as you read. This book, a labor of love, is my first attempt to collate the wealth of knowledge I've encountered. If you find any errors or have suggestions, I warmly welcome your feedback. Your insights will be invaluable in making this a living, evolving guide.

As we conclude this introduction, I want to thank you for choosing to embark on this journey with me. My hope is that "Over 350 Barbara O'Neill Inspired Herbal Healing Home Remedies & Natural Medicine." becomes more than just a book on your shelf; that it becomes a companion on your path to wellness, a source of comfort, and a testament to the incredible healing power of nature.

With all my warmth and kindness,

Margaret Willowbrook

Important information! Why Our Book Does Not Include colored Herb Photos!

Consideration for Cost and Accessibility:

In our commitment to keeping the book affordable, we consciously decided against including color herb photos. This decision directly impacts and lowers the printing costs, making the book more accessible to a broader range of readers. Our priority is to provide comprehensive herbal knowledge at a reasonable price.

Emphasizing the Role of Visual Aids:

Understanding the importance of visual identification in herbal studies, especially for newcomers and in recipe preparation, we recommend for detailed herb images.

https://myplantin.com/plant-identifier/herb

This online resource complements our book perfectly, enabling accurate herb identification and enhancing your herbal learning experience.

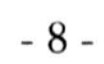

CHAPTER 1: FOUNDATIONS OF HERBAL MEDICINE

This chapter, dedicated to the foundations of herbal medicine, is not merely an introduction to various herbs and their properties. It is a gateway to understanding the profound relationship between humans and the healing powers of the natural world. Herbal medicine, with its ancient roots and modern relevance, offers a unique perspective on health and wellness, emphasizing a harmonious balance between our bodies and the natural environment.

The Historical Context of Herbal Medicine

Herbal medicine is as ancient as humanity itself. From the dawn of civilization, humans have looked to plants and herbs for healing. This traditional knowledge, passed down through generations, forms the bedrock of many contemporary herbal practices. It is a rich tapestry of wisdom, encompassing a deep understanding of the natural properties of plants and their impact on the human body.

This historical perspective is crucial to appreciate fully the value of herbal medicine in our modern context. It provides a lens through which we can view herbal medicine not as a collection of remedies but as a holistic approach to health that has stood the test of time. This historical understanding also highlights the importance of preserving and respecting this ancient knowledge, ensuring its survival and relevance for future generations.

Understanding the Principles of Herbal Medicine

Herbal medicine is grounded in several core principles that guide its practice. Firstly, it is based on the understanding that every plant possesses unique properties that can be harnessed for healing purposes. These properties, ranging from the physical to the energetic, interact with the human body in complex ways.

Additionally, herbal medicine is inherently personalized. It recognizes that each individual has unique health needs and responds differently to various herbs and treatments. This personalized approach is a key differentiator of herbal medicine, allowing for treatments that are tailored to the individual's specific conditions and constitution.

Another fundamental principle is the holistic nature of herbal medicine. Unlike conventional medicine, which often focuses on treating specific symptoms, herbal medicine looks at the individual as a whole. This holistic approach takes into account not only physical symptoms but also emotional, mental, and spiritual well-being.

The Role of Herbs in Human Health

Herbs play a multifaceted role in human health. They are not only used for treating illnesses but also for preventing disease, maintaining wellness, and enhancing physical, mental, and emotional well-being. Herbs can be powerful allies in managing chronic conditions, supporting the body's natural healing processes, and promoting overall health and longevity.

To fully appreciate the role of herbs, one must understand their properties and how they interact with the human body. Each herb contains a unique combination of active compounds that impart specific therapeutic effects. These compounds can work synergistically, enhancing each other's effects, or they can be used individually to target specific health concerns.

The Art and Science of Herbal Medicine

Herbal medicine is both an art and a science. As a science, it requires a deep understanding of botany, chemistry, and human physiology. It involves studying the active constituents of plants, understanding their mechanisms of action, and researching their effects on the human body.

As an art, herbal medicine involves more than just knowledge of herbs and their properties; it requires intuition, wisdom, and a deep connection with the natural world. It also involves understanding the subtle nuances of herbal remedies, knowing how to combine herbs synergistically, and tailoring treatments to the unique needs of each individual.

Cultivating a Relationship with Plants

A key aspect of herbal medicine is cultivating a relationship with plants. This involves more than just using plants for their medicinal properties; it involves developing a deep respect and reverence for them. It's about understanding that plants are living beings with their own energies and spirits and learning to communicate with them.

This relationship with plants is central to the practice of herbal medicine. It involves spending time in nature, observing plants in their natural habitats, and learning to listen to what they have to teach us. This connection with plants enriches the practice of herbal medicine, making it a deeply fulfilling and transformative experience.

One of the most profound aspects of O'Neill's teachings is the deep connection with nature. She advocates for a relationship with the natural world that is based on respect, reverence, and reciprocity. This connection is not just about using nature's resources for our benefit but about understanding our place within the natural ecosystem and our responsibility to care for it.

O'Neill encourages practitioners and students of herbal medicine to spend time in nature, observing and learning from the plants. This immersive experience is seen as essential for developing a deep, intuitive understanding of herbal medicine.

Herbal Medicine in the Modern World

In our modern world, where technology and pharmaceuticals dominate the healthcare landscape, herbal medicine offers a refreshing and vital alternative. It provides a way to reconnect with the natural world, to take control of our health, and to treat our bodies with the respect and care they deserve.

However, integrating herbal medicine into our modern lives requires a thoughtful and informed approach. It involves learning to discern credible information from misinformation, understanding the limitations and risks of herbal remedies, and knowing when to seek professional guidance.

Exploring Herbal Healing Principles

In this exploration of the principles of herbal healing, we immerse ourselves into a world where nature is the healer and we are its willing apprentices. O'Neill's teachings provide a comprehensive framework for understanding and applying the ancient wisdom of herbal medicine in our contemporary lives.

The Holistic Approach

This perspective views the human being not as a collection of separate parts to be treated in isolation but as an integrated whole. In this view, physical ailments are often manifestations of imbalances that could be emotional, spiritual, or environmental in nature. Herbal healing, therefore, is not just about addressing the physical symptoms of a condition but about nurturing the entire being; body, mind, and spirit.

The approach also underscores the importance of prevention over cure. O'Neill teaches that maintaining health is not merely about reacting to illness but about creating a lifestyle that supports overall well-being. This encompasses a balanced diet, regular physical activity, mental and emotional wellness practices, and a harmonious relationship with our environment.

The Synergy of Herbs

O'Neill's teachings emphasize the synergy of herbs, the idea that herbs of different kinds can work together in harmony to produce a more effective healing response than when used individually. This principle is rooted in the understanding that the compounds in herbs can complement and enhance each other's therapeutic effects. The art of creating herbal blends is a key aspect of her teachings, requiring a deep understanding of each herb's properties and how they interact with one another.

In line with this principle, O'Neill encourages practitioners to approach herbal blending with both scientific knowledge and intuitive understanding. This involves not only knowing the active constituents of herbs and their medicinal properties but also understanding the energetic qualities of herbs and how they can harmonize to address the specific needs of an individual.

Understanding the Energetics of Herbs

A unique aspect of O'Neill's approach to herbal healing is the emphasis on the energetics of herbs. This concept goes beyond the biochemical properties of plants to include their energetic qualities, such as warming, cooling, drying, and moistening. These qualities are considered in relation to the individual's constitution and the nature of their condition.

For instance, a person with a naturally warm and dry constitution experiencing inflammation (a hot and often dry condition) may benefit from herbs with cooling and moistening properties. This understanding of energetics allows for a more nuanced and personalized approach to herbal treatment.

The Empowerment of Self-Care

O'Neill's teachings centers on the empowerment of individuals in their health journey. She advocates for self-care and personal responsibility in health and wellness. This involves educating oneself about the principles of herbal medicine, understanding one's own body and its signals, and being proactive in maintaining health.

This empowerment is also about breaking free from the dependency on conventional medical systems and reclaiming the innate power of our bodies to heal. O'Neill teaches that with the right support, our bodies have an incredible capacity for self-healing and that herbs can be powerful allies in this process.

The Integration of Diet and Lifestyle

O'Neill's teachings integrate the use of herbs with dietary and lifestyle modifications. She emphasizes that herbs are most effective when used as part of a holistic approach to health that includes nutritious food, adequate rest, stress management, and regular physical activity.

In her view, diet is not just about nutrition; it's about nourishing the body and soul. It involves choosing foods that are natural, whole, and in alignment with our individual needs. Similarly, lifestyle choices are seen as important to maintaining health and preventing disease. This includes practices like mindfulness, meditation, and spending time in nature, all of which support overall well-being.

A Preview of Different Herb Categories and Their Healing Properties

Embarking on the exploration of various herbs and their healing properties opens us to a world where each leaf, root, and flower holds a story of healing and balance. This is the heart of herbal medicine, exploring the unique characteristics and uses of different herbs. These plants, revered by O'Neill for their medicinal properties, offer a natural pharmacy that can support our health in myriad ways.

The Healing Spectrum of Herbs

Each herb in nature's vast pharmacopeia brings its unique healing properties. O'Neill's teachings shed light on how these properties can be harnessed to address a wide range of health concerns, from the common cold to more complex chronic conditions. Understanding these properties requires not only an awareness of the active constituents of these herbs but also an appreciation for their roles in traditional and contemporary healing practices.

Adaptogenic Herbs for Stress and Balance

Adaptogens, a unique class of herbs, play a pivotal role in O'Neill's herbal repertoire. These herbs, including Ashwagandha, Rhodiola, and Holy basil, are known for their ability to help the body adapt to stress and restore balance. They work at a molecular level to moderate the stress response, enhancing resilience to physical, emotional, and environmental stressors.

Ashwagandha, for instance, has been revered for centuries in Ayurvedic medicine for its restorative and rejuvenating properties. It's known for its ability to support adrenal health, helping to mitigate the effects of stress and fatigue.

Herbs for Digestive Health

Digestive health is another area where O'Neill emphasizes the use of herbs. Herbs like Peppermint, Ginger, and Fennel are celebrated for their ability to soothe digestive discomfort, enhance nutrient absorption, and support gut health.

Peppermint, with its calming and antispasmodic properties, is particularly beneficial in relieving symptoms of indigestion and irritable bowel syndrome. Ginger, known for its warming and anti-inflammatory properties, can alleviate nausea and support healthy digestion.

Herbs for Immune Support

In the realm of immune support, O'Neill highlights the importance of herbs like Echinacea, Elderberry, and Astragalus. These herbs are renowned for their ability to bolster the body's defense mechanisms and enhance overall immunity.

Echinacea, for instance, is widely used for its immune-boosting properties, particularly in the prevention and treatment of colds and flu. Elderberry, rich in antioxidants, has a long history of use in supporting respiratory health.

Herbs for Cardiovascular Health

Cardiovascular health is also a key focus in these teachings. Herbs such as Hawthorn, Garlic, and Ginkgo biloba have been identified for their roles in supporting heart health and circulation. Hawthorn, for example, is known for its cardiotonic properties, improving heart function and promoting healthy circulation.

Herbal Nervines for Mental Well-being

O'Neill also places significance on herbs that support mental and emotional well-being, known as nervines. These include herbs like Lemon Balm, Lavender, and St. John's Wort. Lemon Balm, with its soothing properties, is used to alleviate anxiety and promote calmness. Lavender, renowned for its relaxing aroma, is widely used for stress relief and sleep support.

Herbs for Women's and Men's Health

These teachings also explore herbs specifically beneficial for women's and men's health. For women, herbs like Chaste tree (Vitex), Red raspberry Leaf, and Black Cohosh have been recognized for their efficacy in balancing hormones and addressing menstrual and menopausal issues.

In men's health, herbs such as Saw palmetto and Nettle Root are noted for their supportive role in prostate health and hormonal balance.

Culinary Herbs with Medicinal Properties

The healing power of herbs is not limited to those typically classified as medicinal; many culinary herbs also possess significant health benefits. Herbs like Turmeric, Cinnamon, and Rosemary, commonly used in cooking, are also powerful healers. Turmeric, with its active compound curcumin, is known for its potent anti-inflammatory and antioxidant properties.

The exploration of different herbs and their healing properties is a testament to the diversity and richness of nature's healing capabilities. These herbs, each with its unique profile of benefits, offer a comprehensive approach to health and wellness. They remind us of the interconnectedness of our health with the natural world and the immense potential that lies in understanding and utilizing these natural gifts responsibly and effectively. In the next section, we will further our research by examining the safe gathering and preparation techniques for these medicinal herbs, ensuring their benefits are harnessed to their fullest potential.

CHAPTER 2: HERBAL SAFETY AND CONTRAINDICATIONS

In herbal medicine, as in all forms of healing, the first principle is to do no harm. This chapter teaches the critical aspects of herbal safety and contraindications, an area often overshadowed by the allure of herbal remedies' benefits. Understanding these facets is essential for anyone venturing into the world of herbal medicine, whether as a practitioner, student, or consumer.

The Imperative of Safety in Herbal Medicine

The rising popularity of herbal remedies brings with it the need for a heightened awareness of their safe use. While herbs are natural, it is a misconception that they are inherently safe. Like any therapeutic intervention, they come with their own set of risks and benefits. Safety in herbal medicine involves understanding these risks, knowing how to minimize them, and recognizing when and how to use these remedies effectively.

Understanding Herbal Actions and Constituents

The safety of herbal remedies is deeply tied to their actions and constituents. Herbs contain a variety of active compounds, each with specific effects on the body. For instance, some herbs may have a sedative effect, while others may stimulate the nervous system. Understanding these actions is crucial in predicting how an herb might interact with the body, other herbs, or pharmaceutical medications.

The constituents of herbs, such as alkaloids, glycosides, and flavonoids, also play a significant role in their safety profile. These chemical compounds can have potent physiological effects, beneficial in some contexts and potentially harmful in others. An in-depth understanding of these constituents forms the basis for recognizing contraindications and potential adverse effects.

Identifying and Managing Allergic Reactions

One of the primary safety concerns in herbal medicine is the risk of allergic reactions. Just as with foods and other substances, individuals can have allergic reactions to certain herbs. These reactions can range from mild, such as rashes or itching, to severe, such as anaphylaxis. Identifying and managing these reactions is a vital aspect of safe herbal practice. This involves careful screening for allergies, monitoring for signs of reaction during herbal treatment, and having protocols in place to address any adverse reactions.

Contraindications and Special Populations

Certain populations require special consideration when it comes to herbal treatments. These include pregnant and breastfeeding women, children, the elderly, and individuals with specific health conditions, such as liver or kidney disease. For these groups, certain herbs may be contraindicated, or specific dosages may need to be adjusted. Understanding these contraindications is crucial to prevent harm and ensure the safe use of herbal remedies.

Further, the world of herbal medicine is vast and complex. Herbs, with their myriad of constituents, can interact with our bodies in multifaceted ways. These interactions are not always straightforward and can vary depending on individual factors such as age, genetics, overall health, and concurrent use of medications or other herbs.

This complexity demands a thoughtful and cautious approach to using herbs. It requires us to be diligent in our research and humble in our assertions. Recognizing that our understanding of herbs and their interactions is continually evolving, we must remain open to new information and be willing to adjust our practices accordingly.

Interactions with Pharmaceuticals

As herbal medicine often complements conventional treatments, understanding the potential interactions between herbs and pharmaceutical medications is crucial. Some herbs can potentiate or diminish the effects of certain drugs, leading to increased side effects or reduced therapeutic efficacy. This area of study requires not only a deep knowledge of herbal constituents but also an understanding of pharmacodynamics and pharmacokinetics.

The Importance of Dosage and Formulation

Dosage and formulation are key factors in the safety of herbal medicine. The therapeutic dose of an herb can vary widely depending on the individual, the condition being treated, and the specific herb or herbs being used.

Overdosing can lead to adverse effects, while underdosing may render the treatment ineffective.

The formulation of herbal remedies, including the method of preparation and the part of the plant used, also significantly impacts their safety and effectiveness. Each person's response to a particular herb can also be very unique and must be considered.

Factors like metabolic rate, digestive health, and even emotional state can influence how an individual responds to a herbal remedy. This individuality necessitates a personalized approach to herbal medicine, where remedies are tailored to the specific needs and conditions of the individual.

Reflecting on this individuality also highlights the importance of close observation and communication. Practitioners must be attentive to the responses of their clients and be prepared to modify treatments as necessary. Similarly, individuals using herbs must be attuned to their bodies and communicate any unexpected reactions to their healthcare providers.

Responsible Sourcing and Quality Control

The safety of herbal remedies is not only determined by their inherent properties and how they are used but also by the quality of the herbs themselves. Responsible sourcing and quality control are essential to ensure that herbs are free from contaminants such as pesticides, heavy metals, and adulterants. This includes understanding the origin of herbs, the conditions under which they were grown and harvested, and the processes used in their drying and storage.

The Role of Education and Awareness

A key theme in O'Neill's teachings is the importance of education and awareness in the safe use of herbal remedies. This involves not only educating practitioners and students but also consumers who choose to use these remedies. Increasing awareness about the potential risks, contraindications, and safe practices can empower individuals to make informed decisions about their use of herbal medicine.

This chapter on herbal safety and contraindications is a foundational element of responsible herbal practice. It stresses the need for a balanced approach to herbal medicine, one that respects its power to heal and acknowledges its potential risks. By deepening our understanding of these aspects, we can use herbal remedies not only effectively but safely, ensuring that the practice of herbal medicine continues to be a source of healing and wellbeing.

Reflective Segment on Understanding Herbal Safety

As we practice use of herbal medicine, it becomes imperative to pause and reflect on the concept of herbal safety. This reflective segment aims to deepen our understanding of what it truly means to use herbs safely. It's not merely about following guidelines or adhering to dosages; it's about cultivating a mindset and approach that respects the power of these natural entities and recognizes the intricate ways in which they interact with our bodies and our environment.

The Responsibility of Accurate Information

In an age where information is readily available but not always accurate, the responsibility of disseminating and obtaining correct information about herbal safety is paramount. Misinformation can lead to misuse of herbs, resulting in ineffective treatment or, worse, harm. This responsibility falls on practitioners, educators, and consumers alike.

For practitioners and educators, this means ensuring that the information they share is based on credible sources and is presented in a manner that is understandable and accessible to their audience. For consumers, it involves seeking out reliable information and being discerning about the sources they trust.

Practicing Mindfulness and Intuition

Mindfulness and intuition are invaluable tools in the practice of herbal safety. Being mindful means being fully present and aware during the preparation and use of herbal remedies. It involves paying attention to details, being conscious of the process, and being attuned to the response of the body.

Intuition, while often overlooked in the scientific discourse, plays a significant role in herbal medicine. It involves listening to the subtle cues of the body and the herbs, and trusting one's inner wisdom to guide the healing process. Developing this intuition requires time, experience, and a deep connection with both the self and the natural world.

Navigating the Challenges of Herbal Safety

Navigating the challenges of herbal safety requires a balance of knowledge, experience, and caution. It involves being proactive in learning and staying updated with the latest research while also being cautious in applying this knowledge. It requires being open to learning from mistakes and being willing to adapt and evolve.

Understanding herbal safety is a multifaceted and ongoing process. It involves a deep appreciation of the complexities of herbal interactions, the individuality of responses to herbs, the responsibility of providing and obtaining accurate information, and the importance of education.

Identifying Potential Side Effects and Interactions

In the field of herbal medicine, recognizing and understanding the potential side effects and interactions of herbs is as crucial as acknowledging their healing properties. This subchapter accentuates the vital aspect of identifying potential side effects and interactions associated with herbal remedies. This understanding is not just a precaution but a fundamental component of responsible herbal practice, ensuring that the path to healing remains safe and informed.

Comprehending the Scope of Side Effects

Herbal medicine is often marked by the allure of natural healing. However, it is essential to remember that 'natural' does not automatically imply 'without side effects.' Herbs, like any therapeutic agents, can cause adverse reactions in some individuals. These reactions can range from mild to severe and may manifest as allergies, digestive disturbances, headaches, or more significant complications depending on the individual and the herb in question.

Understanding the scope of these side effects involves more than just a cursory glance at a list of possible reactions. It requires a deep dive into the herb's pharmacology, understanding the mechanisms by which these effects occur.

Monitoring and Managing Side Effects

The proactive monitoring of side effects is a critical component of safe herbal practice. This involves being vigilant about observing any changes that occur after beginning an herbal regimen and being prepared to adjust or discontinue the use of the herb if necessary. It also includes educating individuals about the signs and symptoms to watch for and encouraging open communication about their experiences.

Managing side effects, when they do occur, requires much caution. Depending on the severity and nature of the reaction, this might involve reducing the dosage, changing the method of preparation, or discontinuing the herb altogether. In some cases, supportive treatments may be necessary to alleviate the side effects.

Herb-Drug Interactions: A Critical Consideration

In our modern healthcare landscape, where many individuals are on conventional medications, the potential for herb-drug interactions is a significant concern. These interactions can affect the metabolism of drugs, either increasing their potency and thereby enhancing their side effects or reducing their efficacy.

Navigating herb-drug interactions requires an understanding of pharmacokinetics and pharmacodynamics. It involves knowing how herbs can affect the absorption, distribution, metabolism, and excretion of drugs. O'Neill advocates for careful review and consideration of an individual's medication regimen before recommending or using herbal remedies.

The Importance of Comprehensive Health Assessment

A comprehensive health assessment is critical in identifying potential side effects and interactions. This assessment should include a detailed medical history, an understanding of the individual's current health status, and a thorough review of any medications or supplements they are taking.

This allows practitioners to make informed decisions about which herbs are appropriate and safe for each individual.

Special Precautions for Conditions and Medications

In the intricacy of herbal medicine, special precautions for certain conditions and medications form an essential thread. This aspect of herbal practice demands careful consideration and deep understanding. It involves acknowledging that while herbs offer immense healing potential, they must be used judiciously, especially in the presence of specific health conditions and medications.

Navigating Herbal Use in Chronic Conditions

When dealing with chronic conditions such as heart disease, diabetes, or kidney disorders, the use of herbal remedies requires careful consideration. O'Neill's teachings guide us to approach such scenarios with a blend of wisdom and caution. Herbs that may generally be safe for the average person can have different implications for someone with a chronic condition.

For example, in cardiovascular diseases, herbs that affect blood pressure or heart rate, like Hawthorn or Ginseng, must be used under professional guidance. Their interaction with heart medications or their impact on heart function demands careful monitoring.

In the context of diabetes, herbs that influence blood sugar levels, such as Gymnema or Fenugreek, require cautious use. Their potential to significantly lower blood sugar levels can be a concern, especially when used alongside conventional diabetes medications.

Herbal Use in Pregnancy and Lactation

The use of herbs during pregnancy and lactation is another area where O'Neill's teachings emphasize caution. Many herbs that are typically safe can have contraindications during pregnancy due to their potential to stimulate uterine contractions or affect hormone levels.

For example, herbs like Mugwort or Pennyroyal, while useful in certain contexts, are strongly contraindicated in pregnancy due to their potential to induce miscarriage. Similarly, during lactation, herbs that can be transferred through breast milk and impact the infant, such as Peppermint or Parsley, which can reduce milk supply, must be used with caution.

Age-Related Considerations in Herbal Medicine

O'Neill's approach to herbal safety also considers the age of the individual. Children and the elderly, for instance, have different physiological responses and sensitivities to herbs. In children, the liver and kidneys, responsible for metabolizing and excreting substances, are not fully developed. This factor necessitates lower dosages and the avoidance of certain potent herbs.

In the elderly, decreased liver and kidney function, along with the common presence of multiple medications, calls for a cautious approach. Herbs that may affect hydration levels or interact with medications commonly used by older adults need to be used judiciously.

Mental Health Conditions and Herbal Considerations

When it comes to mental health conditions, such as anxiety, depression, or insomnia, the use of herbs requires a nuanced understanding. While many herbs can support mental health, they can also interact with psychiatric medications.

Herbs like Valerian or Kava, used for their calming effects, may enhance the sedative effect of psychiatric drugs, leading to increased drowsiness or lethargy. Similarly, herbs with mood-enhancing properties should be used carefully in conjunction with antidepressants to avoid excessive serotonin levels, a condition known as serotonin syndrome.

The Complexity of Autoimmune Disorders

In autoimmune disorders, where the body's immune system attacks its tissues, the use of immunomodulating herbs needs careful consideration. Herbs that stimulate the immune system may exacerbate symptoms in autoimmune conditions, with Licorice or Echinacea root being some examples. Conversely, immunosuppressive herbs might offer relief but could also reduce the body's ability to fight infections.

The Impact of Herbs on Liver and Kidney Functions

For individuals with liver or kidney diseases, certain herbs can pose significant risks. Herbs metabolized through the liver or having hepatotoxic potential must be used with extreme caution in liver disorders. Further, alcohol extracts may not be suitable for those with liver problems Similarly, herbs that are diuretics or have high mineral content can strain the kidneys in kidney diseases.

Following special precautions for specific conditions and medications is a cornerstone of safe and effective herbal practice. It involves a thorough understanding of the individual's health status, a deep knowledge of how herbs interact with various conditions and medications, and a commitment to continual learning and adaptation.

CHAPTER 3: BASIC HERBAL PREPARATIONS & DOSAGES

Embarking on the use of herbal remedies involves more than just knowing which herbs to use for which ailments. It encompasses an understanding of the details involved in their preparation and usage. This subchapter focuses on the intricate processes of preparing and using herbal remedies. These processes are crucial for maximizing the efficacy and safety of the herbs, ensuring that their healing potential is fully realized.

Preparation Techniques

The preparation of herbal remedies is an art that requires both knowledge and intuition. O'Neill's teachings cover various preparation methods, including infusions, decoctions, tinctures, and salves.

Infusions, similar to making tea, involve pouring boiling water over the herb and allowing it to steep. This method is suitable for delicate parts of the plant, such as leaves and flowers. Decoctions involve simmering tougher parts, like roots and bark, in water to extract their medicinal properties.

Salves and ointments, made by infusing herbs in oils and then blending with waxes, are used for topical applications. These preparations are beneficial for skin conditions and as healing balms.

Safety Considerations in Preparation

Safety in the preparation of herbal remedies is paramount. This includes understanding the correct dosages and recognizing that some herbs can have potent effects or interact with medications. O'Neill emphasizes the importance of starting with small doses and observing the body's response.

Understanding contraindications is also crucial. Some herbs should not be used during pregnancy or by individuals with certain health conditions. Accurate knowledge and careful consideration of these factors are essential in the safe preparation of herbal remedies.

The gathering and preparation of herbs are practices that require respect, knowledge, and a deep connection with the natural world. These practices are not just about creating remedies but about fostering a relationship with nature that is ethical, sustainable, and mindful.

The Art of Herbal Infusions

Herbal infusions are one of the simplest yet most effective ways to extract the healing properties of herbs. The process involves steeping herbs in hot water, which allows their medicinal compounds to be released. O'Neill emphasizes the importance of temperature and time in this process. For instance, delicate herbs like chamomile and lavender should be infused in just-boiled water for about 5 to 10 minutes to prevent the loss of their volatile oils. In contrast, more robust herbs like nettle or Red raspberry leaf require longer steeping times, typically around 15 to 20 minutes, to fully extract their beneficial properties.

Decoctions for Tougher Plant Materials

Decoctions are ideal for extracting the medicinal properties from tougher plant materials like roots, barks, and seeds. The process involves simmering these parts in water for an extended period, usually ranging from 20 minutes to an hour, depending on the hardness of the material. O'Neill advises that the water should initially be brought to a boil and then reduced to a simmer. This slow process allows for the deep extraction of medicinal compounds. For example, a decoction of burdock root, known for its blood-purifying properties, should be simmered for at least 30 minutes to ensure the extraction of its active constituents.

Topical Applications: Salves and Poultices

For external ailments, O'Neill often recommends the use of salves and poultices. Salves are made by infusing herbs in oils and then blending them with beeswax to create a thick, spreadable ointment. The choice of herbs depends on the condition being treated. For instance, a calendula salve can be used for skin irritations and minor wounds. Poultices involve applying herbs directly to the skin or using a soft cloth soaked in a herbal infusion or decoction. They are particularly useful for localized issues like inflammation or muscle pain.

Herbal Baths and Washes

Herbal baths and washes are another aspect of O'Neill's method, offering a soothing and therapeutic way to use herbs. A herbal bath involves adding a strong infusion or decoction of herbs to bathwater, providing a relaxing and healing experience. Herbal washes, on the other hand, are used to cleanse or treat specific areas of the body. For example, an eye wash made from eyebright or chamomile can help relieve eye irritation or inflammation.

The Importance of Record-Keeping

O'Neill also emphasizes the importance of meticulous record-keeping when preparing and using herbal remedies. Documenting the herbs used, their sources, the methods of preparation, dosages, and the individual's responses, helps in refining treatments and tracking progress over time. This practice is particularly crucial for those who prepare their herbal remedies or for practitioners managing multiple clients.

Mindfulness in Herbal Preparation and Usage

Mindfulness in the preparation and usage of herbal remedies is a key aspect of O'Neill's teachings. This involves being fully present during the process of preparing the remedy, paying close attention to the colors, textures, and scents of the herbs, and being aware of their effects on the body. Such mindfulness enhances the therapeutic experience and deepens the individual's connection to the healing process.

Respecting the Limits of Herbal Medicine

While advocating for the benefits of herbal remedies, O'Neill also stresses the importance of understanding and respecting their limits. This includes recognizing when a condition requires conventional medical intervention and avoiding the use of herbs as a substitute for necessary medical care. Her approach is one of complementary use, where herbal remedies support and enhance overall health and wellbeing, rather than replace conventional treatments.

Dosage and Frequency Tips Recommended by O'Neill

Navigating the world of herbal medicine involves a keen understanding of the appropriate dosage and frequency of herbal medicines. This subchapter digs into the detailed art of determining how much and how often one should consume herbal preparations. These recommendations are not arbitrary; they are derived from a deep understanding of the herbs' properties, the individual's unique constitution, and the specific condition being treated.

The Principle of Start Low, Go Slow

One of the fundamental principles in determining dosage and frequency in herbal medicine, is to start with low doses and gradually increase as needed. This approach allows the body to adjust to the herb and helps in identifying the minimal effective dose; the lowest amount needed to achieve the desired therapeutic effect. This principle is particularly important when working with potent herbs or when treating sensitive individuals, such as children or the elderly.

Dosage Considerations

The determination of the correct dosage depends on several factors, including the age, weight, and health status of the individual, as well as the nature of the herb and the condition being treated. For example, children and elderly individuals generally require smaller doses than healthy adults due to differences in metabolism and body composition.

Additionally, the potency of the herb plays a significant role in dosage determination. Strongly acting herbs, such as those with sedative or laxative properties, typically require smaller doses, while milder herbs may be used in larger quantities.

Frequency of Herbal Intake

The frequency of taking an herbal remedy is as important as the dosage. This factor is influenced by the herb's duration of action and the nature of the condition being treated. Acute conditions, like a cold or an upset stomach, may require more frequent dosing of certain herbs to maintain steady therapeutic levels in the body. Chronic conditions, on the other hand, might benefit from less frequent dosing over a longer period.

O'Neill advises attention to the body's responses when determining frequency. Some individuals may experience relief with less frequent doses, while others may require more regular intake to achieve the desired effects.

Herb-Specific Dosage Guidelines

O'Neill's approach includes specific dosage guidelines for different herbs, recognizing that each herb has its unique profile. For instance, herbs like echinacea, used for immune support, may be taken in higher doses at the onset of symptoms and then reduced as the condition improves. Conversely, tonifying herbs like ashwagandha may be taken in consistent doses over an extended period to build and maintain energy levels.

Adjusting Dosage and Frequency Over Time

An important aspect of O'Neill's methodology is the adjustment of dosage and frequency over time. As the individual's condition changes, so too should the herbal treatment plan. This might mean reducing the dose as symptoms improve or increase it if the desired effect is not achieved.

Additionally, the duration of herbal treatment is a critical consideration. Some herbal remedies are meant for short-term use, while others can be taken safely over longer periods. Understanding the appropriate duration of treatment is essential to prevent potential side effects or tolerance to the herb's effects.

The Role of Personalization in Dosage and Frequency

Personalization is key in O'Neill's approach to dosage and frequency. She emphasizes that herbal medicine is not a one size fits all solution. What works for one individual may not be effective for another, even with the same condition. This variability necessitates a tailored approach, considering the individual's unique physiological makeup, lifestyle, and specific health needs.

Educating on the Importance of Adherence

O'Neill stresses the importance of educating individuals on the significance of adherence to the prescribed dosage and frequency. Adherence ensures the effectiveness of the treatment and reduces the risk of adverse effects. For instance, sporadic intake of an herbal remedy meant to be taken regularly can lead to suboptimal results, while overuse can cause potential harm.

Monitoring and Feedback

Continuous monitoring and feedback are crucial components in adjusting dosage and frequency. O'Neill advises individuals to observe their responses to the herbal treatment closely and communicate any changes or concerns. This feedback loop allows for timely adjustments and ensures that the treatment remains aligned with the individual's evolving health status.

Understanding Herbal Forms and Their Dosages

Different forms of herbal preparations, such as teas, tinctures, capsules, and topicals, require different dosing considerations. O'Neill provides guidance on adjusting dosages based on the form of the herb being used. For example, tinctures are more concentrated than teas and thus require smaller dosages. Understanding these differences is essential for effective and safe herbal treatment.

The Importance of Consistency

Consistency in taking herbal remedies, as per the recommended dosage and frequency, is vital for achieving the desired therapeutic outcomes. O'Neill emphasizes the role of routine in herbal treatment, encouraging individuals to integrate the intake of herbal remedies into their daily schedules in a way that promotes consistent use.

Cautions and Contraindications

O'Neill's teachings also include cautions regarding the contraindications of certain herbs based on dosage and frequency. For instance, herbs that can impact hormonal balance, such as licorice or dong quai, must be used judiciously, considering factors like hormonal status and concurrent use of hormone-related medications.

The Role of Professional Guidance

In O'Neill's practice, the role of professional guidance in determining dosage and frequency is highly valued. Consulting with a knowledgeable herbalist or healthcare provider ensures that the herbal treatment plan is safe, effective, and tailored to the individual's specific needs. This professional input is particularly crucial when dealing with complex health conditions or when using potent herbs.

Balancing Tradition with Modern Understanding

In her approach, O'Neill balances traditional herbal wisdom with modern scientific understanding. This balance is reflected in her recommendations for dosage and frequency, which are grounded in historical use and supported by contemporary research where available.

The determination of appropriate dosage and frequency in herbal medicine is a dynamic and individualized process. It requires a deep understanding of herbal properties, personal health factors, and various herbal forms.

CHAPTER 4: SPECIALIZED HERBAL PLANS AND FORMULATIONS

Herbal medicine extends far beyond general wellness and common ailments. It goes into a deeper, more intricate territory of specialized treatments, where herbs are used not just for their general healing properties but are carefully chosen and combined to address specific health conditions. This chapter explores the art and science of specialized herbal treatments. It is a walk into the heart of therapeutic herbalism, where the true power of herbs is harnessed to provide relief and healing for a range of specific health challenges.

The Essence of Specialized Herbalism

Specialized herbal treatments are based on the premise that each herb possesses unique properties that can be strategically used to target specific health issues. This approach is akin to a master craftsman selecting the perfect tools for a delicate job. It requires an in-depth understanding of each herb's pharmacological profile, including its active constituents, therapeutic actions, and potential side effects and interactions.

This level of understanding allows herbalists to create formulations that are not only effective in alleviating symptoms but also in addressing the underlying causes of health conditions. It is an approach that values the complexity of human health and respects the intricate ways in which our bodies interact with herbal constituents.

A Holistic Approach to Specific Conditions

Herbs are chosen not only for their direct impact on a particular condition but also for their ability to support the body's overall health and balance. This perspective recognizes that the body is an interconnected system, where treating one part affects the whole.

For example, in treating a condition like arthritis, the herbal treatment plan may include anti-inflammatory herbs to reduce joint pain and swelling, but it may also include herbs to support the liver and kidneys, which are vital in managing the body's inflammatory response and in processing the by-products of inflammation.

Addressing Complex Health Issues

Specialized herbal treatments are particularly valuable in addressing complex health issues that do not respond well to conventional treatments or that require a more nuanced approach. Conditions such as chronic fatigue syndrome, autoimmune disorders, and hormonal imbalances are examples where specialized herbal treatments can offer significant relief.

These conditions are often multifaceted and require a comprehensive treatment strategy that addresses various aspects of the condition. Herbs are selected not only for their specific actions related to the condition but also for their ability to support other body systems that may be impacted by the condition or its conventional treatments.

The Role of Diet and Lifestyle

In specialized herbal treatments, the role of diet and lifestyle is emphasized as an integral part of the healing process. Herbs are powerful, but their effects can be enhanced or hindered by the person's diet and lifestyle choices.

For instance, in treating a condition like irritable bowel syndrome, dietary changes to eliminate trigger foods are often necessary alongside herbal treatments to reduce inflammation and support digestive health. Similarly, in conditions like anxiety or insomnia, lifestyle changes such as stress management techniques and establishing a regular sleep routine are essential components of the treatment plan.

Safety and Efficacy in Specialized Treatments

While specialized herbal treatments offer powerful healing possibilities, they also come with a responsibility to ensure safety and efficacy. This involves not only choosing the right herbs but also using them at the right dosages and ensuring they are of high quality.

Herbalists must also be aware of potential contraindications and interactions, particularly when herbs are used alongside conventional medications. Monitoring the person's response to the treatment and making adjustments as necessary is crucial to ensuring the safety and effectiveness of the treatment.

Specialized herbal treatments represent a profound aspect of herbal medicine. They offer the promise of targeted, effective healing for specific health conditions, grounded in a deep understanding of herbal pharmacology, the holistic nature of health, and the unique needs of each individual.

Techniques for Combining Herbs: formulation and synergy

The technique of combining herbs is akin to a culinary chef masterfully blending flavors to create a harmonious dish. Just as in cooking, the practice of combining herbs in therapeutic formulations is a delicate balance of understanding individual properties, interactions, and the desired therapeutic outcome. This subchapter explores the techniques of combining herbs, deep into the principles of herbal synergy, balance, and the creation of effective, holistic remedies.

The Foundation of Herbal Synergy

At the core of combining herbs is the principle of synergy, where the combined effect of the herbs is greater than the sum of their individual parts. O'Neill encourages thoughtfulness to formulation where each herb is selected not only for its own merits but also for how it complements and enhances the actions of other herbs in the blend.

1. **Understanding Herb Categories**: In crafting herbal combinations, it's crucial to understand different categories of herbs such as carminatives (like ginger and fennel), demulcents (such as slippery elm and marshmallow root), adaptogens (like ashwagandha and ginseng), and nervines (such as lemon balm and lavender). Understanding these categories aids in selecting herbs that work harmoniously to target various aspects of a condition.

2. **Complementary Actions**: When combining herbs, it's important to consider how their actions complement each other. For example, in a formula for digestive aid, combining a soothing demulcent like marshmallow root with a carminative like peppermint can address multiple facets of digestive discomfort.

Balancing Herbal Formulas

Balance is key in herbal combinations. This involves considering the energetics of the herbs (warm, cool, dry, moist) and ensuring that the formula is balanced in a way that matches the individual's constitution and the nature of their ailment.

1. **Energetic Balancing**: For instance, if using warming herbs like ginger in a formula, it may be balanced with cooler herbs like peppermint to prevent overheating and irritation, especially in individuals with a warmer constitution.

2. **Dosage Ratios**: Balancing also involves adjusting the ratios of each herb in the formula. More potent herbs may be used in smaller quantities, while milder herbs may form the bulk of the formula.

Harmonizing Herbs and Reducing Adverse Effects

Combining herbs can also serve to harmonize the formula by reducing the potential for adverse effects, and enhancing tolerability.

1. **Mitigating Irritation**: Herbs with potent actions might be combined with soothing herbs to mitigate any potential irritation. This can also tie into herbal energetics, like discussed in the previous section. For instance, a strong laxative herb like senna can be combined with a soothing demulcent like marshmallow to prevent intestinal irritation.

2. **Enhancing Digestibility**: Bitter herbs that stimulate digestion, like gentian, can be combined with carminative herbs like cardamom or fennel to enhance digestibility and prevent potential discomfort like gas or bloating.

Creating Target-Specific Formulas

In creating target-specific formulas, understanding the primary and secondary actions of herbs is essential. This involves choosing a primary herb or herbs that directly address the main symptom or condition and supporting herbs that assist or amplify the primary herb's actions.

1. **Primary and Supportive Herbs**: In a formula for respiratory health, mullein may be the primary herb for its expectorant properties, supported by thyme for its antimicrobial action and licorice for its soothing effect on irritated mucous membranes.

2. **Layered Support**: In addressing a condition like anxiety, a primary herb such as ashwagandha, an adaptogen, can be supported by secondary herbs like passionflower and hops that provide immediate calming effects.

The art of combining herbs is a complex yet immensely rewarding aspect of herbal medicine. It involves a deep understanding of individual herbs, their energetics, actions, and interactions. The techniques of creating synergy, achieving balance, layering effects, harmonizing formulas, and crafting target-specific combinations are essential tools in the herbalist's repertoire.

TAILORING FORMULAS TO INDIVIDUAL NEEDS

The focus on tailoring treatments to meet individual needs is paramount. It involves creating an entire herbal plan. This cancels the one-size-fits-all mentality often found in conventional medicine, recognizing the uniqueness of each individual's body, lifestyle, and health condition.

This subchapter examines the art and science of customizing herbal treatments, a process that requires a deep understanding of the individual as a whole, their environment, and how different herbs can be used synergistically to address specific health concerns.

1. **Comprehensive Health Assessment**: The process begins with a comprehensive health assessment, which includes not only the individual's physical symptoms but also their emotional state, dietary habits, lifestyle, and environmental factors. For instance, in treating insomnia, the approach considers potential stressors, dietary habits, and lifestyle choices alongside physical symptoms.

2. **Personal Health History and Genetic Predispositions**: A detailed personal health history, including any familial health patterns or genetic predispositions, is also taken into account. This information can provide insights into the individual's inherent health strengths and vulnerabilities.

Incorporating Lifestyle and Dietary Considerations

O'Neill stresses that effective herbal treatment goes beyond just prescribing herbs. It involves incorporating lifestyle and dietary changes that support the healing process.

1. **Dietary Modifications**: Nutritional guidance is tailored to support the therapeutic action of herbs and address specific health issues. For example, an anti-inflammatory diet may be recommended alongside herbs for conditions like arthritis.

2. **Lifestyle Adjustments**: Recommendations on lifestyle adjustments such as exercise, sleep, stress management, and exposure to natural environments are integral to the treatment plan. These adjustments are tailored to complement the action of the herbs and enhance overall well-being.

Tailoring Herbal Formulations

Creating a herbal formulation to meet an individual's needs is a nuanced process that involves selecting herbs based on their specific actions and how they interact with each other and the individual's condition.

1. **Selecting Primary and Supportive Herbs**: The formulation typically includes a primary herb that directly addresses the main health concern and supportive herbs that assist in the healing process. For example, in a formula for hypertension, hawthorn may be the primary herb for its cardiovascular benefits, supported by calming herbs like lavender to address stress, a contributing factor to high blood pressure.

2. **Consideration of Herb Energetics**: The energetics of herbs; whether they are warming or cooling, drying or moistening, are considered to ensure the formula aligns with the individual's constitution and current state. A person with a hot, fiery constitution, for instance, may require cooling and calming herbs.

Monitoring and Adjusting Herbal Plans

Tailoring plans to a unique individual is an ongoing process that involves careful monitoring and adjustments as needed.

1. **Regular Follow-ups and Adjustments**: Keeping track of what works, and what doesn't, is essential to assess the effectiveness of the treatment and make any necessary adjustments. The herbal formulation may be modified based on the individual's response and changes in their condition.

2. **Responsive and Dynamic Herbal Plans**: The plan will evolve as the individual's health needs change. This approach ensures that the treatment remains effective and relevant.

Creating unique herbal plans for individual needs is a meticulous and compassionate process. It involves a deep understanding of the individual, thoughtful creation of herbal formulations, and ongoing monitoring and adjustments.

Incorporating Complementary Therapies into Herbal Plans

Holistic treatment plans may also integrate complementary therapies that align with O'Neill's holistic philosophy.

1. **Physical Therapies**: Practices such as massage, acupuncture, or chiropractic care may be included to address physical aspects of health, like pain relief or structural alignment.

2. **Mind-Body Practices**: Mind-body interventions like mindfulness, biofeedback, or guided imagery are often incorporated to support mental and emotional health.

Interactive Elements for Readers to Consider Personalization of Herbal Plans

The personalization of herbal treatments is not just the prerogative of practitioners; it involves active participation from those seeking healing. This subchapter lights up the interactive elements that individuals can consider to personalize their own herbal plans. This process empowers individuals to engage more deeply with their healing journey, integrating their unique needs, experiences, and responses into their treatment plans.

Self-Assessment as a Tool for Personalization

The first step in personalizing herbal treatment is self-assessment. This involves individuals taking stock of their health status, lifestyle, and specific health concerns.

1. **Health and Symptom Journaling**: Keeping a health and symptom journal can be an invaluable tool. This record helps track daily health experiences, symptom patterns, dietary habits, and emotional states. For instance, noting digestive discomfort in relation to meals can help pinpoint triggers and guide the selection of digestive-supportive herbs.

2. **Body Constitution Analysis**: Understanding one's body constitution (such as in Ayurvedic doshas or Traditional Chinese Medicine elements) can guide the choice of herbs. This can also include energetics: determining whether you're a hot /cold or dry / damp individual. One can evaluate their constitution through questionnaires or consultations with practitioners, selecting herbs that balance their specific constitution.

Engaging with Herbal Selection

In personalizing treatment, individuals can engage actively in the selection of herbs, guided by their understanding of their health needs and the properties of different herbs.

1. **Research and Education**: Educating oneself about different herbs and their properties is key. Resources like books, reputable online platforms, and workshops can provide valuable information on herbal actions, indications, and contraindications.

2. **Sensory Engagement with Herbs**: Direct engagement with herbs through sensory experiences: smelling, tasting, and even growing them, can help individuals understand and connect with the herbs they choose to use. This connection can guide intuitive choices in herbal selection While doing this, of course be mindful of safety, allergy, and so on.

Incorporating Lifestyle and Environmental Factors

Personalization also involves considering one's lifestyle and environment, as these can significantly impact the effectiveness of herbal treatments.

1. **Lifestyle Considerations**: Factors such as stress levels, sleep patterns, and physical activity should be considered when choosing herbs. For example, individuals with high stress might benefit from adaptogenic herbs, while those with sleep issues might find nervine herbs more beneficial.

2. **Environmental Influences**: The environment, including climate, pollution levels, and seasonal changes, can influence health and the effectiveness of herbs that are chosen. Individuals can choose herbs that counteract environmental stressors they are exposed to. You can find more on this in our herbal sourcing chapter.

Seeking Professional Guidance When Needed

While personalization encourages self-involvement, recognizing when to seek professional guidance is important, especially from a licensed health professional, naturopath, or herbalist. When taking use of herbs seriously for your health, always pass your decisions by your personal health professional, doctor, or other for safety.

1. Complex Health Conditions: In cases of complex health conditions or when using potent herbs, consulting with a professional herbalist or healthcare provider is advised to ensure safety and effectiveness.

2. **Interpreting Responses**: Professionals can help interpret responses to herbs, especially in distinguishing between healing reactions and adverse effects, and make necessary adjustments in treatment plans.

The personalization of herbal treatments is a deeply interactive process that places individuals at the center of their healing journey. It encompasses a blend of self-assessment, engaged learning, consideration of lifestyle and environmental factors, interactive decision-making, and responsive personalization not only enhances the efficacy of herbal treatments but also fosters a deeper connection with the healing power of herbs and a greater understanding of one's own body and health.

CHAPTER 5: HERBAL DETOXIFICATION AND CLEANSING

The concept of detoxification and cleansing, particularly through the use of herbal remedies, is a fundamental aspect of holistic healing as a whole. This chapter prioritizes the world of herbal detoxification and cleansing with some focus on digestive health, and explores the intricate ways in which herbs can be used to purify and rejuvenate the body, emphasizing the importance of these processes in maintaining health and vitality.

The Philosophy of Detoxification in Herbal Medicine

Detoxification in herbal medicine is based on the principle that the body's natural healing processes can be enhanced by eliminating toxins and impurities that accumulate due to various factors such as diet, environmental pollutants, and stress. It is the ultimate approach to holistic health.

1. **Holistic View of Detoxification**: Unlike the often aggressive detoxification methods popularized in mainstream culture, herbal detoxification is viewed holistically. It is seen not just as a physical cleansing process but as an opportunity to rejuvenate the body, mind, and spirit.

2. **Supporting Natural Body Processes**: The focus is on supporting the body's natural detoxification processes; primarily the liver, kidneys, digestive system, skin, and lungs, rather than forcibly expelling toxins.

3. **Natural Healing Facilitation**: Detoxification is perceived as a facilitator of the body's natural healing processes. By eliminating toxins and waste, it helps clear the path for the body's inherent self-repair mechanisms to function optimally.

4. **Restorative Process**: Beyond removal of toxins, detoxification is also about restoration and rejuvenation. It is seen as a vital process that helps reset the body's systems, enhancing overall vitality and energy.

The Role of Herbal Remedies in Detoxification

Herbal remedies are a central aspect of detoxification, along with regular hydration, persistence, and more.

1. **Herbs for Organ Support**: Specific herbs are identified for their ability to support detoxification organs. For example, milk thistle for liver support or nettle for kidney health.

2. **Herbal Cleanses**: Short-term herbal cleanses, using teas or tinctures made from detoxifying herbs, are often recommended as a way to give the body's detoxification systems a boost.

Detoxification as a Preventative Measure

Detoxification is not only for those who are unwell; it is also seen as a preventive measure to maintain health and prevent disease.

Routine Detox Practices. Incorporating routine detox practices into one's lifestyle, such as regular detox weekends or seasonal cleanses, can help maintain optimal health and prevent the accumulation of toxins.

Holistic Detoxification and Chronic Disease

In cases of chronic disease, detoxification is tailored to support the body's healing processes, taking into consideration the specific needs and limitations of the individual.

1. **Gentle Detoxification**: For individuals with chronic conditions, a gentle approach to detoxification is often advocated, focusing on supporting rather than overburdening the body.

2. **Customized Detox Plans**: Detox plans for chronic disease patients are highly customized, taking into account the individual's condition, treatment regime, and overall health status. See our formulation and herbal treatment chapter.

The role of detoxification is comprehensive and multifaceted in holistic health…but not complicated. It extends beyond the physical realm, encompassing emotional, mental, and environmental aspects of health as well in the effort to restore the body and rid ourselves of toxins.

Understanding Toxins and Their Impact on Health

A comprehensive understanding of what constitutes toxins and how they impact health is crucial in the context of herbal detoxification.

1. **Types of Toxins**: Toxins can come from external sources like pollutants, chemicals, and heavy metals, or internal sources like metabolic by-products. Understanding these sources is key to effectively addressing them through detoxification.

2. **Impact on Health**: Accumulation of toxins can lead to various health issues, including fatigue, digestive problems, skin conditions, and more serious chronic illnesses. The goal of detoxification is to alleviate these conditions holistically by removing the source of the problem: toxins.

Herbs in Detoxification and Cleansing

Certain herbs have properties that make them particularly effective in aiding detoxification and cleansing.

1. **Liver-Supporting Herbs**: Herbs such as milk thistle, dandelion, and turmeric are known for their liver-supporting properties. They help enhance liver function, which is crucial in the detoxification process.

2. **Kidney Cleansing Herbs**: Herbs like uva ursi, cranberry, and nettle support kidney health and assist in the elimination of waste and excess water from the body.

Diet and Nutrition in Herbal Detoxification

Diet plays a significant role in supporting the body's detoxification processes, working in tandem with herbal remedies.

1. **Detoxification Diet**: A diet rich in fruits, vegetables, whole grains, and lean proteins provides the necessary nutrients and antioxidants to support the body during detoxification. Certain foods like leafy greens, beets, and garlic are particularly beneficial in a detox diet.

2. **Hydration**: Adequate hydration is essential during detoxification. Water helps flush out toxins and supports kidney function. Herbal teas can also be a beneficial part of a hydration strategy during detox.

The Role of Digestive Health in Detoxification

A healthy digestive system is key to effective detoxification. Many herbs used in detoxification directly support digestive health. They also help digestive issues such as indigestion, constipation, and diarrhea, common ailments where herbal remedies can be particularly effective, and which can be symptoms of a system in need of detox.

1. **Digestive Aids**: Herbs such as ginger, peppermint, and fennel aid digestion and help alleviate issues like bloating and gas, which can be common during detoxification.

2. **Fiber**: Dietary fiber is essential in a detox diet as it helps bind to toxins and facilitate their elimination through the digestive tract. Herbs with high fiber content, like psyllium husk, can be incorporated into the diet for this purpose.

Customizing Herbal Detoxification Regimens

Herbal detoxification regimens should be tailored to individual needs, taking into account factors such as health status, lifestyle, and personal preferences. Be sure to check back in on our herbal formulation and plans section for more info.

1. **Personalized Herbal Selection**: The selection of herbs for detoxification should be based on the individual's specific health needs and goals. For instance, someone with skin issues might focus on herbs that support skin health in addition to general detoxification herbs.

2. **Duration and Intensity**: The duration and intensity of a detoxification regimen can vary. Short-term, intensive detox programs may be suitable for some, while others may benefit more from a longer, gentler detoxification process.

Methods for Herbal Detox and Cleansing Routines

The practice of detoxification and cleansing is not just a trend, but a profound method of purifying and rejuvenating the body. This subchapter underscores the specific methods for implementing herbal detox and cleansing routine, and specific approaches and preparations.

Let's explore the various ways in which herbs can be utilized in detoxification processes, emphasizing their roles in supporting the body's natural detoxifying organs and systems, and enhancing overall health and vitality.

Herbal Detox Tea Routines

One of the most common methods of herbal detoxification is through the use of detox teas. These teas are formulated with a blend of herbs known for their cleansing properties.

1. **Daily Detox Teas**: A daily detox tea might include herbs like green tea, nettles, and burdock root. This tea can be consumed once or twice daily as a gentle way to support the body's ongoing detoxification.

2. **Targeted Detox Teas**: For more targeted detox needs, such as liver cleansing or supporting a liver condition, a tea blend might include herbs like milk thistle, dandelion root, and artichoke leaf. These teas can be consumed in short cycles, such as a week-long liver cleanse. Be sure to have your doctor or health professional be informed of these approaches if you have a condition.

Herbal Detox Baths

Detox baths are another method of utilizing herbs for detoxification. They are beneficial for not just physical cleansing, but also for relaxation and stress reduction.

1. **Preparing Herbal Detox Baths**: A detox bath can be prepared by adding herbs like lavender, chamomile, or eucalyptus to bath water, either directly or in a muslin bag. Epsom Salts and essential oils may also be added for additional detoxifying and relaxing effects.

2. **Routine and Duration**: Detox baths can be taken once or twice a week as part of a regular detox routine. They are particularly beneficial when taken before bedtime to promote restful sleep.

Herbal Detox Supplements and Capsules

In some cases, herbal detoxification might involve the use of supplements or capsules, especially when specific, concentrated herbal actions are needed.

1. **Supplement Formulations**: Herbal supplements for detox may include concentrated extracts of herbs like turmeric, cilantro, or chlorella, known for their detoxifying properties. These are typically used in cases where a more intense detoxification is needed.

2. **Guidance and Duration**: The use of herbal supplements for detox should be guided by a knowledgeable practitioner, especially regarding dosage and duration, to ensure safety and effectiveness.

Herbal Juices, Smoothies, and Hydration

Incorporating detoxifying herbs into juices and smoothies is a refreshing and nourishing way to cleanse the body. Cold herbal teas and straight water on the regular are also essential to cleansing the body's innate "waterways": the kidneys, lymphatic system, and beyond. Hydration during detoxification is essential.

1. **Herbal Juice Recipes**: Juices can be made using detoxifying herbs and greens like parsley, cilantro, and wheatgrass, combined with fruits and vegetables such as apples, cucumbers, and celery.

2. **Smoothies with Herbal Additions**: Smoothies can include ingredients like spirulina, chlorella, or powdered greens, which offer detoxifying benefits in a more filling form.

3. **Herbal Waters or Infusions:** Staying hydrated is imperative to successful detox. Cucumber or lemon water, cold or light herbal infusions, and simple hydration are highly recommended.

CHAPTER 6: WOMEN'S AND MEN'S HEALTH

Chapter 8 echoes the obscurity of women's and men's health, acknowledging the unique health concerns, challenges, and needs that arise due to differences in anatomy, hormonal fluctuations, and societal roles. This chapter offers an in-depth analysis of gender-specific health strategies, with emphasis on the importance of a personalized, empathetic, and inclusive approach to health care.

Understanding Gender-Specific Health Needs

Women's and men's bodies differ not only anatomically but also in how they react to disease, treatment, and lifestyle factors. Recognizing and addressing these differences is crucial for effective health management.

1. **Biological and Hormonal Variances**: Women and men experience different health risks and challenges due to biological differences, particularly hormonal variations. These differences can significantly impact physical health, mental well-being, and disease risk.

2. **Gender-Specific Diseases and Conditions**: Certain health conditions are unique or more prevalent in either women or men. For example, women face specific reproductive health issues such as menstrual disorders, polycystic ovary syndrome (PCOS), and menopause, while men are more prone to conditions like prostate enlargement and certain heart diseases.

Holistic Health in Women's Care Overview

The holistic approach to women's health encompasses a broad spectrum of care, from reproductive health to general wellness, and acknowledges the impact of life stages such as menstruation, pregnancy, and menopause.

1. **Reproductive Health**: A holistic approach to reproductive health includes not only addressing physical symptoms but also considering emotional and mental health aspects. It involves managing conditions like menstrual irregularities, fertility issues, and menopausal symptoms with a combination of lifestyle modifications, nutritional support, and natural therapies.

2. **Preventive Care and Wellness**: Preventive care in women's health focuses on nutrition, exercise, stress management, and regular health screenings. Lifestyle interventions are tailored to reduce the risk of common

women's health issues like breast cancer, osteoporosis, and autoimmune diseases.

Men's Holistic Health Overview: Beyond the Physical

In men's health, a holistic approach extends beyond physical ailments to encompass mental and emotional well-being, often addressing the societal stigma around men's emotional health.

1. **Prostate Health and Cardiovascular Disease**: Key areas in men's health include prostate health, where conditions like benign prostatic hyperplasia (BPH) and prostate cancer are of concern, and cardiovascular health, as men are at a higher risk for heart diseases.

2. **Mental Health and Stress Management**: Acknowledging and addressing mental health issues, which are often underreported in men, is crucial. Stress management, emotional well-being, and addressing lifestyle factors like alcohol consumption and smoking are integral parts of a holistic men's health strategy.

Nutrition and Dietary Needs

The nutritional needs of women and men vary based on hormonal differences, metabolic rates, and risk of certain diseases. Tailoring diet to these needs is a key aspect of holistic health.

1. **Women's Nutritional Focus**: For women, dietary focus may include calcium and iron due to risks of osteoporosis and anemia, particularly during certain life stages like pregnancy and post-menopause.

2. **Men's Nutritional Focus**: Men's diets may need to emphasize heart-healthy foods rich in omega-3 fatty acids, fiber, and plant sterols to mitigate the risk of heart disease.

Exercise and Physical Activity

Physical activity is essential for both women and men, but the focus and type of exercise might differ based on specific health goals and physiological differences.

1. **Exercise for Women**: Exercise routines for women might focus more on strength training to combat the risk of osteoporosis, along with cardiovascular exercises for overall heart health.

2. **Exercise for Men**: Men's exercise regimens may emphasize cardiovascular health, weight management, and muscle building, considering the higher prevalence of obesity and heart disease.

Lifestyle Factors Influencing Men's and Women's Health

Lifestyle factors play a significant role in both women's and men's health, impacting everything from hormonal balance to mental well-being.

1. **Stress and Its Management**: Understanding and managing stress is vital, as it can exacerbate gender-specific health issues such as hormonal imbalances in women and hypertension in men.

2. **Work-Life Balance**: Achieving a balance between work and personal life is essential for maintaining overall health and wellness. This balance helps mitigate stress, improve mental health, and enhance life satisfaction.

3. **Emotional Health in Women**: Women might benefit from support systems that address the emotional aspects of menstrual health, childbirth, menopause, and balancing societal roles.

4. **Emotional Health in Men**: For men, creating safe spaces for expressing emotions and addressing mental health issues is key. This approach challenges the traditional norms that often discourage men from seeking help for emotional issues.

By integrating gender-specific nutritional needs, exercise regimens, lifestyle factors, and emotional health considerations, this approach provides a more effective and personalized pathway to health and wellness.

HERBAL SOLUTIONS FOR HORMONAL BALANCE AND REPRODUCTIVE HEALTH

Hormonal balance and reproductive health are pivotal aspects of overall well-being, deeply influencing physical, emotional, and mental health. Herbal solutions play a significant role in nurturing and maintaining this delicate balance. Here, we assess the integration of traditional wisdom and modern herbal practices, highlighting how specific herbs can be utilized to address a spectrum of hormonal and reproductive issues, with a focus on safety, efficacy, and the holistic harmony of the body.

Understanding Hormonal Balance

Hormonal balance is a dynamic and complex aspect of health, involving a delicate interplay of various hormones that regulate bodily functions.

1. **The Role of Hormones**: Hormones, acting as chemical messengers, play crucial roles in regulating metabolism, growth and development, tissue function, sexual function, reproduction, sleep, and mood.

2. **Consequences of Imbalance**: Hormonal imbalances can lead to a myriad of health issues, ranging from menstrual irregularities, infertility, weight gain, to mood swings and decreased energy levels.

Herbal Remedies for Women's Hormonal Health

In addressing women's hormonal health, specific herbs are known for their efficacy in balancing hormones and addressing reproductive health issues.

1. **Chaste tree Berry (Vitex)**: Traditionally used for regulating menstrual cycles, Vitex is renowned for its ability to balance estrogen and progesterone levels, making it beneficial for conditions like premenstrual syndrome (PMS) and menopausal symptoms.

2. **Red raspberry Leaf**: Often used to strengthen the uterine lining and improve menstrual health, this herb is also popular among pregnant women for its uterine toning properties.

Herbs for Men's Hormonal Health

Men's hormonal health, particularly concerning testosterone levels and prostate health, can also be supported through specific herbs.

1. **Saw palmetto**: Widely used for prostate health, Saw palmetto can help in reducing the symptoms of benign prostatic hyperplasia (BPH) and may contribute to balancing testosterone levels.

2. **Nettle Root**: Nettle root supports prostate health and urinary functions. It is also thought to help in balancing male hormones and can be beneficial in reducing symptoms of BPH.

Supporting Fertility with Herbal Remedies

Fertility issues, affecting both men and women, can be addressed through a range of herbal remedies designed to enhance reproductive health.

1. **Maca Root**: Known for its hormone-balancing effects, Maca root is used to enhance fertility in both men and women. It is believed to improve sperm quality and quantity in men and regulate menstrual cycles in women.

2. **Shatavari**: Traditionally used in Ayurvedic medicine, Shatavari is considered a potent fertility-enhancing herb for women, believed to nourish the reproductive system and regulate menstrual cycles.

Managing Menopause and Andropause

Menopause in women and andropause in men are significant hormonal transition periods that can be managed effectively with herbal remedies.

1. **Black Cohosh**: Black Cohosh is commonly used for managing menopausal symptoms like hot flashes, mood swings, and sleep disturbances. It's thought to have estrogenic effects, helping to mitigate the decline in estrogen levels during menopause.

2. **Ginseng**: Ginseng is beneficial in managing andropause symptoms in men, including fatigue and decreased libido. It is also known for its overall energy-boosting properties.

The management of hormonal balance and reproductive health through herbal remedies, offers a natural, effective, and empathetic approach to healthcare. By imbibing the power of these natural remedies, individuals can navigate the complexities of hormonal and reproductive health with greater ease and efficacy.

Real-Life Examples Illustrating the Application in Gender-Specific Health Issues

Exploring gender-specific health issues through the lens of real-life examples provides invaluable insights into the practical application of holistic health strategies. This subchapter avails a series of case studies and anecdotal experiences that illuminate the efficacy of tailored approaches in addressing health concerns unique to women and men. These narratives point out the role of personalized treatment, including herbal remedies, dietary adjustments, and lifestyle interventions. They offer a vivid illustration of how individualized care can lead to significant improvements in gender-specific health conditions.

Case Studies in Women's Health

1. **Polycystic Ovary Syndrome (PCOS)**: Sarah, a 28-year-old woman, struggled with irregular menstrual cycles, weight gain, and acne, classic symptoms of PCOS. Her treatment involved a combination of dietary changes, including a low-glycemic diet and increased intake of whole foods, along with herbal remedies like Chaste tree Berry and Saw palmetto. This integrative approach not only regularized her menstrual cycles but also alleviated her acne and helped her manage her weight more effectively.

2. **Menopause Management**: Linda, a 52-year-old experiencing severe menopausal symptoms such as hot flashes, mood swings, and insomnia, found relief through a holistic regimen. Her plan included Black Cohosh and Evening Primrose Oil to manage hot flashes and mood swings, along with lifestyle modifications like regular yoga and mindfulness practices. These interventions significantly improved her quality of life during menopause.

Examples in Men's Health

1. **Benign Prostatic Hyperplasia (BPH)**: John, a 60-year-old man, faced urinary difficulties and discomfort due to BPH. His treatment included Saw palmetto and Nettle Root to alleviate urinary symptoms, complemented by dietary adjustments to include more vegetables and omega-3 fatty acids. Regular moderate exercise, particularly walking, also played a key role in his symptom management.

2. **Cardiovascular Health**: Mark, a 45-year-old with a family history of heart disease, integrated Hawthorn Berry into his routine as a preventive measure. Alongside, he adopted a heart-healthy diet rich in fiber, lean proteins, and healthy fats, and incorporated daily cardiovascular exercises into his lifestyle. His proactive approach led to improved cardiovascular health markers.

Integrating Herbal and Lifestyle Approaches

1. **Stress-Related Insomnia**: Emily, a 35-year-old woman, experienced insomnia linked to her high-stress job. Incorporating stress management techniques such as meditation and deep breathing, alongside herbal remedies like Valerian Root and Lemon Balm, she achieved significant improvements in her sleep quality and overall stress levels.

2. **Weight Management**: Alex, a 40-year-old man struggling with obesity, followed a holistic weight management plan. This included dietary changes focusing on reducing processed foods and sugars, increasing physical activity, and using herbs like Green Tea and Cayenne Pepper for their metabolic-boosting properties. His commitment to this comprehensive approach resulted in a sustainable weight loss.

Addressing Fertility Issues

1. **Female Fertility**: Rachel, a 30-year-old trying to conceive, faced irregular ovulation. Her holistic treatment plan involved dietary changes to balance hormones, regular acupuncture sessions, and herbs like Maca Root and Shatavari. These interventions helped normalize her ovulation and eventually led to a successful pregnancy.

2. **Male Fertility**: David, a 33-year-old with low sperm count, adopted a holistic approach to improve his fertility. This included dietary adjustments to increase antioxidants, regular exercise to boost testosterone levels, and herbs like Ashwagandha and Ginseng. Over time, his sperm count improved, aiding in his and his partner's journey to parenthood.

Holistic Approaches to Mental Health

1. **Depression in Women**: Anna, a 38-year-old woman, dealt with depression. Her holistic treatment included St. John's Wort for its mood-lifting properties, coupled with Omega-3 supplements and a diet rich in fruits and vegetables. Regular engagement in group fitness classes also provided her with both physical and social support.

2. **Anxiety in Men**: Kevin, a 42-year-old, experienced high levels of anxiety. His regimen included herbal remedies such as Passionflower and Kava, alongside mindfulness meditation and cognitive-behavioral therapy. These combined strategies helped him manage his anxiety more effectively.

These real-life examples demonstrate the profound impact of holistic health approaches in addressing gender-specific health issues. They illustrate that solutions tailored to individual needs, incorporating a blend of herbal remedies, dietary interventions, and lifestyle changes, can lead to significant health improvements. These narratives validate the principles of personalized care, maximizing the importance of understanding and addressing the unique health challenges faced by women and men.

CHAPTER 7: CHILDREN'S HERBAL REMEDIES

The utilization of herbal remedies in pediatric care presents a unique approach to addressing the health concerns of children. Unlike adults, children require more specialized and gentle care, considering their developing bodies and specific health needs. Chapter 9 investigates children's herbal remedies, drawing upon the principles of safety, efficacy, and age-appropriateness. The chapter aims to provide a comprehensive guide to using herbal treatments for common childhood ailments, balancing traditional wisdom with modern understanding.

The Distinctiveness of Children's Physiology

Children are not miniature adults; their bodies function differently and are in a continuous state of growth and development. This distinctiveness necessitates a careful approach when considering herbal remedies.

1. **Developing Immune System**: A child's immune system is still developing, making them more susceptible to infections but also offering a unique opportunity for building long-term immunity.

2. **Metabolic Rate and Dosage Considerations**: Children have a higher metabolic rate compared to adults, which affects how they process substances, including herbs. This necessitates careful consideration of dosages and formulations of herbal remedies.

Safe Use of Herbal Remedies in Children

Safety is paramount when using herbal remedies in pediatric care. The delicate nature of children's bodies requires a cautious approach to avoid any potential adverse effects.

1. **Choosing Safe Herbs**: Selecting herbs that are known for their safety and mildness in children is crucial. Herbs like Chamomile, known for its soothing properties, and Echinacea, used for immune support, are commonly used due to their safety profiles.

2. **Professional Guidance**: Consulting with a pediatrician or a qualified herbalist before administering herbal remedy for children is essential. They

can provide guidance on appropriate herbs, dosages, and formulations suitable for children.

Collaboration with Healthcare Professionals

Collaboration with pediatricians or professional herbalists is crucial when using herbal treatments, especially for more serious or chronic conditions.

1. **Integrative Approach**: Working with healthcare professionals ensures that the herbal treatments are part of an integrative approach, complementing any other medical treatments the child may be receiving.

2. **Professional Oversight**: Regular check-ups and consultations with healthcare professionals help in monitoring the child's progress and adjusting treatments as needed.

3. **Consulting with Pediatricians**: Regular consultations with a pediatrician ensure that the herbal treatments align with the child's overall healthcare plan.

4. **Collaboration with Herbalists**: Involving a professional herbalist can provide additional insights into the appropriate use of herbal remedies, ensuring they are tailored to the child's specific needs.

Age-Appropriate Herbal Formulations

The formulation of herbal remedies for children must consider not only the appropriate dosages but also the palatability and administration method.

1. **Dosages for Children**: Herbal dosages for children are typically lower than for adults and need to be adjusted according to the child's age, weight, and health condition.

2. **Palatable Preparations**: Children are more likely to accept herbal remedies in pleasant-tasting forms, such as herbal syrups, glycerites, or teas sweetened with Honey (for children over one year of age).

Preventive and Acute Use Herbal Remedies

In addition to treating specific ailments, herbal remedies can be used preventively in children to bolster their natural defenses and promote overall well-being.

1. **Immune Support**: Regular use of certain immune-supportive herbs, especially during cold and flu season, can help in building a child's resistance to infections in a preventive way.

2. **Gut Health**: Herbs that support digestive health can be used as a preventive measure, particularly for children with a tendency towards digestive issues.

3. **Respiratory Infections**: For common colds and mild respiratory infections, herbs like Elderberry, known for its immune-boosting properties, and Thyme, with its natural expectorant qualities, are often used. These herbs can be administered in the form of syrups or mild teas.

4. **Digestive Issues**: Digestive complaints such as colic, indigestion, and mild constipation in children can be managed with gentle herbs like Chamomile, known for its calming effect on the digestive system, and Fennel, which can relieve gas and bloating.

This chapter emphasizes the importance of understanding the unique physiological and developmental needs of children when using herbal treatments. Through careful selection, safe formulation, and appropriate integration with diet and lifestyle, herbal remedies offer a natural and effective approach to addressing a wide range of childhood health issues. This serves as a guide for parents and caregivers in harnessing the gentle power of nature to nurture and maintain their child's health, underscoring the critical role of informed, cautious, and loving care in pediatric herbal therapy.

Preparations Suitable for Children

The form in which an herb is administered is as important as the herb itself, especially in pediatric care.

1. **Herbal Syrups and Glycerites**: These are often preferred for children due to their palatable taste. Herbal syrups can be made from a variety of herbs, depending on the condition being treated, and are sweetened in a natural and healthy manner.

2. **Infusions and Mild Teas**: Herbal teas, made from gentle herbs and sufficiently diluted, can be a comforting and effective way to administer herbal treatments to children.

Adjusting Dosages and Formats for Pediatric Use

The adjustment of dosages and formats to suit the unique needs of children is a critical aspect of safe and effective treatment. The emphasis here is on understanding how children's physiology differs from adults and the implications this has for herbal medicine.

Fundamentals of Pediatric Herbal Dosage

Determining the correct dosage of herbal remedies for children is far more complex than simply reducing adult dosages. It requires an understanding of children's metabolic rate, body weight, age, and overall health.

1. **Age-Based Adjustments**: Dosage guidelines often vary significantly depending on the child's age. Infants and toddlers, for instance, require much lower doses compared to older children, given their smaller body size and developing organ systems.

2. **Weight Considerations**: In many cases, dosages are calculated based on the child's weight. This approach ensures that the dosage is proportional to the child's physical size, a critical factor in the effective and safe use of herbal medicine.

Integrating Herbal Remedies into Children's Routines

Incorporating herbal remedies into a child's daily routine can enhance their acceptability and efficacy.

1. **Mealtime Integration**: Administering herbal remedies with meals or snacks can improve compliance in children. It can also aid in the digestion and absorption of the herbs.

2. **Creating Positive Associations**: Making the process of taking herbal remedies a positive experience can encourage adherence. This might involve creating a routine around remedy administration or pairing it with a favored activity.

Herbal Medicine as Part of a Holistic Health Approach

In pediatric care, herbal remedies are most effective when used as part of a holistic health approach, which includes diet, lifestyle, and emotional well-being.

1. **Balanced Diet**: A nutritious diet that supports a child's overall health can enhance the effectiveness of herbal remedies. This includes a diet rich in fruits, vegetables, whole grains, and adequate proteins.

2. **Healthy Lifestyle**: Adequate sleep, regular physical activity, and a stress-free environment contribute to the overall health of the child and the efficacy of the herbal treatments.

Discussion on Common Misconceptions and O'Neill's Approach to Pediatric Herbal Care

In pediatric herbal care, misconceptions abound, often stemming from a lack of understanding or misinformation about the nature and efficacy of herbal remedies for children. Addressing these misconceptions is crucial for fostering a safe and informed approach to pediatric herbalism. This subchapter aims to dispel these myths and elucidate the principles of safely incorporating herbal remedies into children's health care. By exploring O'Neill's approach, we gain a clearer understanding of how to effectively and responsibly use herbal treatments in pediatric care.

Common Misconceptions in Pediatric Herbalism

There are several widespread misconceptions regarding the use of herbal remedies in children, often leading to either undue skepticism or inappropriate use.

1. **"Herbs Are Completely Safe Because They Are Natural"**: One of the most prevalent myths is that all herbal remedies are inherently safe because they are natural. However, like all treatments, herbs can have side effects and interact with other medications, and have strong effects on children. Recognizing that natural does not always equate to safe is crucial in pediatric herbal care.

2. **"Adult Herbal Remedies Can Be Directly Translated to Children"**: Another common misconception is that children can safely consume adult herbal remedies in smaller doses. This overlooks the specific physiological and developmental needs of children, potentially leading to ineffective or harmful dosing.

O'Neill's Approach to Dispelling Myths

Barbara O'Neill's approach to pediatric herbal care offers valuable insights into addressing these misconceptions.

1. **Emphasis on Safety and Appropriateness**: O'Neill stresses the importance of understanding the safety profile of each herb used in children, including potential side effects and interactions. Her approach involves thoroughly researching and understanding the herbs before recommending them for pediatric use.

2. **Customization of Herbal Remedies for Children**: O'Neill advocates for the customization of herbal remedies to suit the unique needs of children. This includes consideration of age-appropriate dosages, suitable formats for administration, and the child's specific health condition and overall constitution.

Responsible Use of Herbs in Children

Responsible use of herbal remedies in children involves several key practices.

1. **Start with the Least Invasive Options**: O'Neill's approach often involves starting with the least invasive herbal options, particularly those known for their gentle action and minimal side effects.

2. **Use of Culinary Herbs**: Incorporating common culinary herbs, which are generally milder and well-tolerated, can be an effective and safe way to introduce herbal treatments to children.

Overcoming Skepticism with Evidence-Based Practices

To overcome skepticism and build trust in pediatric herbal care, reliance on evidence-based practices is vital.

1. **Research and Clinical Evidence**: O'Neill encourages the use of herbs backed by research and clinical evidence, particularly those with a proven track record of safety and efficacy in children.

2. **Case Studies and Anecdotal Evidence**: Sharing successful case studies and anecdotal evidence, while not a substitute for scientific research, can provide practical insights into the effective use of herbs in pediatric care.

Herbal Education for Families

Educating families about the benefits and proper use of herbal remedies is a cornerstone of O'Neill's approach.

1. **Workshops and Resources**: Providing workshops, literature, and online resources can empower parents with the knowledge needed to safely use herbal remedies at home.

2. **Encouraging Informed Decision-Making**: Empowering parents to make informed decisions regarding their child's health care, including the use of herbal remedies, is a key aspect of O'Neill's educational approach.

Addressing common misconceptions in pediatric herbal care is crucial for the safe and effective use of herbal remedies in children. Barbara O'Neill's approach, characterized by an emphasis on safety, customization, and education, offers valuable guidance in this area. By dispelling myths, educating parents, and integrating herbal treatments with conventional care, a responsible and informed approach to pediatric herbalism can be achieved.

CHAPTER 8: MENTAL AND EMOTIONAL WELL-BEING

The pursuit of mental and emotional well-being is as vital as maintaining physical health, yet it often remains shrouded in less clarity and understanding. This chapter explores the world of mental and emotional health, recognizing it as an integral part of overall well-being. The focus here is on understanding, nurturing, and maintaining mental and emotional wellness through various natural and holistic methodologies. This exploration emphasizes the interconnectedness of the mind, body, and spirit, acknowledging that true health encompasses all aspects of human experience.

The Complexity of Mental and Emotional Health

Mental and emotional well-being is multifaceted, encompassing our thoughts, emotions, behaviors, and overall psychological state. It's a dynamic continuum, influenced by various internal and external factors.

1. **Understanding Emotional Health**: Emotional health refers to how well we manage our emotions and express them appropriately. It involves awareness, understanding, and acceptance of our feelings, and the ability to handle stress, adapt to change, and overcome challenges.

2. **Mental Health Spectrum**: Mental health includes our emotional, psychological, and social well-being. It influences how we think, feel, act, handle stress, relate to others, and make choices. Its state can range from flourishing to struggling to clinical mental illness.

Herbal Remedies in Mental Health

The use of herbal remedies in supporting mental and emotional well-being has been a practice for centuries. Rooted in traditional knowledge, these natural treatments offer an alternative or complement to conventional methods.

1. **Herbs for Stress and Anxiety**: Herbs such as Ashwagandha, Lavender, and Lemon Balm are renowned for their stress-relieving properties. They can be used to create a calming effect, reduce anxiety, and promote relaxation.

2. **Natural Mood Enhancers**: St. John's Wort, Rhodiola, and Saffron are some of the herbs known for their mood-enhancing properties. They have been traditionally used to alleviate symptoms of depression and improve emotional well-being.

Emotional Well-being in Different Life Stages

Mental and emotional health needs can vary significantly across different stages of life, requiring tailored approaches for children, adolescents, adults, and the elderly.

1. **Childhood and Adolescence**: During these formative years, the focus is on fostering healthy emotional development, resilience, and coping skills. Addressing issues like bullying, self-esteem, and academic stress is crucial.

2. **Adulthood and Aging**: In adults, managing work-life balance, family responsibilities, and societal pressures are key for mental health, while for the elderly, issues like loneliness, loss of independence, and cognitive decline take precedence.

The Role of Community and Social Connections

The impact of community and social connections on mental and emotional health cannot be overstated. A sense of belonging, community involvement, and strong social support networks are essential components of emotional well-being.

1. **Building Strong Social Ties**: Engaging in community activities, nurturing friendships, and maintaining close family ties can provide emotional support and a sense of belonging.

2. **Addressing Loneliness and Isolation**: In a world where loneliness and social isolation are increasing, creating opportunities for meaningful social interactions is more important than ever.

Overcoming Challenges to Mental Wellness

Confronting the challenges to mental and emotional health involves recognizing the barriers, be they societal stigma, lack of resources, or personal struggles, and finding ways to overcome them.

1. **Combating Stigma**: One of the biggest challenges in addressing mental health is the stigma associated with it. Education, open conversations, and advocacy are key to breaking down these barriers.

2. **Access to Resources**: Ensuring access to mental health resources, including counseling, therapy, and support groups, is essential for those struggling with mental and emotional issues.

Chapter 10 offers a comprehensive insight into the vast and complex domain of mental and emotional well-being. It underscores the necessity of a holistic approach that encompasses not just medical or therapeutic interventions but also considers lifestyle, nutrition, herbal remedies, social connections, and the overarching environment.

Exploring Herbs and lifestyle approaches for Mental Health and Stress RELIEF

The use of herbs for mental health and stress relief is pivotal. This subchapter looks into the depth of herbalism, focusing on herbs that have been traditionally and scientifically acknowledged for their benefits in enhancing mental well-being and alleviating stress. This exploration reveals how specific herbs can be incorporated into daily routines to support mental health, mitigate stress, and foster a balanced emotional state, all within the framework of holistic well-being.

Herbs for Alleviating Anxiety and Stress

Certain herbs are specifically valued for their calming and anxiolytic properties.

1. **Lavender (Lavandula angustifolia)**: Renowned for its soothing scent, Lavender is widely used for its ability to reduce anxiety and induce relaxation. Its essential oil, used in aromatherapy, or the dried herb in teas, can provide a calming effect on the nervous system.

2. **Chamomile (Matricaria recutita)**: Traditionally used as a mild relaxant, Chamomile is effective in soothing stress and easing anxiety. Its gentle nature makes it suitable even for children, often used to calm restlessness or anxiety.

Herbs for Depression and Mood Imbalances

Certain herbs have been recognized for their potential in managing depression and mood swings, offering natural alternatives or adjuncts to conventional treatment.

1. **St. John's Wort (Hypericum perforatum)**: Widely known for its antidepressant properties, St. John's Wort has been used for centuries to alleviate symptoms of mild to moderate depression. It is thought to work by increasing the levels of neurotransmitters in the brain.

2. **Rhodiola Rosea**: Rhodiola is an adaptogen, aiding the body in adapting to stress, and is known for its ability to enhance mood and alleviate depression. Its role in balancing the stress hormones makes it particularly useful for stress-induced mood swings.

Seasonal Affective Disorder (SAD) and Herbal Remedies

The reduced sunlight in winter can lead to Seasonal Affective Disorder, a type of depression related to changes in seasons. Certain herbs can help alleviate its symptoms.

1. **St. John's Wort**: Known for its antidepressant properties, St. John's Wort can be beneficial for those experiencing mild to moderate SAD symptoms.

2. **Rhodiola Rosea**: An adaptogen, Rhodiola can help enhance mood and combat fatigue, making it suitable for combating the lethargy often associated with SAD.

Herbs for Cognitive Function and Mental Clarity

Enhancing cognitive function and mental clarity is another area where herbal remedies can be significantly beneficial.

1. **Ginkgo biloba**: Ginkgo is well-known for its ability to enhance cognitive function. It improves blood flow to the brain, which can help with memory retention, focus, and overall mental clarity.

2. **Gotu kola (Centella asiatica)**: Traditionally used in Ayurvedic and Chinese medicine, Gotu kola is reputed for its ability to improve mental function and is often used as a tonic for memory and concentration.

Adaptogenic Herbs for Stress Management

Adaptogenic herbs have a unique capacity to help the body resist and adapt to stress and exert a normalizing effect upon bodily processes.

1. **Ashwagandha (Withania somnifera)**: Ashwagandha is highly revered for its stress-relieving properties. It helps the body cope with external stresses such as toxins in the environment and internal stresses such as anxiety and insomnia.

2. **Holy basil (Tulsi)**: Holy basil, known as Tulsi in Ayurvedic medicine, is another adaptogen that helps the body adapt to stress and maintain mental balance. It is also revered for its spiritual significance in many cultures.

Addressing Sleep Disorders with Herbs

Poor sleep quality is a common issue affecting mental health. Certain herbs can be effective in promoting restful sleep.

1. **Valerian Root (Valeriana officinalis)**: Valerian is often used for its sedative properties, effective in treating insomnia and improving sleep quality.

2. **Passionflower (Passiflora incarnata)**: Passionflower is another herb used for its sleep-inducing properties. It is particularly beneficial for those with insomnia related to anxiety.

The exploration of herbs for mental health and stress relief offers a comprehensive approach to managing mental well-being. By understanding and utilizing the therapeutic properties of specific herbs, and integrating them into a balanced lifestyle, one can effectively support mental and emotional health.

Integrating Natural Therapies Together

The use of natural therapies, including herbal remedies, aromatherapy, and others, is a key aspect of improving mental and emotional wellness in a holistic way.

1. **Herbal Remedies**: Herbs like St. John's Wort, Ashwagandha, and Lavender can be used under professional guidance to address symptoms of stress, anxiety, and mild depression.

2. **Aromatherapy**: The use of essential oils, either through diffusers, baths, or topical application, can have a calming and uplifting effect on the mind and emotions.

Mind-Body Practices

Mind-body practices are central to O'Neill's holistic approach, emphasizing the interconnectedness of physical health with mental and emotional well-being.

1. **Yoga and Tai Chi**: These practices not only improve physical fitness but also enhance mental clarity, emotional balance, and stress resilience.

2. **Biofeedback and Mindfulness-Based Stress Reduction (MBSR)**: Techniques such as biofeedback and MBSR enable individuals to become more aware of their body's responses to stress and learn how to control them effectively.

Embracing Creativity and Recreation

Participation in creative and recreational activities is often overlooked but is vital in enhancing mental and emotional wellness.

1. **Creative Expressions**: Activities like painting, writing, or playing music provide an outlet for expressing emotions and can be incredibly therapeutic.

2. **Outdoor Activities and Nature Exposure**: Spending time in nature and engaging in outdoor activities can have a rejuvenating effect on both the mind and emotions.

Cultivating Positive Mindsets

O'Neill emphasizes the power of positive thinking and cultivating mindsets that support mental and emotional wellness.

1. **Practicing Gratitude**: Regularly practicing gratitude can shift focus from negative to positive aspects of life, enhancing overall emotional well-being.

2. **Cognitive Reframing**: Learning to reframe negative thoughts and perceptions into positive ones can significantly impact emotional health and resilience.

The methods for improving mental and emotional wellness offer a comprehensive and multi-faceted approach. This approach integrates physical health, stress management, social connections, natural therapies, mind-body practices, restful sleep, creative outlets, and positive mindsets into a cohesive strategy for mental and emotional health.

Reflective Questions or Exercises Applying Teachings to Personal Mental Health Scenarios

In the quest for mental and emotional well-being, self-reflection plays a pivotal role. This subchapter emphasizes the importance of reflective questions and exercises in applying teachings to personal mental health scenarios. These introspective practices are designed to deepen self-awareness, uncover underlying emotional patterns, and foster a proactive approach to mental health.

The Power of Self-Reflection in Mental Health

Self-reflection is a powerful tool in understanding and managing one's mental and emotional well-being. It involves looking inward, examining thoughts, feelings, and behaviors, and understanding their impact on one's life.

1. **Awareness of Emotional States**: Regular self-reflection helps in recognizing and acknowledging current emotional states, whether they are stress, anxiety, contentment, or joy. This awareness is the first step in managing emotions effectively.

2. **Understanding Thought Patterns**: Reflective practices aid in identifying recurrent thought patterns that may be contributing to mental health issues, such as tendencies toward negative or catastrophic thinking.

Reflective Questions for Personal Insight

Reflective questions are designed to provoke thought and insight into one's mental and emotional processes. They can be used as a part of daily journaling or during meditation.

1. **What are the predominant emotions I felt today, and what triggered them?**: This question helps individuals track their emotional responses and the triggers, enhancing emotional regulation.

2. **What thoughts tend to recur in my mind, and how do they affect my mood and behavior?**: This prompts introspection into habitual thought patterns and their impact on one's emotional state.

Exercises for Applying Holistic Teachings

Applying holistic teachings to one's life involves practical exercises that integrate these teachings into daily routines.

1. **Gratitude Journaling**: Keeping a gratitude journal, where one writes down things they are thankful for each day, can shift focus from negative to positive, enhancing overall well-being.

2. **Mindfulness Practice**: Engaging in mindfulness practices, such as mindful breathing or mindful walking, helps in staying present and reduces tendencies to ruminate on past or future worries.

Visualization and Affirmations

Visualization and affirmations are powerful tools in molding one's mental state and fostering a positive mindset.

1. **Positive Visualization**: Practicing visualization, where one imagines a positive outcome or a peaceful scenario, can have a calming effect and help in developing a positive outlook on life.

2. **Affirmations**: Repeating positive affirmations daily can help in rewiring the brain towards positive thinking and self-empowerment.

Reflective Exercises for Stress Management

Managing stress is crucial for mental health, and reflective exercises can be highly effective in this regard.

1. **Stress Diary**: Keeping a stress diary, where one notes down moments of high stress and their responses to these situations, can help in identifying patterns and triggers of stress.

2. **Relaxation Techniques**: Practicing relaxation techniques, such as progressive muscle relaxation or guided imagery, especially during times of high stress, can provide immediate relief and enhance long-term stress management skills.

Developing Emotional Resilience

Emotional resilience is the ability to adapt and bounce back from stress and adversity. Reflective exercises can help in building this resilience.

1. **Challenge and Change Perspective**: Encouraging oneself to view challenges as opportunities for growth and learning helps in developing resilience.

2. **Journaling for Resilience**: Writing about past challenges and how one overcame them can reinforce a sense of strength and resilience.

Self-Compassion Exercises

Self-compassion is fundamental to mental health, involving treating oneself with the same kindness and understanding as one would treat a friend.

1. **Self-Compassion Breaks**: Taking short breaks during the day to speak to oneself compassionately, especially during times of failure or difficulty, can enhance self-esteem and reduce self-criticism.

2. **Loving-Kindness Meditation**: Practicing loving-kindness meditation, where one directs feelings of love and kindness towards themselves and others, can foster an attitude of compassion and interconnectedness.

Addressing Mental Blocks and Barriers

Reflective questions and exercises can also help in identifying and addressing mental blocks and barriers that hinder emotional well-being.

1. **Identifying Limiting Beliefs**: Questions like "What beliefs are holding me back?" can help in recognizing and challenging limiting beliefs.

2. **Exploring Solutions**: Reflecting on questions like "What steps can I take to overcome these barriers?" encourages proactive problem-solving.

Reflective questions and exercises form an essential component of holistic mental health care. They offer a pathway for individuals to engage deeply with their emotional and mental processes, apply holistic teachings to their personal scenarios, and foster growth and healing. These practices encourage a journey of self-discovery, awareness, and transformation, leading to improved mental and emotional wellness.

Chapter 9: Seasonal Herbal Remedies

The concept of aligning healthcare practices with the rhythms of nature is deeply rooted and widely respected. This recognizes the dynamic interplay between our bodies and the changing seasons, advocating for the use of seasonal herbal remedies as a way to harmonize our internal health with the external environment. Chapter 11 offers a profound exploration into the world of seasonal herbal remedies, drawing from traditional wisdom and modern holistic practices. This involves the intricacies of selecting, preparing, and utilizing herbs that are particularly beneficial at different times of the year, thereby optimizing health and wellness in alignment with nature's cycles.

The Significance of Seasonal Changes in Health

Human health and wellness are intrinsically linked to the cycles of nature. Each season brings with it unique environmental changes that can impact physical and mental well-being.

1. **Impact of Seasons on Health**: The changing seasons can influence various aspects of health, including immune system function, mood, energy levels, and even susceptibility to certain health conditions. For instance, winter can bring about challenges in immune health and mood, while summer might stress hydration and heat-related issues.

2. **Seasonal Adaptation of the Body**: The human body naturally undergoes certain adaptations in response to seasonal changes. Understanding and supporting these adaptations through the use of appropriate herbal remedies can enhance health and well-being.

Spring: Detoxification and Renewal

Spring is often associated with renewal and detoxification, making it an ideal time to cleanse and rejuvenate the body after the winter months.

1. **Herbs for Detoxification**: Herbs like Dandelion, Nettle, and Milk Thistle are renowned for their detoxifying properties. They support liver function, aid in the elimination of toxins, and provide a refreshing start to the new

season. Check out our previous section that focuses on detoxification and digestive health.

2. **Supporting Allergy Relief**: Spring is also the season of allergies for many. Herbs like Butterbur and Quercetin can be effective in easing allergy symptoms.

Summer: Energy, Hydration, and Vitality

During the warm summer months, the focus shifts to maintaining hydration, protecting the skin, and sustaining energy levels in the face of increased outdoor activity.

1. **Herbs for Hydration and Cooling**: Herbs such as Hibiscus, Mint, and Cucumber are perfect for their cooling and hydrating properties. They can be used in teas or infused waters to keep the body cool and hydrated.

2. **Natural Sun Protection and Skin Care**: Herbs like Green Tea and Aloe vera offer protective and soothing properties for the skin, which can be beneficial in addressing sun exposure and promoting skin health during summer.

Autumn: Immune Boosting and Preparation for Winter

Autumn is a transitional period, where strengthening the immune system becomes a priority in preparation for the colder months.

1. **Immune-Boosting Herbs**: Echinacea, Elderberry, and Astragalus are excellent for bolstering the immune system. Their use during autumn can help prepare the body for the upcoming winter.

2. **Herbs for Respiratory Health**: With the onset of colder weather, respiratory health becomes crucial. Herbs like Mullein, Thyme, and Licorice can support lung health and aid in respiratory function.

Winter: Immune Support and Mood Enhancement

Winter challenges include maintaining immune function and coping with reduced sunlight and its effects on mood and energy.

1. **Supporting Immune Health**: Continuing the use of immune-supportive herbs like Elderberry, Garlic, and Ginger can help maintain health during the winter months.

2. **Mood and Energy Support**: Herbs like St. John's Wort and Rhodiola can be particularly useful in addressing seasonal affective disorder (SAD) and low energy levels often associated with the shorter days and longer nights of winter.

Understanding Seasonal Diet and Herbal Integration

The integration of seasonal diets with herbal remedies is a key aspect of holistic health. Eating according to the season and complementing it with corresponding herbal remedies can optimize health.

1. **Seasonal Foods**: Consuming foods that are naturally available in each season can provide the body with nutrients that are particularly needed during that time.

2. **Harmonizing Diet with Herbs**: For example, incorporating light, detoxifying foods and herbs in spring aligns with the body's natural inclination towards cleansing after winter.

The Role of Environmental Factors

The change in environmental conditions with each season significantly impacts our health. Adjusting herbal remedies according to environmental changes is crucial for maintaining balance.

1. **Adapting to Humidity and Dryness**: In humid summers, astringent herbs like Witch hazel can be useful, while in dry winters, moisturizing herbs like Marshmallow root can be beneficial.

2. **Coping with Seasonal Allergens**: In seasons where allergens are prevalent, herbs that support the respiratory system and immune response can be particularly helpful.

Herbal Preparations According to Seasons

The method of preparing and consuming herbs can also vary with seasons to match the body's needs.

1. **Cold Infusions in Summer**: Cold infusions or herbal iced teas are ideal for summer, providing hydration and cooling effects.

2. **Warm Decoctions in Winter**: In winter, warm herbal decoctions and hot teas can provide warmth and boost immunity.

The use of seasonal herbal remedies, as part of a broader holistic approach to health, offers a profound way to align our bodies with the natural rhythms of the earth. By understanding and respecting the unique requirements of each season, and by utilizing herbs, diet, and lifestyle practices that resonate with these natural cycles, we can optimize our physical, mental, and emotional well-being throughout the year.

Adapting Herbal Treatments According to the Changing Seasons

The philosophy of adapting herbal treatments to the changing seasons is a fundamental aspect of holistic health care. This is a recognition that our health needs to evolve with the changing seasons, and therefore, the herbs we use for treatment and wellness should also vary correspondingly. Embracing the cyclical nature of the earth and its correlation with human health, this subchapter explores the adaptation of herbal treatments to different seasons and how this practice not only aligns with the body's natural rhythms but also enhances the efficacy of herbal remedies in promoting health and preventing illness.

The Rationale Behind Seasonal Herbal Adaptation

Understanding why and how the body's needs change with the seasons is key to effectively adapting herbal treatments.

1. **Seasonal Health Needs**: Each season brings with it unique environmental factors; temperature changes, humidity levels, allergens, and varying amounts of sunlight, all of which impact health differently. For instance, winter's cold can increase susceptibility to respiratory illnesses, while summer heat might stress hydration and skin health.

2. **Aligning with Natural Rhythms**: Adapting herbal treatments according to the seasons is about aligning with the body's natural rhythms. This approach helps in maintaining balance and harmony in the body, reducing the risk of seasonal health issues.

Understanding Herbal Energetics in Seasonal Context

Herbal energetics, the warming, cooling, drying, or moistening nature of herbs; play a crucial role in seasonal adaptation.

1. **Matching Energetics to Seasonal Needs**: Using herbs with energetics that match the seasonal needs of the body can enhance health and well-being. For example, cooling herbs are more suited for summer, while warming herbs are beneficial in winter.

2. **Individual Energetics**: It's also important to consider the individual's unique energetics and constitution when selecting herbs, as personal needs may vary even within a given season. For instance, some individuals may require more moistening herbs in winter if they have a naturally dry constitution.

Seasonal Changes and Mental Health

The changing seasons also affect mental and emotional well-being, and adapting herbal treatments accordingly can be highly beneficial.

1. **Winter Blues and Herbal Mood Lifters**: In winter, shorter daylight hours can lead to Seasonal Affective Disorder (SAD). Herbs like St. John's Wort and Rhodiola can be helpful in uplifting mood.

2. **Stress and Relaxation**: During stressful seasons, such as the end-of-year holidays, herbs like Valerian and Chamomile can aid relaxation and stress relief.

Incorporating Seasonal Foods and Herbs

Integrating seasonal foods with herbal treatments enhances their effectiveness and supports overall health.

1. **Eating with the Seasons**: Consuming fruits and vegetables that are in season ensures a diet rich in necessary nutrients and aligns with the body's seasonal needs.

2. **Cooking with Herbs**: Incorporating culinary herbs and spices that are suited to the season, such as Basil in summer or Rosemary in winter, adds both flavor and health benefits to meals.

Cultural Practices and Seasonal Wellness

Many cultural practices around the world embrace the concept of aligning health practices with the seasons, offering valuable insights.

1. **Traditional Seasonal Practices**: Practices such as Ayurvedic seasonal routines or Traditional Chinese Medicine's alignment with seasonal energies can provide a deeper understanding of how to live in harmony with nature's rhythms.

2. **Community and Seasonal Festivities**: Participating in seasonal festivities and community activities can foster a sense of connection and well-being, aligned with the season's spirit.

Adapting herbal treatments and lifestyle practices according to the changing seasons is a profound way to maintain balance and harmony in both physical and mental health. This advocates for a responsive and dynamic way of caring for health. By tuning into the unique demands of each season and utilizing specific herbs, foods, and lifestyle practices, individuals can optimize their health and well-being throughout the year.

Chapter 10: Incorporating Herbs into Daily Life

Incorporating herbs into daily life is a practice that dates back to ancient times, reflecting a deep connection between human health and the natural world. This chapter examines the art and science of integrating herbal remedies into everyday routines, a concept that is gaining renewed interest in modern holistic health practices. It addresses the practical aspects of selecting, preparing, and using herbs in a way that is both effective and harmonious with contemporary lifestyles.

The Relevance of Herbs in Modern Life

In the modern world, herbs offer not only health benefits but also serve as a means to slow down, reconnect with nature, and nurture a more mindful approach to health.

1. **Preventive Health**: Herbs offer a natural way to support the body's defenses, improve resilience to stress, and enhance overall vitality, aligning well with the preventive health paradigm.

2. **Accessibility and Sustainability**: With a growing emphasis on sustainable living, incorporating herbs into daily life also represents an environmentally friendly approach to health and wellness.

Incorporating Herbs into Family Health

Herbs can be safely and effectively incorporated into family health practices, offering natural options for everyday ailments.

1. **Children and Herbs**: Introducing mild and safe herbs to children, such as Chamomile for calming or Echinacea for immune support, can be a gentle way to address common health concerns.

2. **Educating Family Members**: Educating family members about the benefits and safe use of herbs encourages a holistic approach to health within the household.

Everyday Uses of Herbs for Health and Wellness Following O'Neill's Lifestyle Recommendations

The use of herbs in daily life involves integrating these natural remedies into various aspects of our daily routines for health and wellness. This subchapter explores the practical, everyday applications of herbs. It emphasizes the philosophy that maintaining health is not just about reactive treatments but is deeply rooted in the proactive, daily integration of natural remedies and practices.

Herbal Supplements for Daily Health

For those seeking more concentrated benefits or specific therapeutic effects, herbal supplements can be incorporated into daily health routines.

1. **Daily Herbal Capsules or Tablets**: Supplements like turmeric capsules for inflammation, milk thistle for liver health, or ashwagandha for stress relief can be taken as part of a daily supplement regimen.

2. **Quality and Source Considerations**: When choosing herbal supplements, it's important to consider the quality and source, opting for products that are organic and sustainably sourced.

Herbal Teas for Hydration and Wellness

Herbal teas offer a delightful and healthful way to stay hydrated while enjoying the therapeutic benefits of various herbs.

1. **Custom Tea Blends**: Creating custom tea blends based on personal health needs and preferences can be a rewarding practice. For example, a blend of peppermint, ginger, and chamomile can aid digestion and soothe the stomach.

2. **Regular Tea Rituals**: Establishing a routine of herbal tea consumption, such as a calming chamomile tea before bed or a refreshing green tea in the morning, can be an enjoyable and healthful daily ritual.

Herbal Approaches to Immune Support

Strengthening the immune system is a key focus of holistic health, and daily use of certain herbs can be beneficial.

1. **Daily Immune Tonics**: Herbs like echinacea, astragalus, and elderberry can be used as tonics to boost the immune system, particularly during times when it is under stress, such as the cold and flu season.

2. **Incorporating Immune-Boosting Herbs in Meals**: Garlic, onions, and medicinal mushrooms can be included in daily meals for their immune-enhancing properties.

Herbs for Energy and Vitality

For those seeking natural ways to boost energy and vitality, certain herbs can be particularly effective.

1. **Adaptogenic Herbs for Energy**: Adaptogens like ginseng and rhodiola can help improve energy levels and resilience to stress.

2. **Herbal Smoothies and Juices**: Adding powdered or fresh herbs like spirulina, wheatgrass, or maca to smoothies or juices can provide a natural energy boost.

Herbs in Mindfulness and Meditation Practices

Integrating herbs into mindfulness and meditation practices can enhance their benefits.

1. **Burning Herbal Incense**: Herbs such as sage, cedar, and sweetgrass can be used as incense during meditation or mindfulness practices, aiding in grounding and focus.

2. **Herbal Essential Oils in Meditation**: Applying or diffusing essential oils during meditation can help deepen the practice and promote relaxation.

Incorporating herbs into daily life is a practice that enhances overall wellness, offering natural solutions for a range of health concerns. By weaving herbs into nutrition, stress management, immune support, and other aspects of daily living, individuals can tap into the vast healing potential of the plant world.

This represents a shift from reactive healthcare to a more balanced, holistic way of living, where health is nurtured daily through natural, simple, and effective means. By adopting this, individuals can foster a lifestyle that is in harmony with nature, sustainable, and deeply enriching.

Start Incorporating Herbs Daily

Incorporating herbs into daily life is a practice that can significantly enhance overall health and well-being. However, for many individuals, knowing where to start can be a challenge. This subchapter provides a clear and actionable plan to guide readers in integrating herbal remedies into their daily routines. The aim is to make the use of herbs accessible, practical, and effective, enabling readers to harness the full potential of these natural healers in a way that is sustainable and enjoyable. This comprehensive guide outlines step-by-step methods to seamlessly incorporate herbs into various aspects of daily life, from dietary habits to wellness routines, ensuring a holistic approach to health.

Step 1: Understanding Herbal Basics

Before integrating herbs into daily life, gaining a basic understanding of different herbs and their properties is essential.

1. **Research Common Herbs**: Start by researching common herbs and their health benefits. Familiarize yourself with herbs like ginger for digestion, lavender for relaxation, and echinacea for immune support.

2. **Learn About Herbal Safety**: Educate yourself on the safe usage of herbs, understanding potential side effects and interactions, especially if you are taking prescription medications.

Step 2: Setting Intentions and Goals

Define clear intentions and goals for incorporating herbs into your life. This will guide your choices and help you stay focused.

1. **Identify Health Goals**: Determine what health aspects you want to improve with herbs; whether it's boosting immunity, improving sleep, managing stress, or enhancing digestion.

2. **Set Realistic Expectations**: Understand that herbs are a complementary approach and may take time to show results. Set realistic expectations for your herbal journey.

Step 3: Starting with Simple Herbal Integrations

Begin by integrating herbs into your daily routines in simple, manageable ways.

1. **Herbal Teas**: Start your day with a cup of herbal tea suited to your health goals. For example, peppermint tea can be refreshing and aid digestion, while chamomile tea can be calming.

2. **Cooking with Herbs**: Incorporate culinary herbs like rosemary, thyme, and basil into your cooking. Use turmeric and ginger liberally for their anti-inflammatory properties.

Step 4: Incorporating Herbal Supplements

If specific health needs require more potent herbal interventions, consider herbal supplements.

1. **Choose Quality Supplements**: Opt for high-quality, organic herbal supplements from reputable sources.

2. **Start with Low Doses**: Begin with lower doses to see how your body responds and gradually increase as needed.

Step 5: Developing a Daily Herbal Routine

Establish a daily routine that incorporates herbal practices consistently.

1. **Morning Rituals**: Include herbal tonics or smoothies in your morning routine. Consider Aloe vera juice for digestive health or a green smoothie with spirulina for energy.

2. **Evening Wind-Down**: Create an evening routine with relaxing herbal teas or a warm bath infused with lavender or Epsom Saltss for relaxation.

Step 6: Personalizing Herbal Choices

Tailor your herbal selections to your unique health needs and preferences. Be sure to check out our herbal plan and formulation chapter for more information on this.

1. **Consider Personal Health Conditions**: Choose herbs that specifically address your individual health concerns. For instance, if you have chronic stress, adaptogenic herbs like ashwagandha may be beneficial.

2. **Preference and Taste**: Select herbs that you enjoy in terms of taste and aroma. This increases the likelihood of you sticking with your herbal routine.

Step 7: Creating Herbal Infusions and Decoctions

Learn to make basic herbal infusions and decoctions to extract the maximum benefits from herbs.

1. **Making Herbal Teas**: Steep herbs like chamomile or peppermint in hot water to make soothing teas.

2. **Preparing Decoctions**: For tougher herbs like roots and bark, simmer them in water for a longer period to make a decoction.

Step 8: Exploring Topical Applications

Explore the use of herbs topically for skin and hair care, as well as for muscle and joint health.

1. **Herbal Oils and Salves**: Create or purchase herbal oils and salves for topical application. For example, use arnica oil for bruises or aches, and calendula salve for skin irritations.

2. **Herbal Baths and Soaks**: Add herbs or essential oils like Epsom Saltss, lavender, or rosemary to baths for a relaxing and therapeutic experience.

Step 9: Integrating Herbs into Household Products

Replace some chemical-laden household products with herbal alternatives for a healthier living environment.

1. **Natural Cleaning Products**: Use herbs like thyme and lavender in homemade cleaning products for their natural antiseptic properties.

2. **Herbal Air Fresheners**: Create natural air fresheners using essential oils or dried herbs to enhance the ambiance of your home.

Step 10: Growing Your Own Herbs

If space allows, growing your own herbs can be a rewarding way to ensure a fresh, readily available supply.

1. **Starting a Herb Garden**: Begin with easy-to-grow herbs like basil, mint, and parsley. Even a small windowsill garden can provide a range of herbs.

2. **Harvesting and Storing**: Learn how to harvest and store herbs correctly to maintain their potency and freshness.

Step 11: Keeping an Herbal Journal

Documenting your herbal journey can be insightful and help track progress and responses.

1. **Record Experiences and Observations**: Note down how you feel after using certain herbs, any changes in health conditions, and recipes or preparations you've tried.

2. **Adjusting and Refining**: Use your journal insights to adjust your herbal routines and choices, refining them to better meet your health goals.

Step 12: Continual Learning and Adaptation

The world of herbal medicine is vast. Continual learning and adaptation are key to fully harnessing the benefits of herbs.

1. **Educational Resources**: Utilize books, online courses, workshops, and seminars to expand your knowledge of herbal medicine.

2. **Staying Updated**: Keep abreast of the latest research and developments in the field of herbalism to refine your practices and choices.

Step 13: Seeking Professional Guidance When Necessary

Consult with herbalists or healthcare providers for personalized advice, especially for specific health conditions or when using potent herbs.

1. **Professional Consultations**: Seek advice for developing a personalized herbal regimen, especially if you are dealing with specific health issues or taking medications.

2. **Safety First:** Always prioritize safety, especially when integrating herbs with other medications or treatments.

By following these steps, individuals can create a holistic herbal routine that not only addresses specific health needs but also contributes to a broader sense of well-being. This is not just about the physical benefits of herbs; it's also about fostering a deeper connection with nature and embracing a lifestyle that prioritizes natural, preventive healthcare. By this, individuals embark on a path of natural wellness that is enriching, sustainable, and deeply aligned with the body's innate healing capabilities.

CHAPTER 11: SUSTAINABLE AND ETHICAL SOURCING OF HERBS

In an era where the global demand for herbal products is steadily rising, the sustainable and ethical sourcing of herbs has become a topic of paramount importance. By opening up various aspects of sustainable and ethical sourcing, from cultivation and harvesting to fair trade and ecological considerations, this chapter aims to guide readers through the complexities of responsibly procuring herbs in a way that is both environmentally sound and socially equitable.

The Importance of Sustainable Sourcing

Sustainable sourcing of herbs is crucial to ensure the long-term viability of medicinal plants and the ecosystems in which they thrive, and this should also apply to how herbs are grown and produced

1. **Preservation of Biodiversity**: Many herbs are harvested from the wild, and unsustainable practices can lead to the depletion of native populations and loss of biodiversity. Sustainable sourcing ensures that these plants can regenerate and that their habitats are preserved.

2. **Impact on Local Ecosystems**: Responsible sourcing practices consider the broader ecological impact of herb cultivation and harvesting, including soil health, water use, and the well-being of local wildlife.

3. **Organic Farming**: This approach avoids the use of synthetic pesticides and fertilizers, focusing instead on natural methods to maintain soil health and control pests, which is crucial for the sustainability of herb cultivation.

4. **Biodynamic Farming**: Biodynamic agriculture goes a step further, viewing the farm as a cohesive ecosystem and integrating cosmic rhythms and holistic principles into farming practices.

5. **Diverse Crop Cultivation**: Support suppliers who practice crop diversity, which helps in maintaining soil health, controlling pests naturally, and preserving a wide range of plant species.

6. **Permaculture and Agroforestry Practices**: These sustainable agricultural practices mimic natural ecosystems, promoting biodiversity and ecological harmony.

The Role of Certifications in Verifying Sustainability

Certifications can play a critical role in ensuring the sustainability and ethical standards of herb sourcing.

1. **Organic Certification**: This verifies that herbs are grown without synthetic pesticides and fertilizers, in a way that supports ecological balance.

2. **Fair Trade Certification**: Fair trade certifications ensure that herbs are sourced under conditions that uphold social and economic equity for workers.

Ethical Considerations in Herbal Sourcing

Ethical sourcing extends beyond environmental concerns, encompassing the fair treatment of workers and respect for indigenous knowledge.

1. **Fair Labor Practices**: Ethical sourcing ensures that workers involved in the cultivation, harvesting, and processing of herbs are paid fair wages and work under safe conditions.

2. **Respecting Indigenous Rights**: Many medicinal herbs are tied to indigenous cultures and traditions. Ethical sourcing involves respecting these cultural connections and ensuring that indigenous communities are fairly compensated and not exploited.

Conservation of Endangered Species

Certain herbs are classified as endangered or threatened due to overharvesting and habitat loss.

1. **Avoiding Endangered Herbs**: Be aware of and avoid using herbs that are on endangered lists unless they are cultivated in a manner that does not harm wild populations.

2. **Supporting Conservation Efforts**: Support conservation efforts by choosing suppliers who actively participate in or contribute to the conservation of endangered species and their habitats.

Wildcrafting: Sustainable Harvesting from the Wild

Wildcrafting is the practice of harvesting herbs directly from their natural habitats, and it requires careful management to be sustainable.

1. **Responsible Wildcrafting Practices**: These include harvesting herbs in a way that allows the plant population to regenerate, avoiding overharvesting, and ensuring that the ecological balance of the habitat is maintained.

2. **Legal and Ethical Considerations**: Wildcrafting must also adhere to legal regulations and ethical guidelines, ensuring that wild herb populations are protected and conserved.

Traceability and Transparency in Herb Sourcing

Traceability and transparency are key to ensuring that herbs are sustainably and ethically sourced. Be sure to look into these practices and processes with each supplement or herbal product company you buy from.

1. **Tracking the Supply Chain**: Knowing where and how herbs are sourced, right from the farm to the final product, is crucial in ensuring sustainability and ethical practices.

2. **Consumer Awareness**: Educated consumers can make informed decisions and support brands and products that adhere to sustainable and ethical sourcing practices, thereby encouraging a broader shift in the industry.

3. **Testing for Contaminants**: Ensure that herbs are tested for contaminants like heavy metals, pesticides, and microbes, which can be harmful to health.

4. **Research Suppliers**: Take the time to research suppliers' practices and policies regarding sustainability and ethics. This can include looking into their sourcing methods, certifications, and company ethos.

5. **Transparency**: Choose suppliers who are transparent about their sourcing locations, methods, and the steps they take to ensure sustainability and ethical practices.

Sustainable Packaging and Shipping

The sustainability of herb sourcing extends to packaging and shipping practices.

1. **Eco-friendly Packaging**: Look for suppliers who use biodegradable, recyclable, or minimal packaging to reduce environmental impact.

2. **Reducing Carbon Footprint in Shipping**: Prefer suppliers who adopt environmentally friendly shipping practices, such as carbon-neutral shipping or bulk shipping options to minimize carbon emissions.

Consumer Responsibility and Education

As consumers, educating ourselves and making informed decisions are crucial steps in supporting sustainable and ethical herb sourcing.

1. **Continuous Learning**: Stay informed about issues related to herb sourcing, including environmental concerns, ethical dilemmas, and new sustainability initiatives.

2. **Making Informed Choices**: Use your purchasing power to support businesses and suppliers who align with sustainable and ethical practices, and encourage others to do the same.

Sustainable and ethical sourcing of herbs is an endeavor that encompasses environmental stewardship, social responsibility, and respect for traditional knowledge. By adhering to the guidelines outlined in this chapter, individuals can contribute to a more sustainable and equitable system of herb production and consumption.

Supporting Local Herbal Communities and Considering Environmental IMPACTS

The ethos of supporting local herbal communities and considering environmental impacts in the sourcing and use of herbs is a cornerstone of sustainable and ethical herbalism. This does not only foster the preservation and propagation of medicinal plants but also supports the livelihoods of local growers and communities, reinforcing the symbiotic relationship between humans and nature. The guidance offered here emphasizes the interconnectedness of health, community well-being, and environmental stewardship.

Engaging with Local Herbalists and Growers

Building relationships with local herbalists and growers can provide access to high-quality, fresh herbs while supporting the local economy.

1. **Purchasing Locally Grown Herbs**: Buying herbs directly from local farmers or herbalists ensures freshness and supports local agriculture.

2. **Participating in Community Herbal Events**: Engaging in local herbal fairs, markets, and workshops can foster community connections and enhance one's understanding of herbs.

Advocating for Ethical Wildcrafting

Ethical wildcrafting ensures that wild herbs are harvested sustainably, protecting them from overexploitation and preserving their natural habitats.

1. **Responsible Harvesting Practices**: Supporting harvesters who adhere to ethical wildcrafting guidelines, such as taking only what is needed and leaving enough for regeneration, is essential.

2. **Educating About Sustainable Foraging**: Providing education on sustainable foraging practices can help protect wild herb populations and their ecosystems.

Fostering Community-Based Herbal Projects

Community-based projects can empower local communities, preserve traditional knowledge, and promote sustainable practices.

1. **Community Gardens and Herbal Co-ops**: Establishing community herb gardens or cooperatives can provide access to medicinal plants while fostering community involvement and education.

2. **Conservation and Restoration Projects**: Participating in or supporting local conservation and restoration projects for medicinal plants can help maintain biodiversity and ecological health.

Advocating for Policy and Regulatory Support

Advocating for supportive policies and regulations is essential for the sustainable development of the herbal sector.

1. **Lobbying for Supportive Legislation**: Engaging in advocacy efforts to lobby for legislation that supports sustainable and ethical herbal practices, such as organic certification, fair trade, and conservation policies.

2. **Participation in Regulatory Processes**: Participating in regulatory processes to ensure that policies and regulations are informed by the needs and perspectives of the local herbal community.

Supporting local herbal communities and considering environmental impacts in herb sourcing encompasses environmental stewardship, social responsibility, cultural preservation, and economic sustainability. Through collective efforts and shared responsibility, we can ensure that the benefits derived from herbal resources are sustainable, equitable, and beneficial for all stakeholders, including future generations.

Discussion AND Reflection on the Importance of Sustainability in Herbal Practice

Sustainability in herbal encompasses a broad spectrum of practices, from the cultivation and harvesting of herbs to their processing and distribution. This subchapter opens a discussion and reflection on the critical importance of sustainability in herbal practice, underscoring how it aligns with the ethics of natural medicine and the broader context of environmental stewardship and social responsibility in a global context. The focus here is to foster a deeper understanding and commitment among practitioners, consumers, and enthusiasts towards sustainable practices in the field of herbal medicine.

Sustainable Sourcing and Its Challenges

While the intent to source herbs sustainably is commendable, it often comes with challenges that need addressing.

1. **Navigating Certification and Standards**: Understanding and navigating various certifications and standards for sustainable sourcing can be complex.

2. **Balancing Cost and Accessibility**: Often, sustainably sourced herbs can be more costly, posing challenges in making herbal medicine accessible to a broader population.\

Reflecting on the Global Impact of Local Practices

The practice of herbal medicine at a local level has a global impact. Reflecting on this interconnectedness is crucial for understanding the role of sustainability.

1. **Understanding the Global Herbal Market**: Recognizing how local practices contribute to global supply chains can foster a deeper understanding of the importance of sustainable practices.

2. **Responsibility to Global Communities**: Herbal practitioners and consumers have a responsibility to consider how their choices affect communities and environments worldwide.

Sustainable Herbalism as an Ethos

Sustainable herbalism is more than a set of practices; it's an ethos that encompasses respect for nature, social responsibility, and a commitment to the health of future generations.

1. **Living the Principles**: Practitioners of sustainable herbalism embody the principles in their personal and professional lives, serving as examples for others.

2. **Commitment to Continuous Learning**: Engaging in continuous learning and adaptation is essential to stay abreast of best practices in sustainable herbalism.

Sustainability in herbal practice is a multi-dimensional concept that extends beyond environmental conservation to encompass social equity, economic viability, and ethical responsibility. As practitioners, consumers, and advocates of herbal medicine, understanding and implementing sustainable practices is imperative to ensure the longevity and efficacy of herbal remedies while protecting the planet and supporting communities.

CHAPTER 12: HERBAL PREPARATION, SOURCING, PRESERVATION AND STORAGE

The art of herbal medicine extends far beyond the mere identification of herbs and their properties. It encompasses a deep understanding of how to safely gather and prepare these natural gifts, as well as how to preserve and store them for use over the long-term.

This subchapter digs into the practices essential for ensuring the potency and safety of herbal remedies though such techniques. These practices are not only crucial for maximizing the healing benefits of herbs but also embody a deeper respect for nature and its resources.

The Ethics of Herbal Gathering

Before going into the technicalities of gathering herbs, it is crucial to understand the ethics that guide these practices. Ethical gathering is rooted in a profound respect for nature and its ecosystems. It involves taking only what is needed, ensuring that the harvesting of herbs does not deplete natural populations or disturb their natural habitat. This respect extends to seeking permission from landowners and recognizing the cultural significance of certain plants to indigenous communities.

O'Neill outlines the importance of sustainable gathering practices. This includes understanding the life cycle of plants, gathering at the appropriate time in the season to ensure regeneration, and being mindful of the impact of harvesting on the local ecosystem. For example, when gathering roots, one should only take a portion of the root system, leaving enough to allow the plant to recover and continue its growth cycle.

Identification and Quality

Accurate identification of herbs is a fundamental aspect of safe herbal gathering. Misidentification can lead to the use of the wrong herb, potentially causing harm. O'Neill advises the use of reliable field guides and, if possible, learning from experienced herbalists.

Assessing the quality of herbs is equally important. This involves examining the plants for signs of health and vitality. Healthy plants are more likely to have a higher concentration of beneficial compounds. Factors such as color, aroma, and texture can provide clues to the quality of the herb. For instance, vibrant colors and strong, fresh scents are often indicators of good quality.

Harvesting Techniques

Proper harvesting techniques are essential for preserving the integrity and medicinal properties of herbs. Different parts of the plant; leaves, flowers, roots, seeds, require different harvesting techniques. O'Neill teaches that leaves and flowers should be harvested when the plant is in its peak flowering stage, as this is when the concentration of active constituents is highest.

When harvesting roots, it is typically done in the fall when the plant's energy has moved back into the root system. Seeds are collected when they are fully mature and have begun to dry on the plant. The techniques of harvesting also include gentle handling to prevent bruising and damage to the plant tissues.

Drying and Storage

Once harvested, the proper drying and storage of herbs are crucial for maintaining their medicinal qualities. O'Neill's guidelines suggest that herbs should be dried quickly to prevent the growth of mold and the degradation of active compounds. Methods of drying include air drying, using a dehydrator, or in some cases, oven drying at a low temperature.

The storage of dried herbs is equally important. Herbs should be stored in airtight containers away from direct sunlight and moisture. Glass jars with tight-fitting lids are ideal for this purpose. Properly dried and stored herbs can retain their potency for up to a year.

Techniques for Preserving and Storing Herbs

In herbal medicine, the preservation and storage of herbs are as crucial as their cultivation and sourcing. The process of preserving and storing herbs involves understanding the unique properties of each herb and employing methods that best retain their medicinal qualities. This chapter aims to guide enthusiasts, practitioners, and consumers of herbal medicine through various techniques and considerations for effective preservation and storage. By doing so, it ensures that the integrity and healing power of herbs are maintained from harvest to use, aligning with the holistic approach of maximizing therapeutic benefits while minimizing waste and loss of quality.

The Importance of Proper Preservation and Storage

The significance of preserving and storing herbs correctly cannot be overstated. It is a critical step in maintaining the therapeutic properties of herbs.

1. **Retention of Medicinal Properties**: Proper preservation techniques ensure that the active constituents of herbs are retained, thereby guaranteeing their effectiveness when used for medicinal purposes.

2. **Preventing Degradation and Spoilage**: Improper storage can lead to degradation of herbs due to factors like moisture, light, and temperature, resulting in spoilage and loss of medicinal qualities.

Understanding the Basics of Herbal Preservation

Herbal preservation involves a variety of techniques, each suited to different types of herbs and their specific properties. Read further into this chapter to get a deeper dive into these storage and preservation approaches.

1. **Drying**: Drying is one of the most common methods of preserving herbs. It involves removing moisture from the herbs, thereby inhibiting the growth of microorganisms that cause decay.

2. **Freezing**: Freezing is another effective method, especially for preserving the flavor and medicinal properties of fresh herbs.

Factors Influencing Herbal Preservation

Several factors influence the effectiveness of herbal preservation, and understanding these is key to choosing the right method.

1. **Moisture Content**: Herbs with high moisture content, like basil or mint, may require different preservation techniques compared to those with lower moisture content.

2. **Herb Type and Form**: The preservation method may vary depending on whether the herb is a leaf, flower, root, or seed.

Storing Preserved Herbs

Once preserved, proper storage of herbs is crucial to maintaining their quality over time.

1. **Airtight Containers**: Herbs should be stored in airtight containers to protect them from moisture and air, which can lead to spoilage.

2. **Cool, Dark, and Dry Storage**: Herbs are best stored in cool, dark, and dry places to prevent degradation from light and heat.

Labeling and Organization

Proper labeling and organization of stored herbs are important for ease of use and maintaining effectiveness.

1. **Labeling with Date and Name**: Each container of preserved herbs should be labeled with the herb's name and the date of preservation to track freshness and potency.

2. **Organized Storage System**: Organizing herbs systematically, perhaps alphabetically or by type, can facilitate easy access and ensure that older herbs are used first.

Special Techniques for Specific Herbs

Certain herbs may require special preservation techniques due to their unique properties.

1. **Preserving Volatile Oils**: Herbs with volatile oils, such as peppermint or eucalyptus, may require quick drying or freezing methods to retain their essential oils.

2. **Storing Roots and Barks**: Roots and barks often require different preservation techniques, such as slicing and drying at specific temperatures, to ensure their medicinal constituents are maintained.

Impact of Preservation on Herbal Efficacy

The method of preservation can impact the efficacy of herbs, making it crucial to choose methods that align with the intended use of the herb.

1. **Retention of Active Constituents**: Preservation methods should be chosen based on their ability to retain the active constituents relevant to the herb's medicinal use.

2. **Considerations for Therapeutic Use**: The intended therapeutic use of the herb should guide the choice of preservation method to ensure maximum efficacy.

Sustainable and Ethical Considerations in Preservation

Sustainability and ethics should also guide the preservation and storage of herbs, reflecting a holistic approach to herbalism.

1. **Environmentally Friendly Methods**: Preference should be given to preservation methods that have a minimal environmental impact, such as air drying or using energy-efficient dehydrators.

2. **Ethical Sourcing and Preservation**: Ethical considerations should extend to preservation, ensuring that the methods used do not negatively impact the environment or local communities.

The preservation and storage of herbs is critical for maintaining the herbs' medicinal properties and ensuring their longevity. These techniques are not just about prolonging the shelf life of herbs but are deeply intertwined with the philosophy of maximizing their therapeutic benefits. This subchapter reiterates various methods and techniques for preserving and storing herbs. It offers detailed insights into the best practices that ensure herbs retain their potency, flavor, and healing properties over time.

Drying Herbs

Drying is one of the most traditional and effective methods for preserving herbs. It involves removing moisture from the herbs, which prevents the growth of bacteria and mold.

1. **Air Drying**: This is a simple and natural method, suitable for most herbs, especially leafy ones like basil, oregano, and mint. Herbs are tied in small bundles and hung upside down in a warm, dry, and well-ventilated area away from direct sunlight.

2. **Oven Drying**: For quicker drying, herbs can be placed on a baking sheet in a low-temperature oven. This method requires careful monitoring to prevent burning and ensure even drying.

3. **Using Dehydrators**: Dehydrators are ideal for controlling temperature and air flow, making them suitable for drying a variety of herbs. They are particularly useful in humid climates where air drying is less effective.

Freezing Herbs

Freezing preserves the flavor and some of the medicinal properties of herbs, particularly those with high moisture content.

1. **Freezing in Water**: Herbs can be chopped and frozen in ice cube trays with water. This method is great for herbs used in cooking, as the cubes can be directly added to dishes.

2. **Freezing in Oil**: Herbs can also be frozen in oil, which is ideal for herbs used in sautéing and frying. The oil helps preserve the flavor and texture of the herbs.

3. **Blanching Before Freezing**: For some herbs, blanching before freezing can help retain color and flavor. This involves briefly boiling the herbs and then plunging them into ice water before freezing.

Creating Herbal Infused Oils

Infused oils are another way to preserve the medicinal properties of herbs, especially those with volatile oils.

1. **Cold Infusion Method**: Herbs are soaked in oil, such as olive or almond oil, for several weeks in a warm, sunny spot, then strained and stored.

2. **Heat Infusion Method**: For a quicker process, herbs and oil can be gently heated over a double boiler for a few hours, then strained and stored.

Preserving Herbs in Vinegar and Honey

Vinegar and Honey are also effective mediums for preserving certain herbs.

1. **Herbal Vinegars**: Herbs can be steeped in vinegar to create flavorful and medicinal preparations. Apple cider vinegar is commonly used due to its own health benefits.

2. **Herbal Honeys**: Soaking herbs in Honey not only preserves their properties but also creates a pleasant medicinal product. This is particularly useful for herbs used in soothing sore throats and coughs.

Long-term Preservation Strategies

For long-term storage, some additional strategies can be employed.

1. **Vacuum Sealing**: Vacuum-sealed bags can extend the shelf life of dried herbs by protecting them from air and moisture.

2. **Silica Gel Packs**: Including silica gel packs in herb containers can help absorb any excess moisture and keep the herbs dry.

Quality Checks and Routine Monitoring

Regular monitoring is key to ensuring the herbs maintain their quality over time.

1. **Periodic Quality Checks**: Regularly check stored herbs for any signs of degradation, such as changes in color, smell, or texture.

2. **Rotating Stock**: Use a first-in, first-out system to ensure older stocks are used before newer ones, maintaining the freshness and potency of the herbs.

Sustainable Practices in Preservation and Storage

Sustainability should also be considered in the preservation and storage of herbs.

1. **Eco-friendly Packaging**: Opt for environmentally friendly packaging materials, such as glass or recyclable plastics.

2. **Energy Efficiency**: When using methods like dehydrating or freezing, consider the energy efficiency of appliances to minimize the environmental impact.

Effective preservation and storage of herbs are foundational to the practice of herbal medicine, ensuring that the full therapeutic potential of herbs is available when needed. By understanding and applying the various techniques of drying, freezing, tincturing, and oil infusion, as well as proper storage methods, practitioners and enthusiasts can ensure the longevity and efficacy of their herbal remedies.

Practical Tips and 'Homework' for Implementing Effective Preservation Techniques

Implementing effective preservation techniques for herbs requires more than just an understanding of various methods; it demands practical application and consistent practice. This subchapter is dedicated to providing hands-on tips and actionable 'homework' assignments for individuals looking to integrate effective herb preservation techniques into their routine. These practical exercises are designed to deepen one's skills and knowledge in herbal preservation, ensuring that the medicinal properties of herbs are maintained for their optimal use.

Practical Tip 1: Establishing a Drying Routine

A consistent drying routine is fundamental for preserving many types of herbs.

Homework Assignment:

- Identify three commonly used herbs in your kitchen or herbal practice.

- Research the optimal drying method for each herb (air drying, oven drying, dehydrating).

- Practice drying each herb using the identified method and document the process, including time taken and changes observed in the herbs.

Practical Tip 2: Creating Your Own Herbal Tinctures

Making herbal tinctures is an excellent way to preserve herbs' medicinal properties.

Homework Assignment:

- Follow a step-by-step guide to create your tincture, label it with the date and contents, and monitor the tincture over a four to six-week period, shaking it daily.

Practical Tip 3: Experimenting with Freezing Techniques

Freezing herbs is a quick way to preserve their freshness, especially for culinary use.

Homework Assignment:

- Select two herbs with high moisture content, such as basil or cilantro.

- Experiment with different freezing techniques: freezing in water, oil, and as a pesto or puree.

- Document the flavor and texture of these herbs after thawing and use them in a cooking recipe to evaluate their preserved quality.

Practical Tip 4: Vacuum Sealing Dried Herbs

Vacuum sealing can significantly extend the shelf life of dried herbs.

Homework Assignment:

- After drying a batch of herbs, use a vacuum sealer to package them.

- Store these herbs for a month, then open and evaluate their condition compared to non-vacuum sealed herbs in terms of aroma, texture, and color.

Practical Tip 5: Making and Storing Herbal Infused Oils

Herbal oils are both therapeutic and can be used in cooking.

Homework Assignment:

- Choose a herb and a carrier oil (like olive or almond oil) to create an infused oil.

- Use either the cold infusion method or the heat infusion method to prepare your herbal oil.

- Store the oil in a cool, dark place and use it within a specified time, noting any changes in its properties.

Practical Tip 6: Building a Herbal Storage System

Proper storage is as important as the preservation method itself.

Homework Assignment:

- Designate a storage area in your home that is cool, dark, and dry.

- Organize your preserved herbs, tinctures, and oils in this area using airtight containers, proper labeling, and a first-in, first-out system.

- Regularly check this area for any signs of spoilage or degradation.

Practical Tip 7: Utilizing Natural Antioxidants in Preservation

Natural antioxidants can enhance the shelf life of oil-based herbal preparations.

Homework Assignment:

- Research natural antioxidants such as Vitamin E or rosemary extract.

- Add these antioxidants to one of your herbal oil preparations.

- Compare the shelf life and quality of this preparation with another batch without antioxidants over a period.

Practical Tip 8: Learning Through Observation

Observation is a key aspect of mastering herbal preservation.

Homework Assignment:

- Select several herbs with different preservation needs (such as leafy herbs, roots, and flowers).

- Apply a suitable preservation method to each (drying, freezing, tincturing, etc.) and closely observe and record the changes over time, noting aspects like color, texture, scent, and any signs of spoilage.

Practical Tip 9: Experimenting with Herbal Vinegars and Honeys

Herbal vinegars and Honeys are not only medicinal but also culinary delights.

Homework Assignment:

- Create a herbal vinegar using Apple cider vinegar and a herb of your choice. Let it infuse for 4-6 weeks, shaking it regularly.

- Similarly, prepare a herbal Honey by infusing raw Honey with a different herb.

- Use these preparations in cooking or as a remedy and note their flavors, effectiveness, and shelf life.

Practical Tip 10: Implementing a Rotational System for Herb Use

A rotational system ensures that herbs are used while they are most potent.

Homework Assignment:

- Organize your herbs and herbal preparations according to their preservation dates.

- Plan to use the oldest items first and rotate stock regularly.

- Keep track of the usage and replenishment of your herbs to maintain a fresh and effective supply.

Practical Tip 11: Engaging in Continuous Learning

The field of herbal preservation is ever-evolving, and continuous learning is key.

Homework Assignment:

- Subscribe to herbal journals, join online forums, or participate in workshops focused on herbal preservation.

- Implement at least one new preservation technique you learn every few months.

- Share your learnings and experiences with a community of herbal enthusiasts.

Practical Tip 12: Sustainability in Herbal Preservation

Sustainability should be a guiding principle in your preservation practices.

Homework Assignment:

- Audit your current preservation methods for their environmental impact.

- Research and implement at least one more eco-friendly preservation method, such as using solar dehydrators or recycling jars for tinctures.

- Evaluate the changes and consider their long-term sustainability benefits.

Mastering the art of preserving and storing herbs is a vital skill in herbalism, ensuring that the healing properties of herbs are available whenever needed. Through these practical tips and hands-on homework assignments, individuals can develop a deeper understanding and proficiency in various herbal preservation techniques. As each herb is unique in its preservation needs, the continuous application and refinement of these techniques are essential.

CHAPTER 13: HERBAL FIRST AID KIT

The concept of an herbal first aid kit takes a central stage in health and wellness, offering a natural and effective alternative to conventional first aid methods. This chapter provides an in-depth explanation of creating and utilizing a herbal first aid kit, a vital component for anyone seeking to integrate natural remedies into their healthcare practices.

The herbal first aid kit is a testament to the power and versatility of herbs in addressing a wide range of common ailments and emergencies. This comprehensive guide depicts the selection of herbs, preparation of remedies, and practical applications, ensuring that individuals are well-equipped to handle minor health issues with natural, effective solutions.

The Essence of a Herbal First Aid Kit

The essence of a herbal first aid kit lies in its ability to offer immediate, accessible, and natural remedies for various common health concerns.

1. **Natural and Holistic Approach**: A herbal first aid kit embodies the principles of natural medicine, offering remedies that work in harmony with the body's natural healing processes.

2. **Empowerment through Self-Care**: Equipping oneself with a herbal first aid kit is an empowering step towards taking charge of one's health and well-being, reducing reliance on synthetic medications for minor ailments.

Selecting Herbs for the First Aid Kit

The selection of herbs for a first aid kit is a thoughtful process, guided by the herbs' medicinal properties and the types of ailments they can address.

1. **Broad-Spectrum Herbs**: Including herbs with broad-spectrum healing properties, such as calendula for skin issues or chamomile for digestive discomfort, is crucial.

2. **Specific Remedies for Common Ailments**: Herbs like peppermint for headaches, Aloe vera for burns, or echinacea for immune support, are essential in a well-rounded kit.

Preparation of Herbal Remedies

The preparation of herbal remedies is a key aspect of building a first aid kit, involving various forms such as tinctures, salves, oils, and teas.

1. **Tinctures for Longevity**: Preparing tinctures of certain herbs ensures that their medicinal properties are preserved for longer periods and are readily available for use.

2. **Salves and Ointments for Topical Application**: Creating salves and ointments for external use, such as comfrey salve for bruises or Tea tree oil ointment for antiseptic needs.

Practical Applications of Herbal Remedies

Understanding the practical applications of each herb and remedy in the kit is vital for effective first aid.

1. **Knowledge of Herbal Actions**: Familiarity with the actions of herbs, such as anti-inflammatory, antiseptic, or analgesic properties, allows for their appropriate application in various situations.

2. **Method of Application**: Knowing how to apply each remedy, whether it be a poultice, a compress, or an oral administration, is essential for the efficacy of the treatment.

Safety and Precautions

While herbal remedies are generally safe, understanding their proper use and potential contraindications is crucial.

1. **Allergies and Sensitivities**: Being aware of potential allergic reactions or sensitivities to certain herbs and testing them before widespread use.

2. **Interactions with Medications**: Knowledge of any possible interactions between herbal remedies and prescription medications.

Customizing the Herbal First Aid Kit

Customizing the first aid kit to suit individual or family needs ensures that it is tailored to specific health requirements and preferences.

1. **Personalization Based on Lifestyle**: Including remedies that align with one's lifestyle, activities, and common health issues faced.

2. **Family-Specific Needs**: Adjusting the kit to include remedies suitable for children or elderly family members, considering their specific health needs.

Portability and Accessibility

Designing the first aid kit for portability and ease of access is important, especially for those who travel or spend a lot of time outdoors.

1. **Compact and Travel-Friendly Design**: Organizing the kit in a compact, portable container that can easily fit in a backpack or car.

2. **Labeling and Organization**: Clearly labeling each remedy and organizing the kit in a way that makes it easy to find what is needed quickly in an emergency.

Education and Training

Possessing the knowledge and skills to use the herbal first aid kit effectively is as crucial as the kit itself.

1. **Learning Herbal First Aid Techniques**: Acquiring knowledge through books, courses, or workshops on how to use each herb and remedy in the kit.

2. **Practice and Familiarization**: Regularly practicing the preparation and application of remedies to become comfortable and efficient in using the kit.

Sustainable and Ethical Sourcing of Herbs

Ensuring that the herbs and ingredients in the first aid kit are sourced sustainably and ethically aligns with the principles of holistic health.

1. **Choosing Ethically Sourced Herbs**: Opting for herbs that are grown and harvested sustainably, respecting environmental and social ethics.

2. **Supporting Local Herb Suppliers**: Where possible, sourcing herbs from local growers or suppliers to support community businesses and reduce the ecological footprint.

Regular Maintenance of the Kit

Regular maintenance of the herbal first aid kit ensures that its contents remain effective and safe to use.

1. **Checking Expiry Dates**: Regularly checking and replacing any remedies that have expired or lost their potency.

2. **Restocking and Updating**: Keeping the kit stocked and updating it with new remedies or herbs as needed.

Incorporating Complementary Tools and Supplies

In addition to herbal remedies, incorporating other complementary tools and supplies can enhance the functionality of the first aid kit.

1. **Essential Tools**: Including items such as scissors, tweezers, cotton swabs, and bandages to assist in the application of remedies.

2. **Educational Materials**: Carrying a small guide or notes on the use of each herb and remedy for quick reference.

Addressing a Range of Health Concerns

A well-prepared herbal first aid kit can address a range of health concerns from minor injuries to common ailments.

1. **Minor Injuries**: Including herbs and remedies for cuts, bruises, insect bites, and sprains.

2. **Common Ailments**: Having remedies on hand for issues like indigestion, headaches, stress, or insomnia.

Creating and maintaining a herbal first aid kit is a rewarding endeavor that enhances one's ability to respond to health concerns with natural, effective solutions. The herbal first aid kit is not only a toolkit for wellness but also a symbol of a lifestyle that values and utilizes the healing power of nature, reflecting a deep understanding and respect for the ancient wisdom of herbalism.

Building a Basic Kit of Herbal Remedies for Immediate Needs

Creating a basic herbal first aid kit involves a thoughtful selection of herbs and natural remedies targeted at addressing immediate and common health concerns. This subchapter searches deeper into the the importance of choosing a range of herbs that are versatile, effective, and safe for various situations, from minor injuries to everyday health complaints.

Essential Herbs for Immediate Needs

Certain herbs are particularly useful for immediate needs due to their specific healing properties.

1. **Calendula**: Known for its skin-healing properties, calendula is ideal for cuts, scrapes, and mild burns. It can be included in the kit as a cream, ointment, or tincture.

2. **Peppermint**: Useful for digestive issues, headaches, and as a cooling agent, peppermint can be included as tea or oil.

Tools and Supplies for the Herbal Kit

In addition to herbal remedies, certain tools and supplies are essential for a well-equipped first aid kit.

1. **Application Tools**: Include items such as cotton balls, swabs, and small spatulas for applying salves and ointments.

2. **Storage Containers**: Opt for small, durable containers that protect the remedies from light and air, such as amber glass bottles for tinctures and metal tins for salves.

Simple Home Preparations

Some effective first aid remedies can be prepared easily at home, providing a cost-effective and personalized approach to herbal first aid.

1. **Aloe vera Gel**: Fresh Aloe vera gel, extracted from the leaves of the aloe plant, is excellent for burns, sunburn, and skin irritation.

2. **Herbal Teas**: Packets of dried herbs like chamomile or ginger can be included for making teas to address issues like stress or indigestion.

Addressing Common Ailments

The kit should contain remedies that address a variety of common ailments, from skin issues to respiratory problems.

1. **Respiratory Relief**: Herbs like thyme, known for its expectorant properties, or eucalyptus oil for inhalation, can be included for respiratory concerns.

2. **Pain and Fever**: Willow bark, nature's aspirin, can be used for pain relief and fever reduction.

Organizing and Maintaining the Kit

A well-organized and regularly maintained kit is essential for ensuring the remedies are effective when needed.

1. **Organization**: Organize the remedies in a way that makes them easy to find and use. Grouping them by type (such as tinctures, salves, teas) or by the ailment they address can be helpful.

2. **Regular Checks**: Regularly check the contents of the kit for expiration dates, potency, and condition. Replace any items that are past their prime or have been used up.

Educational Components

Including educational materials in the kit can provide valuable information on how to use the remedies effectively.

1. **Herbal First Aid Guide**: Create or include a small guidebook or pamphlet that provides basic information on each herb and remedy in the kit.

2. **Emergency Contacts**: List contacts for emergency medical help and advice, as well as contacts for local herbalists or naturopaths for non-emergency queries.

Building a basic herbal first aid kit is a proactive step towards embracing natural health solutions for common ailments and emergencies. It requires careful selection, preparation, and organization of a variety of herbal remedies, each chosen for its specific healing properties and ease of use. Such a kit reflects a commitment to a holistic and natural approach to health and wellness.

Quick Reference Guide for Emergency Herbal Treatments

In emergency situations, having a quick reference guide for herbal treatments can be invaluable. This subchapter focuses on developing a comprehensive, easy-to-navigate guide that outlines the use of herbal remedies for various emergency scenario. Such a guide is a resource that empowers individuals to respond with confidence and knowledge when faced with health crises, using natural and effective remedies.

Understanding Herbal Emergency Treatments

Before diving into the specific remedies, it's essential to understand the role and scope of herbal treatments in emergencies.

1. **Role of Herbal Remedies in Emergencies**: Herbal remedies can provide immediate relief for various conditions and support the body's natural healing process.

2. **Limitations and When to Seek Medical Help**: Recognize the limitations of herbal remedies and understand when it's crucial to seek professional medical assistance.

Creating the Quick Reference Guide

Developing a guide that is easy to use and understand is key to its effectiveness in emergencies.

1. **Clear Layout and Organization**: Organize the guide by types of emergencies (e.g., cuts, burns, allergic reactions) for quick access.

2. **Simple and Direct Instructions**: Provide clear, concise instructions on how to prepare and use each remedy.

Remedies for Cuts and Wounds

In the case of minor cuts and wounds, certain herbs can play a crucial role in cleaning and aiding the healing process.

1. **Calendula for Healing**: Known for its antiseptic and healing properties, calendula can be applied as a salve or wash.

2. **Yarrow to Stop Bleeding**: Yarrow is effective in stopping bleeding and can be applied directly to the wound.

Herbal Treatments for Allergic Reactions

Allergic reactions can be sudden and uncomfortable, and certain herbs can provide quick relief.

1. **Nettle for Allergies**: Nettle is known to relieve allergic symptoms and can be taken as a tea or tincture.

2. **Chamomile for Skin Reactions**: Chamomile, applied topically as a compress, can soothe skin reactions like hives.

Handling Digestive Emergencies

Digestive emergencies like nausea, indigestion, or diarrhea can be alleviated with specific herbal remedies.

1. **Ginger for Nausea**: Ginger is effective in treating nausea and can be taken as tea or chewed raw.

2. **Peppermint for Indigestion**: Peppermint tea can relieve indigestion and soothe the stomach.

Respiratory Issues and Herbal Solutions

In cases of minor respiratory issues like coughs or congestion, certain herbs can offer relief.

1. **Eucalyptus for Congestion**: Eucalyptus steam inhalation can clear nasal congestion and ease breathing.

2. **Thyme for Coughs**: Thyme has expectorant properties and can be used in a tea to relieve coughs.

Stress and Anxiety Relief

Herbs can play a significant role in managing sudden stress and anxiety.

1. **Lavender for Calming**: Lavender, used in aromatherapy or as a tea, can have a calming effect on the nerves.

2. **Lemon Balm for Anxiety**: Lemon balm, known for its mild sedative properties, can be taken as a tea to alleviate symptoms of anxiety.

Herbal First Aid for Headaches

Headaches, whether tension-related or migraines, can be effectively managed with certain herbs.

1. **Peppermint Oil for Tension Headaches**: Applied topically, peppermint oil can provide relief from tension headaches.

2. **Feverfew for Migraines**: Feverfew is a well-known herb for preventing and treating migraines and can be taken in capsule or tea form.

Dealing with Insomnia and Sleep Issues

Herbs can offer a natural solution for insomnia and other sleep disturbances.

1. **Valerian Root for Insomnia**: Valerian root, known for its sedative qualities, can be taken as a tincture or tea for inducing sleep.

2. **Chamomile for Restless Sleep**: A cup of chamomile tea before bed can promote a restful and peaceful sleep.

Treating Muscle Aches and Pain

For muscle aches and pains, certain herbs can provide soothing relief.

1. **Comfrey for Muscle Pain**: Comfrey, used as a poultice or salve, can relieve muscle pain and speed up healing.

2. **Cayenne Pepper for Topical Pain Relief**: Cayenne pepper, used in a salve, can help reduce muscle soreness and joint pain.

Bites and Stings: Herbal Interventions

Herbal remedies can be effective in treating insect bites and stings.

1. **Plantain for Bites and Stings**: Plantain, applied as a fresh poultice, can reduce itching and swelling from insect bites.

2. **Witch hazel for Inflammation**: Witch hazel can be used as a soothing agent for bites, reducing inflammation and discomfort.

Safety Considerations and Disclaimer

The guide should include safety considerations and a disclaimer, emphasizing the importance of understanding each herb's properties and potential interactions.

1. **Highlight Allergy Warnings**: Include warnings about potential allergic reactions to certain herbs.

2. **Emphasis on Professional Medical Advice**: Remind users to seek professional medical advice for serious or uncertain conditions.

Regular Updates and Review

Keeping the guide updated with the latest information and research ensures its continued relevance and effectiveness.

1. **Annual Review of Contents**: Regularly review and update the guide to include new findings, additional herbs, or revised recommendations.

2. **Feedback and Improvement**: Encourage users to provide feedback on the guide, facilitating continuous improvement and refinement.

A quick reference guide for emergency herbal treatments is an invaluable resource for anyone embracing a holistic approach to health. As users become more familiar with the guide and its contents, they develop greater confidence and skill in utilizing herbal remedies.

Chapter 14: Empowering Yourself through Herbal Knowledge

In this age of information overload and quick-fix solutions, taking the time to understand and embrace the wisdom of herbal medicine offers a pathway to deeper health insights and a more attuned way of living. This chapter is dedicated to exploring how individuals can empower themselves through the acquisition and application of herbal knowledge. This exploration aims to inspire and equip readers with the tools and confidence to integrate herbal knowledge into their daily lives, fostering a sense of autonomy and connection with the natural world.

Tools and Resources for Continuing Education in Herbal Medicine Reflecting O'Neill's Commitment

This subchapter outlines the various tools and resources available for those seeking to deepen their knowledge and practice in herbal medicine. Here, we will launch into a range of educational tools and resources, from traditional methods to modern digital platforms, each offering unique opportunities for growth and learning in the field of herbalism. This guide aims to provide readers with a comprehensive understanding of how to continuously expand their herbal knowledge and skills, aligning with O'Neill's vision of empowering individuals through education and self-awareness in natural health.

Comprehensive Herbal Texts and Books

Building a library of herbal texts is foundational for anyone serious about their education in herbal medicine.

1. **Classic Herbal Medicine Books**: Start with the classics - texts that have stood the test of time and provide a solid foundation in herbal knowledge.

2. **Modern Herbal Publications**: Supplement your library with modern publications that offer the latest research, clinical studies, and contemporary applications of herbal medicine.

Enrolling in Herbal Medicine Courses

Structured courses provide a systematic approach to learning, from basic to advanced levels.

1. **Local Workshops and Classes**: Participate in workshops and classes offered by local herbalists or health centers. These often provide hands-on experience with herbs.

2. **Online Herbal Medicine Courses**: Leverage the flexibility and diversity of online courses, which can range from introductory lessons to specialized topics in herbalism.

Herbal Medicine Schools and Institutes

For those seeking a more formal and comprehensive education, attending a school or institute dedicated to herbal medicine is a significant step.

1. **Accredited Herbal Programs**: Research and consider enrolling in accredited programs that offer certifications or degrees in herbal medicine. Apprenticeships are also out there.

2. **Specialized Training**: Some institutions offer specialized training in areas like ethnobotany, herbal pharmacology, or clinical herbalism.

Utilizing Digital Platforms and Resources

The digital age has opened up a wealth of resources for herbal education.

1. **Online Forums and Communities**: Engage with online forums and communities where herbalists, both novice and experienced, share insights, ask questions, and offer advice.

2. **Webinars and Online Lectures**: Attend webinars and online lectures hosted by experts in the field. These can provide up-to-date information and new perspectives on various herbal topics.

Field Work and Botanical Studies

Practical experience is invaluable in herbal education. Engaging in field work and botanical studies deepens understanding and appreciation for plants.

1. **Herb Walks and Botanical Tours**: Participate in guided herb walks or botanical tours to learn about plant identification, habitats, and traditional uses.

2. **Botanical Gardens and Herbariums**: Visit botanical gardens and herbariums to study a wide variety of plants and their characteristics.

Mentorship and Apprenticeships

Learning under the guidance of an experienced herbalist through mentorship or apprenticeships can be profoundly impactful.

1. **Seeking a Mentor**: Connect with an experienced herbalist who can provide personalized guidance, share practical wisdom, and offer insights from their own journey.

2. **Apprenticeship Programs**: Consider apprenticeship programs that offer immersive learning experiences, from harvesting herbs to preparing remedies and understanding their application.

Herbal Conferences and Symposia

Attending conferences and symposia is a great way to stay abreast of the latest developments in herbal medicine and network with professionals in the field.

1. **National and International Conferences**: Attend conferences that bring together herbalists, healthcare professionals, researchers, and educators from around the world.

2. **Specialized Symposia**: Look out for symposia focusing on specific areas of herbal medicine, such as women's health, herbal pharmacology, or integrative medicine practices.

Self-Study and Independent Research

Self-motivated study and research are crucial for deepening one's understanding of herbal medicine.

1. **Independent Research Projects**: Undertake independent research projects on specific herbs, their uses, or herbal medicine practices.

2. **Staying Informed on Scientific Research**: Regularly read scientific journals and articles related to herbal medicine to stay informed about new findings and perspectives.

Integrating Technology in Herbal Learning

Utilizing technology can enhance the learning experience and provide access to a wide range of resources.

1. **Herbal Medicine Apps**: Use apps related to herbal medicine for quick reference, plant identification, or dosage calculations.

2. **Online Research Databases**: Access online databases and libraries for scholarly articles and research papers on herbal medicine.

Empowering oneself through continuous education in herbal medicine offers profound insights into health, healing, and the natural world. This contributes to the broader community by preserving and spreading the invaluable knowledge of herbal medicine.

CONCLUSION OF THE BOOK

As we reach the conclusion of this enlightening journey through the world of herbal medicine and natural remedies, it is essential to pause and reflect on the profound insights and knowledge we have garnered. This book has not only been a guide to the myriad uses of herbs and their benefits but also a testament to the power of nature in healing and maintaining health.

In this concluding chapter, we synthesize the key learnings, reiterate the core principles of herbal medicine, and envisage the future of this ancient yet ever-evolving practice. This is not just an end but a beacon that lights the way forward for those who seek to continue exploring the vast, verdant world of herbalism.

Synthesis of Key Learnings

Throughout this book, we have traversed various aspects of herbal medicine, from the fundamentals of herbal properties to the intricate methods of preparation and application.

1. **Holistic Understanding**: We've gained a holistic understanding of herbs; not just as mere ingredients but as entities imbued with healing properties, deeply connected to our health and the environment.

2. **Practical Knowledge**: Practical knowledge in preparing and using herbal remedies has been a key focus, empowering readers to take an active role in their health and well-being.

Reiterating Core Principles of Herbal Medicine

The core principles of herbal medicine, which have been the backbone of this book, deserve a final emphasis.

1. **Nature's Wisdom**: The principle that nature offers profound healing wisdom, and that by aligning with this wisdom, we can achieve better health and balance.

2. **Individualized Approach**: The understanding that herbal medicine is highly individualized; what works for one may not work for another, underscoring the importance of personalization in treatment.

The Role of Herbal Medicine in Modern Healthcare

In the context of modern healthcare, herbal medicine plays a complementary role, offering natural alternatives and adjuncts to conventional treatments.

1. **Integrative Approach**: The growing trend of an integrative approach to health, where herbal remedies are used alongside conventional medicine to optimize health outcomes.

2. **Preventive Healthcare**: Herbal medicine's strong emphasis on prevention, promoting wellness rather than merely treating disease.

The Future of Herbal Medicine

Looking forward, the realm of herbal medicine is poised for growth, with increasing recognition and scientific validation.

1. **Scientific Research and Validation**: The future promises more scientific research into herbal remedies, providing a stronger evidence base for their use.

2. **Global Integration:** The global integration of diverse herbal traditions, leading to a richer, more inclusive understanding of herbal medicine.

This book, in essence, is a gateway to a world where health is viewed through the lens of nature's simplicity and profundity. It invites readers to continue exploring, experimenting, and embracing the rich tapestry of herbal medicine.

Journeying through herbal medicine a path that leads to a deeper understanding of ourselves and our intrinsic connection with the natural world. As we integrate these teachings into our lives, we become part of a larger movement; one that values wellness, sustainability, and the wisdom of nature.

Summarizing O'Neill's Teachings as Interpreted by Willowbrook

As we draw the curtains on this insightful exploration of herbal medicine, it is fitting to culminate by summarizing and reflecting upon the teachings of Barbara O'Neill as interpreted through the practical and intuitive lens of Margaret Willowbrook. This subchapter sublimes the essence of O'Neill's philosophy, as seen through Willowbrook's perspective, encapsulating the fundamental principles, practices, and beliefs that have shaped their approach to natural health and healing.

The Holistic View of Health

Central to O'Neill's teachings is the holistic view of health, which Willowbrook embraces and advocates. This approach considers the whole person; body, mind, and spirit, in the quest for optimal health.

1. **Interconnectedness of Body Systems**: Willowbrook echoes O'Neill's emphasis on the interconnectedness of body systems, advocating for treatments that address the underlying causes of illness rather than just symptoms.

2. **Emotional and Spiritual Health**: The recognition of emotional and spiritual factors in physical health is a key element in O'Neill's teachings, as reflected in Willowbrook's holistic practices.

Herbal Medicine and Natural Remedies

At the heart of O'Neill's teachings are herbal medicine and natural remedies, areas where Willowbrook's expertise and experience shine through.

1. **Use of Medicinal Herbs**: Willowbrook's approach reflects O'Neill's advocacy for the use of medicinal herbs, harnessing their natural healing properties for various health conditions.

2. **DIY Remedies and Self-Sufficiency**: Both practitioners emphasize the importance of preparing one's own remedies and encourage self-sufficiency in managing health.

Prevention over Treatment

The principle of prevention over treatment is a cornerstone in O'Neill's teachings, a theme consistently evident in Willowbrook's approach.

1. **Proactive Health Measures**: Emphasis on proactive measures to prevent illness, such as maintaining a healthy diet, regular exercise, and stress reduction techniques.

2. **Early Intervention**: The importance of early intervention in health issues, recognizing signs and symptoms, and addressing them naturally before they escalate, is a key tenet shared by both O'Neill and Willowbrook.

Holistic Approaches to Common Health Issues

O'Neill's approach to common health issues, which Willowbrook has adopted and adapted, involves viewing these issues through a holistic lens, considering all contributing factors.

1. **Natural Approaches to Chronic Diseases**: Methods for managing chronic diseases such as diabetes, heart disease, and arthritis using natural remedies and lifestyle changes are a focal point.

2. **Mental Health and Herbal Support**: The use of herbal remedies and lifestyle interventions to support mental health, including anxiety and depression, is a significant aspect of their teachings.

Final Thoughts and Future Directions

As Willowbrook interprets and carries forward O'Neill's teachings, she also looks to the future, considering how these principles can be adapted and expanded upon.

1. **Evolving Practices**: Recognizing that the field of herbal medicine and natural health is continually evolving, and staying abreast of new research and developments is essential.

2. **Expanding Reach and Influence**: The hope and intention to expand the reach of these teachings, influencing a broader audience to embrace natural health practices and herbal medicine.

In summarizing Barbara O'Neill's teachings through the interpretive lens of Margaret Willowbrook, we see a rich throng of holistic health principles, deeply rooted in the wisdom of nature and refined through practical application and modern understanding. These teachings go beyond mere treatments; they represent a way of life, a philosophy that intertwines health, wellness, and harmony with nature.

Final Reflections from Margaret Willowbrook, Drawing on O'Neill's Wisdom

In the concluding remarks of this comprehensive journey through the realms of herbal medicine and natural healing, Margaret Willowbrook offers her final reflections, deeply rooted in the wisdom imparted by Barbara O'Neill. This subchapter is a contemplative synthesis of the journey, encapsulating the essence of the teachings and the profound impact they have had on Willowbrook's perspective and practices. Here, Willowbrook not only reiterates the core principles she has embraced but also shares her insights on how these teachings can be integrated into our lives, shaping our approach to health, wellness, and our relationship with the natural world.

The Journey of Learning and Healing

Willowbrook begins by reflecting on her journey, a path that has been both enlightening and transformative.

1. **Personal Transformation**: She shares her experiences of personal growth and healing, attributing her profound understanding of health and wellness to the teachings of O'Neill.

2. **The Role of the Teacher**: Willowbrook emphasizes the importance of having a mentor like O'Neill, whose teachings have been instrumental in guiding her and many others on the path of natural healing.

Embracing Nature's Rhythms

Willowbrook's reflections bring into focus the significance of living in harmony with nature's rhythms.

1. **Seasonal Living**: She talks about the impact of aligning one's lifestyle with the changing seasons, and how this has deepened her connection with the natural world.

2. **Learning from Nature's Cycles**: Willowbrook shares insights on how observing and understanding nature's cycles can provide valuable lessons for personal health and well-being.

The Power of Simplicity

In her reflections, Willowbrook underscores the power of simplicity, a key principle she learned from O'Neill.

1. **Simplicity in Remedies**: She emphasizes the effectiveness of simple, time-tested remedies over complex formulations, advocating for the use of easily available, common herbs.

2. **Minimalism in Lifestyle**: Willowbrook also touches on the benefits of a minimalist lifestyle, reducing reliance on material things and focusing on the essentials for health and happiness.

Reflections on Personal Growth and Contribution

Willowbrook concludes with personal reflections on her growth as a practitioner and her contributions to the field.

1. **Journey of Self-Discovery**: She shares her journey of self-discovery through the study and practice of herbal medicine, describing how it has shaped her worldview and approach to life.

2. **Contribution to Community and Nature:** Willowbrook reflects on her contributions to her community and the environment, highlighting her efforts to promote sustainable practices and natural wellness.

In these final reflections, Margaret Willowbrook, inspired by the teachings of Barbara O'Neill, invites us to view our health and well-being through the lens of nature's wisdom. Her insights refine the importance of a holistic approach, the power of simplicity, and the necessity of sustainable practices in our pursuit of health. We are reminded that the journey of learning in herbal medicine is endless, filled with opportunities for growth, discovery, and deeper connection with the natural world. Willowbrook's reflections serve as a guide towards a future where natural healing is not just a practice but a way of life, deeply ingrained in our daily routines and embraced by our communities.

Last Words

As we reach the conclusion of this journey through the world of herbal remedies, I want to extend my heartfelt congratulations and gratitude to you, the reader, for embarking on this path of natural healing and holistic wellness. Your commitment to exploring and embracing the wisdom encapsulated in these pages is not only commendable but a vital step towards a more harmonious and balanced way of life.

This book, inspired by the teachings of Barbara O'Neill and the timeless wisdom of herbal medicine, is more than just a collection of recipes; it is a testament to the power of nature in healing and nurturing our bodies and minds. Each remedy, carefully crafted and detailed, is a drop in the vast ocean of natural healing practices that humanity has cultivated over millennia.

As you close this book, remember that it is not meant to be tucked away and forgotten. Let it be a living resource, a companion in your ongoing journey towards wellness. Keep it within reach, for the wisdom it contains is meant to be revisited, whether to find a remedy for a specific ailment or to seek inspiration for maintaining daily health and vitality.

The world of herbal medicine is dynamic and ever evolving, and so should be your relationship with these remedies. Feel encouraged to adapt and tailor these recipes to suit your unique needs and circumstances. Listen to your body, for it speaks a language older than any text, guiding you towards the herbs and preparations that resonate most with your personal journey to health.

Remember, each step you take in incorporating these natural remedies into your life is a step towards a deeper connection with the natural world and a more profound understanding of your own body. The path to wellness is as much about nurturing the spirit and mind as it is about healing the body.

In closing, let this book serve as your gateway to an empowered and informed approach to health, where you are the steward of your own well-being, inspired by the enduring wisdom of nature. Congratulations on completing Volume 1 of your journey through the art of herbal remedies. I hope it has been both enriching and enlightening, filled with moments of health and happiness.

To delve even deeper into the world of natural wellness, I invite you to turn the page and begin Volume 2, where over 300 meticulously detailed recipes await you. With precise instructions and specific ingredient amounts, your journey into herbal mastery will continue to flourish.

With warm regards and best wishes for your continued health and wellness,

Margaret Willowbrook.

INDEX

Note: As you are reading this book on Kindle, unfortunately, the index and the locations of herbs and ailments will not work as expected due to the unique formatting of digital pages compared to a physical book. We apologize for this inconvenience, as there is no technical solution available for this issue.

REFERENCES

1. **"The Herbal Apothecary: 100 Medicinal Herbs and How to Use Them"** by JJ Pursell (2015)

2. **"The Herbal Medicine-Maker's Handbook: A Home Manual"** by James Green (2000)

3. **"Making Plant Medicine"** by Richo Cech (2000)

4. **"The Complete Herbal Tutor"** by Anne McIntyre (2010)

5. **"Rosemary Gladstar's Medicinal Herbs: A Beginner's Guide"** by Rosemary Gladstar (2012)

6. **"Back To Eden"** by Jethro Kloss (1939)

7. **"Common Herbs for Natural Health"** by Juliette de Bairacli Levy (1974)

8. **"Complete Earth Medicine Handbook"** by Susanne Fischer-Rizzi (1996)

9. **"Herbal: 100 Herbs from the World's Healing Traditions"** by Mimi Prunella Hernandez (2021)

10. **"The Way of Herbs"** by Michael Tierra (1998)

11. **"Alchemy of Herbs"** by Rosalee de la Forêt (2017)

12. **"Herbal Recipes for Vibrant Health"** by Rosemary Gladstar (2008)

13. **Books and lectures** from Barbara O'Neill.

Bonus Page: Video Short Tutorials by Barbara O'Neill

Thank you for joining us on this journey through the world of herbal healing and natural medicine. To enrich your learning experience, we're thrilled to offer you exclusive access to a collection of video short tutorials featuring Barbara O'Neil. These tutorials, extracted directly from her lectures, provide practical, visual guidance on implementing the natural health practices discussed in this book.

By subscribing, you'll not only gain instant access to our current video library but also be updated with new videos as we continue to add to our collection. This is a fantastic way to stay connected with the latest in herbal healing and natural medicine, ensuring you're always equipped with the knowledge to support your wellness journey.

How to Access:

Simply scan the QR code below or follow the provided link to subscribe and unlock your access. This is our way of saying thank you and enhancing your journey toward holistic health with the invaluable wisdom of Barbara O'Neill.

https://www.instagram.com/infinitewellnesswave

As new tutorials become available, you'll be the first to know, allowing you to continuously expand your understanding and application of natural health principles.

We hope these video tutorials serve as a valuable resource in your quest for wellness, bringing the teachings of Barbara O'Neill to life in a new and engaging way. Your feedback and suggestions are always welcome as we grow this library together.

A MESSAGE FROM THE PUBLISHER:

Are you enjoying the book? We would love to hear your thoughts!

Many readers do not know how hard reviews are to come by and how much they help a publisher. We would be incredibly grateful if you could take just a few seconds to write a brief review on Amazon, even if it's just a few sentences!

Please be aware that this is an ongoing project, and we are continuously improving the book's content thanks to your feedback. While it may not be perfect yet, your support greatly helps us!

Please go here to leave a quick review:

https://amazon.com/review/create-review?&asin=B0CSDCGZFK

We would greatly appreciate it if you could take the time to post your review of the book and share your thoughts with the community. If you have enjoyed the book, please let us know what you loved the most about it and if you would recommend it to others. Your feedback is valuable to us, and it helps us to improve our services and continue to offer high-quality literature to our readers.

www.abetteryoueveryday.com
Email: info@abetteryoueveryday.com

Over 350 Barbara O'Neill Inspired Herbal Healing Home Remedies & Natural Medicine.

Volume 2

A Better You Everyday Publications
Email: info@abetteryoueveryday.com

Disclaimer
The information provided in this book is for educational and informational purposes only and is not affiliated with, authorized, endorsed by, or in any way officially connected with Barbara O'Neill or her affiliates or subsidiaries. The use of Barbara O'Neill's name in this book is for explanatory, educational, and reference purposes only, to discuss and provide insight into the theories and practices she has publicized through her teachings and public appearances. The views and interpretations presented in this book solely reflect those of the author and have not been reviewed or approved by Barbara O'Neill or her representatives.

The content within this book is not intended as medical advice and should not be taken as such. The author, Margaret Willowbrook, is not a medical professional. This book should not replace consultation with a qualified healthcare professional. It is essential that before beginning any new health practice, you consult with your physician, especially if you have any pre-existing health conditions.

While every effort has been made to verify the information provided in this book, the field of natural health is dynamic, and as such, the content may not reflect the most recent research or medical consensus. The author and publisher assume no responsibility for errors, omissions, or contrary interpretations of the subject matter herein.

Readers are encouraged to confirm the information contained within this publication through independent research and professional advice. Any perceived slights of specific people or organizations are unintentional. By reading this book, you agree that the author and publisher are not responsible for the success or failure of your health decisions related to any information presented.

A Better You Everyday Publications
Email address info@abetteryoueveryday.com

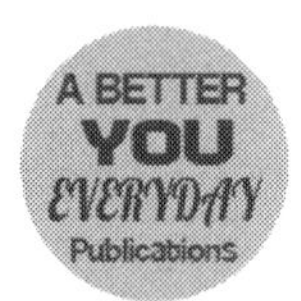

www.abetteryoueveryday.com

Printed or published to the highest ethical standard.

Over 350 Barbara O 'Neill Inspired Herbal Healing Home Remedies & Natural Medicine

Holistic Approach to Organic Health, Natural Cures and Nutrition for Sustaining Body and Mind Healing

Volume 2

By Margaret Willowbrook

USA
2024

CONTENTS

Glimpse into the Chapters Ahead.

Margaret Willowbrook invites you on a journey deeper into nature's embrace, inspired by Barbara O'Neill. This narrative begins with a transformative experience, highlighting the profound impact of herbal remedies. It sets the foundation for a book that goes beyond mere recipes, emphasizing a reconnection with nature's inherent healing power.

Chapter 1: Nutritional Wellness & Antioxidants. Explore the essence of maintaining and enhancing overall health through nature's bounty. Discover remedies that fortify general well-being, boost energy, and support the immune system, laying the groundwork for a life of vitality.

Chapter 2: Mental and Emotional Health. Navigate the delicate landscape of mental and emotional wellness with herbal allies. Learn about natural solutions for stress, anxiety, and sleep disorders, offering pathways to mental clarity and emotional balance.

Chapter 3: Digestive and Excretory Systems. Discuss the herbal wisdom that nurtures the digestive system and maintains excretory health. From liver detoxification to kidney and urinary tract health, uncover herbal strategies for internal cleansing and optimization.

Chapter 4: Cardiovascular and Respiratory Systems. Uncover heart-healthy remedies and respiratory system supports, addressing everything from cardiovascular health to breathing ease. This chapter emphasizes herbs that nourish and protect these vital systems.

Chapter 5: Musculoskeletal and Nervous Systems. Focus on herbs that alleviate pain, reduce inflammation, and support musculoskeletal health. Identify botanicals that bolster the nervous system, ensuring strength and resilience from bone to brain.

Chapter 6: Specific Health Concerns for Men and Women. Address unique health issues faced by men and women with targeted herbal remedies. From hormonal balance to reproductive health, find nature's answers to gender-specific concerns.

Chapter 7: External Body Health and Care. Conclude with external wellness, exploring herbal remedies for skin, hair, eye, and oral health. This section is dedicated to using herbal solutions for external healing and care, showcasing nature's capacity to nurture from the outside in.

Join Margaret Willowbrook as she deepens the exploration into herbal healing, inspired by the teachings of Barbara O'Neill, and discover the powerful connection between nature's remedies and holistic health.

FOREWORD.

Welcome, cherished readers, to "Over 350 Barbara O'Neill Inspired Herbal Healing Home Remedies & Natural Medicine: Volume 2." As we journey further into natural healing, this second volume was conceived from a pressing need for space, a dedicated place to expand upon the intricate recipes and remedies that the first volume could only briefly introduce. The initial collection, spanning over 150 pages, touched upon the surface of herbal wisdom. To search deeper, adding another 290 pages to provide extended explanations and applications, would not only challenge the practicality of printing but also the usability of such a vast tome. A book surpassing 340 pages becomes unwieldy, detracting from the very essence of this work, accessibility and application.

Hence, Volume 2 was born, focusing solely on the detailed exploration of recipes and remedies for a multitude of health concerns. This decision allows us to offer you a comprehensive guide without compromise, ensuring each page is a step towards mastery in herbal healing. Herein lies knowledge, awaiting your discovery and destined to enrich your journey towards holistic health.

This volume is a companion in your exploration of nature's bounty, knowing it exists because of our shared commitment to nurturing wellness through the wisdom of the earth. Let us continue to walk this path together, armed with deeper insights and a broader spectrum of healing modalities, all inspired by the enduring teachings of Barbara O'Neill.

With gratitude for your continued trust and companionship on this journey,
Margaret Willowbrook.

Attention!

Before you dive into this captivating book, we have an exclusive offer just for you! A fantastic FREE Bonus:

Get Your Ready-to-Print Herbal Reference Guide Bonuses!

Remedy Recipes (6 pages)

EXPLORE A VARIETY OF NATURAL, EASY-TO-PREPARE REMEDY RECIPES FOR DAILY HEALTH NEEDS, SPANNING STRESS RELIEF TO IMMUNE SUPPORT.

Herbal First Aid (4 pages)

ACCESS DETAILED HERBAL SOLUTIONS FOR COMMON HEALTH ISSUES, PROVIDING NATURAL EMERGENCY CARE ALTERNATIVES.

Herb Directory (6 pages)

DELVE INTO AN EXTENSIVE DIRECTORY OF MEDICINAL HERBS, COMPLETE WITH USES, BENEFITS, AND PREPARATION TIPS.

These printable guides, crafted after extensive research and dedication, offer quick, easy access to a wealth of herbal remedies, recipes, and first aid information. Designed for fast reference, they cover everything from specific herbs in our 'Herb Directory', to swift recipes in 'Remedy Recipes', and practical emergency care in 'Herbal First Aid'. Though we plan to sell them separately in the future, we're currently offering these guides for free as our appreciation for your book purchase, as a way of saying thank you and adding extra value to your reading experience.

For instant delivery, simply chat with our Facebook bot via the link below or scan the accompanying QR code.

http://tinyurl.com/Herbalbonuses

Alternatively, you can request the guides by emailing us at: info@abetteryoueveryday.com.

Enjoy your reading and these additional resources!

Introduction: Deepening the Journey with Remedies and Recipes.

Welcome to "Over 350 Barbara O'Neill Inspired Herbal Healing Home Remedies & Natural Medicine: Volume 2," a continuation of our exploration into the healing potential of nature. This volume is devoted entirely to offering detailed remedies and recipes, going through the depths of practical application of herbal wisdom for a variety of health concerns. Unlike Volume 1, which laid the foundational principles of herbal medicine, safety guidelines, and introduced broader concepts such as the importance of mental and emotional well-being, incorporating herbs into daily life, and methods for herbal preservation and storage, Volume 2 zeroes in on providing exhaustive recipes and remedies.

Volume 1 remains an essential read, covering critical topics that we do not revisit in this volume, such as "Foundations of Herbal Medicine," "Herbal Safety and Contraindications," "Women's and Men's Health," "Seasonal Herbal Remedies," "Children's Herbal Remedies," and more. These chapters are pivotal for understanding the holistic approach we advocate, ensuring safe practice and laying the groundwork for the deeper explorations contained herein.

In Volume 2, our focus is to enrich your herbal practice with a comprehensive compendium of specific treatments, designed to empower you with the knowledge to address health concerns directly through nature's offerings. While Volume 1 introduced you to the vast world of herbal healing and its principles, Volume 2 is your detailed guide to action, bringing those principles to life through direct application.

As we go through this volume, let it serve not only as a reference but as a testament to the depth and breadth of herbal medicine's capacity to heal and nurture. Whether you are seeking to enhance general wellness, address specific physical ailments, or support mental and emotional health, this book provides the tools and insights needed to harness the power of herbs for holistic healing.

Embark on this detailed journey with an understanding of the importance of the foundational knowledge provided in Volume 1 and let Volume 2 guide you further down the path of natural wellness and healing. Together, these volumes embody a comprehensive approach to living in harmony with nature's rhythms, offering a source of wisdom for a healthier, more balanced life.

With anticipation for the discoveries, we'll make together,

Margaret Willowbrook.

HOW THIS BOOK IS STRUCTURED.

Here begins our journey through over 320 detailed recipes for treating common conditions, each inspired by the profound teachings of Barbara O'Neill. These remedies draw from the vast, natural pharmacy of herbs, combining traditional wisdom with practical insights for today's health challenges. Categorized for your convenience, this collection offers a hands-on guide to crafting effective, natural treatments. Whether you're addressing digestive discomfort, seeking mental clarity, or bolstering your immune system, these recipes are designed to empower you with holistic solutions for enhancing wellness across various aspects of health.

In the forthcoming sections, we embark on an in-depth exploration of over 320 meticulously crafted recipes and remedies, each embodying the essence of Barbara O'Neill's holistic teachings. For every remedy and recipe presented, we meticulously outline an introduction that sets the context, a comprehensive list of ingredients, detailed instructions for preparation, guidelines on usage, necessary cautions to ensure safety, and an explanation of what users can anticipate in terms of benefits and outcomes. This methodical arrangement guarantees both clarity and thoroughness, providing readers with the tools needed to implement O'Neill's herbal wisdom effectively and safely into their daily lives. Through detailed explanations, we aim to dispel any ambiguity, allowing for an enriched understanding and application of each treatment.

Important information! Why Our Book Does Not Include colored Herb Photos!

Consideration for Cost and Accessibility:

In our commitment to keeping the book affordable, we consciously decided against including color herb photos. This decision directly impacts and lowers the printing costs, making the book more accessible to a broader range of readers. Our priority is to provide comprehensive herbal knowledge at a reasonable price.

Emphasizing the Role of Visual Aids:

Understanding the importance of visual identification in herbal studies, especially for newcomers and in recipe preparation, we recommend for detailed herb images.

https://myplantin.com/plant-identifier/herb

This online resource complements our book perfectly, enabling accurate herb identification and enhancing your herbal learning experience.

CHAPTER 1: NUTRITIONAL WELLNESS & ANTIOXIDANTS.

SPIRULINA AND CHLORELLA SMOOTHIE FOR NUTRITIONAL BOOST.

The Spirulina and Chlorella Smoothie combines two powerhouse algae, spirulina and chlorella, known for their dense nutrient profiles, including vitamins, minerals, and proteins, offering a significant nutritional boost.
Ingredients:

- 1 teaspoon spirulina powder
- 1 teaspoon chlorella powder
- 1 cup of your preferred liquid base (water, almond milk, coconut water)
- Optional: fruits (banana, apple, berries) for taste and additional nutrients

Instructions:

- In a blender, combine 1 teaspoon each of spirulina and chlorella powder with 1 cup of your chosen liquid base. Add any optional fruits for flavor and extra nutritional benefits.
- Blend until smooth.
- Taste and adjust the ingredients as necessary. If the smoothie is too thick, add more liquid to reach your desired consistency.

What to Expect:
This smoothie provides a rich source of vitamins (including B vitamins and vitamin C), minerals (such as iron and magnesium), and plant-based protein, contributing to improved energy levels, immune function, and overall health. Its vibrant green color reflects its phytonutrient content, which can support detoxification processes and promote antioxidant protection.

SPIRULINA AND WHEATGRASS SMOOTHIE FOR NUTRITIONAL BOOST.

The Spirulina and Wheatgrass Smoothie is a powerhouse drink, blending the intense nutritional profiles of spirulina and wheatgrass. This smoothie is an excellent way to start your day or replenish your body after a workout with a dense dose of vitamins, minerals, and antioxidants.
Ingredients:

- 1 teaspoon spirulina powder
- 1 teaspoon wheatgrass powder
- 1 cup of your choice of liquid (water, almond milk, coconut water, etc.)
- Optional: fruits (banana, berries, apple) for added flavor and nutrients

Instructions:

- Add 1 teaspoon each of spirulina and wheatgrass powder to a blender.
- Pour in 1 cup of your chosen liquid. Add any optional fruits for sweetness and extra vitamins.
- Blend until smooth and fully combined.

What to Expect:

This smoothie offers a concentrated source of nutrients, including iron, calcium, magnesium, and vitamins A, C, E, and B vitamins. Drinking it can support energy levels, immune function, and detoxification processes. The natural plant-based proteins in spirulina and wheatgrass also make it an excellent supplement for muscle repair and growth.

Apple Cider Vinegar and Honey Tonic for Overall Wellness.

The Apple Cider Vinegar and Honey Tonic is a health-boosting concoction that combines the digestive benefits of apple cider vinegar with the soothing properties of honey, diluted in warm water for a gentler impact on the stomach. Consuming this tonic daily can aid in promoting digestive health and overall wellness.

Ingredients:

- 1 tablespoon apple cider vinegar
- 1 tablespoon honey
- 1 cup warm water

Instructions:

- In a cup, mix 1 tablespoon of apple cider vinegar with 1 tablespoon of honey.
- Add 1 cup of warm water to the mixture and stir until the honey is fully dissolved.

What to Expect:

This tonic supports digestive health by improving gut flora and encouraging healthy digestion. Apple cider vinegar can also help regulate blood sugar levels and support weight management, while honey provides antioxidants and a natural energy boost. Drinking this tonic daily can contribute to a feeling of overall well-being and vitality.

Sea Buckthorn Berry Juice for Antioxidant Support.

Sea Buckthorn Berry Juice is a vibrant and nutrient-dense drink, packed with antioxidants, vitamins, and essential fatty acids. Consuming this juice supports overall health and vitality by providing a powerful boost to the body's antioxidant defences.

Ingredients:

- Pure sea buckthorn berry juice (available as a ready-to-drink juice or concentrated form)

Instructions:

- If using concentrated sea buckthorn berry juice, dilute according to the package instructions, typically with water or another juice for taste adjustment.
- Consume the juice as is if you have the ready-to-drink variety.

What to Expect:

Sea buckthorn berry juice is high in vitamins C and E, omega-7 fatty acids, and other antioxidants that contribute to healthy skin, improved immunity, and reduced inflammation. Its regular consumption can aid in protecting against cellular damage and chronic diseases, promoting a state of well-being and enhanced energy levels.

Green Tea and Lemon Elixir for Antioxidant Boost.

The Green Tea and Lemon Elixir is a revitalizing beverage that combines the antioxidant-rich qualities of green tea with the vitamin C and detoxifying benefits of fresh lemon juice. This elixir is perfect for daily consumption to support overall health and vitality.

Ingredients:

- 1 bag of green tea or 1 tablespoon of loose-leaf green tea
- Juice of ½ lemon
- 1 cup hot water

Instructions:

- Steep the green tea in 1 cup of hot water for 3 to 5 minutes, depending on desired strength.
- Remove the tea bag or strain the loose-leaf tea.
- Stir in the juice of ½ lemon into the brewed tea.

What to Expect:

Drinking this elixir regularly can provide a significant antioxidant boost, thanks to the polyphenols in green tea and the vitamin C in lemon. This combination can help protect against oxidative stress, support immune function, and promote healthy skin. The elixir can also aid in hydration and digestion, making it a beneficial addition to your daily routine for promoting wellness.

Moringa Leaf Powder for Nutritional Supplement.

Moringa Leaf Powder is a highly nutritious supplement made from the dried leaves of the Moringa oleifera tree. Known as a "miracle tree" for its medicinal and health benefits, the powder is rich in vitamins, minerals, proteins, antioxidants, and amino acids, making it an excellent addition to your diet for boosting nutritional intake.

Ingredients:

- 1-2 teaspoons moringa leaf powder
- 1 cup of water, juice, or your preferred smoothie ingredients

Instructions:

- Mix 1-2 teaspoons of moringa leaf powder into a cup of water or juice for a quick and nutritious drink. Alternatively, blend the powder into your favorite smoothie recipe to enhance its nutritional value.
- Stir or blend well to ensure the powder is fully dissolved or integrated.

What to Expect:

Regular consumption of Moringa Leaf Powder can provide a significant boost to your overall health. It supports immune function, reduces inflammation, helps to manage blood sugar levels, and improves energy levels. Its high antioxidant content also promotes skin health and protects against oxidative stress. Due to its comprehensive range of nutrients, moringa is an excellent supplement for those looking to increase their dietary intake of essential vitamins and minerals.

MORINGA AND WHEATGRASS NUTRIENT-RICH BLEND.

The Moringa and Wheatgrass Nutrient-Rich Blend combines the powerful nutritional profiles of moringa leaf powder and wheatgrass powder, creating a superfood supplement that's packed with vitamins, minerals, antioxidants, and chlorophyll. This blend is an excellent way to enhance your daily nutrient intake, supporting overall health and vitality.

Ingredients:

- 1 teaspoon moringa leaf powder
- 1 teaspoon wheatgrass powder
- 1 cup of your preferred liquid (water, almond milk, coconut water)

Instructions:

- In a glass or blender, mix 1 teaspoon of moringa leaf powder with 1 teaspoon of wheatgrass powder.
- Add 1 cup of your chosen liquid. If using a blender, you can also add fruits or vegetables to enhance the flavor and nutritional content of your smoothie.
- Stir well or blend until the powders are fully dissolved and the mixture is smooth.

What to Expect:

This blend provides a comprehensive range of health benefits, including improved energy levels, enhanced immune function, and support for detoxification processes. Moringa is known for its high levels of vitamins A,

C, and E, minerals, and amino acids, while wheatgrass offers a significant amount of chlorophyll, which is beneficial for blood health and detoxification. Consuming this blend regularly can help fill nutritional gaps in your diet, promote overall well-being, and support a healthy lifestyle.

SEA MOSS GEL FOR MINERAL BOOST.

Sea Moss Gel is a versatile and nutrient-dense supplement made from sea moss, a type of seaweed that boasts a high mineral content, including iodine, calcium, potassium, and magnesium. Taking sea moss gel can provide a natural mineral boost to support overall health and wellness.

Ingredients:

- 1 cup raw sea moss
- Water for soaking
- 2 cups filtered water (for blending)

Instructions:

- Thoroughly rinse 1 cup of raw sea moss under cold water to remove any debris or sea salt.
- Soak the cleaned sea moss in enough water to cover it completely. Let it soak for 12-24 hours at room temperature until it expands and becomes softer.
- After soaking, drain off the water and rinse the sea moss again.
- Place the soaked sea moss in a blender. Add 2 cups of filtered water, or adjust the amount of water to achieve your desired gel consistency.
- Blend until smooth and creamy.
- Transfer the sea moss gel to an airtight container and refrigerate. The gel will thicken further as it cools.

How to Use:

- Consume 1-2 tablespoons of sea moss gel daily, either directly or by adding it to smoothies, teas, soups, or other dishes as a nutritional supplement.

What to Expect:

Having sea moss gel in your diet can provide a significant mineral boost, supporting thyroid function, digestion, joint health, and skin health. Its mucilaginous texture also makes it a soothing remedy for irritated mucous membranes. Regular consumption can contribute to improved energy levels and overall vitality, thanks to its comprehensive nutritional profile.

SCHISANDRA BERRY AND LICORICE ROOT ADAPTOGENIC TONIC.

The Schisandra Berry and Licorice Root Adaptogenic Tonic is a synergistic blend that combines the adaptogenic properties of schisandra berry extract with the soothing and harmonizing effects of licorice root powder. This tonic is designed to support stress resilience, enhance vitality, and promote overall well-being when added to warm water or tea.

Ingredients:

- ½ teaspoon schisandra berry extract
- ½ teaspoon licorice root powder
- 1 cup warm water or your favorite herbal tea

Instructions:

- In a cup, mix ½ teaspoon of schisandra berry extract with ½ teaspoon of licorice root powder.
- Add 1 cup of warm water or brewed herbal tea to the mixture. Stir well until the powders are fully dissolved.
- Enjoy this tonic warm, ideally in the morning or early afternoon for an adaptogenic boost.

What to Expect:

Consuming the Schisandra Berry and Licorice Root Adaptogenic Tonic can help enhance your body's ability to adapt to stress, support liver health, and promote hormonal balance. Schisandra berry is known for its ability to increase resistance to stress and boost energy without overstimulating, while licorice root can help harmonize the body's systems and improve digestion. This tonic is a gentle yet effective way to support your body's adaptogenic response, making it a valuable addition to a holistic wellness regimen.

Kelp and Spirulina Thyroid Support Smoothie.

The Kelp and Spirulina Thyroid Support Smoothie is a nutrient-dense beverage designed to support thyroid health through the natural iodine content found in both kelp and spirulina. This smoothie not only aids in maintaining healthy thyroid function but also provides a wealth of vitamins, minerals, and antioxidants.

Ingredients:

- 1 teaspoon kelp powder
- 1 teaspoon spirulina powder
- 1 banana (for natural sweetness and creaminess)
- 1 cup of spinach or kale (for added nutrients)
- 1 cup almond milk, coconut water, or water (for blending)
- Optional: ½ apple or pear for extra sweetness

Instructions:

- Add 1 teaspoon each of kelp powder and spirulina powder to a blender.
- Add the banana, spinach or kale, and your choice of liquid. Include the optional apple or pear if desired for additional sweetness.
- Blend all the ingredients until the mixture is smooth.

- Taste the smoothie and adjust sweetness if necessary by adding more fruit or a natural sweetener like honey.

What to Expect:
Consuming this smoothie can support thyroid function thanks to the iodine-rich kelp and spirulina, essential for the production of thyroid hormones. Regular intake may help regulate energy levels, support metabolism, and contribute to overall well-being. This smoothie also offers anti-inflammatory benefits and boosts immune health due to the antioxidants and vitamins provided by the added fruits and greens.

Seaweed and Miso Soup for Thyroid Support.

Seaweed and Miso Soup is a nourishing and flavorful dish that combines the rich iodine content of seaweed with the probiotic benefits of miso, creating a powerful support for thyroid health. This soup is easy to prepare and can be customized with various thyroid-supportive ingredients for additional health benefits.
Ingredients:

- 4 cups water or vegetable broth
- 1 cup seaweed (kelp, nori, or wakame), rinsed and chopped
- 2-3 tablespoons miso paste (adjust to taste)
- ½ cup tofu, diced (optional, for protein)
- 2 green onions, thinly sliced
- 1 tablespoon ginger, grated (for anti-inflammatory properties)
- Optional: Mushrooms, carrots, or other vegetables for added nutrients

Instructions:

- In a large pot, bring 4 cups of water or vegetable broth to a simmer.
- Add the chopped seaweed and simmer for 5-10 minutes, or until the seaweed is tender.
- In a small bowl, mix the miso paste with a little bit of the warm broth until it becomes a smooth mixture. This step prevents clumping and ensures the miso blends well into the soup.
- Add the miso mixture, diced tofu, sliced green onions, and grated ginger to the pot. If using additional vegetables, add them now as well.
- Allow the soup to simmer for another 5 minutes, making sure not to boil it as boiling can reduce the probiotic benefits of miso.
- Taste and adjust the seasoning, adding more miso paste if needed for flavor.

What to Expect:

Consuming Seaweed and Miso Soup regularly can support thyroid function due to the iodine-rich seaweed, which is essential for the production of thyroid hormones. The miso provides probiotics that support gut health, an important factor in overall hormonal balance. The additional ingredients like ginger add anti-inflammatory benefits, while tofu and vegetables contribute to the soup's nutritional profile, making it a wholesome and supportive meal for thyroid health and general wellness.

HIBISCUS AND ROSEHIP ANTIOXIDANT TEA.

Hibiscus and Rosehip Antioxidant Tea is a vibrant and refreshing beverage packed with antioxidants. The combination of tangy hibiscus flowers and nutrient-rich rosehips creates a delicious tea that supports overall health by fighting oxidative stress and inflammation.

Ingredients:

- 1 tablespoon dried hibiscus flowers
- 1 tablespoon dried rosehips
- 1 cup hot water

Instructions:

- Mix 1 tablespoon of dried hibiscus flowers with 1 tablespoon of dried rosehips in a tea infuser or directly in a cup.
- Pour 1 cup of boiling water over the hibiscus and rosehips, allowing them to steep for 5 to 10 minutes, depending on your taste preference for strength and tartness.
- If you've used a tea infuser, remove it from the cup. If the flowers and rosehips were added directly, strain the tea into another cup to remove them.

What to Expect:

Drinking Hibiscus and Rosehip Antioxidant Tea offers a delightful taste experience along with a boost in antioxidants, particularly vitamin C, which supports immune health and skin vitality. Hibiscus has been shown to help lower blood pressure and promote liver health, while rosehips contribute to joint health and may aid in reducing inflammation. This tea is perfect for enjoying any time of day when you need a refreshing and healthful pick-me-up.

SPIRULINA AND BLUEBERRY SUPERFOOD SMOOTHIE.

The Spirulina and Blueberry Superfood Smoothie is a powerhouse of nutrition, blending the rich, earthy goodness of spirulina with the sweet, antioxidant-packed blueberries and the creamy texture of banana. This smoothie is an excellent choice for anyone looking to boost their energy levels and nutrient intake in a delicious and convenient way.

Ingredients:

- 1 teaspoon spirulina powder
- 1 cup blueberries (fresh or frozen)
- 1 ripe banana
- 1 cup milk of choice (almond milk, coconut milk, oat milk, or dairy milk)

Instructions:

- Add 1 teaspoon of spirulina powder, 1 cup of blueberries, 1 ripe banana, and 1 cup of your chosen milk to a blender.
- Blend on high until the mixture is smooth and creamy. If the smoothie is too thick, you can add more milk or a bit of water to reach your desired consistency.
- Taste the smoothie and adjust the sweetness if necessary. You can add a touch of honey, maple syrup, or a pitted date for natural sweetness if needed.

What to Expect:

This Spirulina and Blueberry Superfood Smoothie offers a nutrient-rich blend that's not only energizing but also supports overall health. Spirulina provides a concentrated source of protein, vitamins, minerals, and antioxidants, while blueberries add fiber and additional antioxidants to the mix. Bananas bring natural sweetness and potassium, making this smoothie a balanced, healthful treat. It's perfect for a quick breakfast, a midday energy boost, or a post-workout replenishment.

SPIRULINA AND CHLORELLA SUPERFOOD SUPPLEMENT.

The Spirulina and Chlorella Superfood Supplement is a powerful blend of two of the most nutrient-dense algae known for their high content of vitamins, minerals, and antioxidants. This supplement offers a comprehensive boost to overall health, supporting immune function, detoxification, and energy levels.

Ingredients:

- 1 teaspoon spirulina powder
- 1 teaspoon chlorella powder
- 1 cup water or your preferred smoothie ingredients

Instructions:

- In a glass, mix 1 teaspoon of spirulina powder and 1 teaspoon of chlorella powder with 1 cup of water. Stir well until the powders are completely dissolved. For a more flavorful option, blend these powders into your favorite smoothie instead of water. Use fruits like bananas, berries, or apples, and liquids like almond milk or coconut water for a delicious and nutritious drink.

- If blending into a smoothie, add all ingredients, including the spirulina and chlorella powders, into a blender. Blend until smooth.

What to Expect:

Incorporating the Spirulina and Chlorella Superfood Supplement into your daily routine can significantly enhance your nutrient intake, providing a wide array of essential vitamins and minerals, including B vitamins, vitamin C, magnesium, iron, and zinc. These algae are also known for their high chlorophyll content, which can aid in detoxification processes and promote a healthy immune system. The combination of spirulina and chlorella can help improve energy levels, support detoxification, and enhance overall well-being. Due to their concentrated nutrient content, starting with a small dose and gradually increasing it based on your tolerance is recommended.

SEA BUCKTHORN AND ACAI BERRY ANTIOXIDANT SMOOTHIE.

The Sea buckthorn and Acai Berry Antioxidant Smoothie is a vibrant and nutrient-dense drink that combines the exceptional antioxidant properties of sea buckthorn and acai berry powders with the natural sweetness and vitamins of fruits. This smoothie is an excellent choice for boosting your antioxidant intake, supporting immune health, and promoting overall vitality.

Ingredients:

- 1 teaspoon sea buckthorn powder
- 1 teaspoon acai berry powder
- 1 banana, for sweetness and creaminess
- ½ cup mixed berries (blueberries, strawberries, raspberries), fresh or frozen
- 1 cup spinach or kale, for added nutrients
- 1 cup almond milk, coconut water, or water, for blending
- Optional: 1 tablespoon honey or maple syrup, for added sweetness

Instructions:

- Add 1 teaspoon each of sea buckthorn powder and acai berry powder to a blender.
- Add the banana, mixed berries, spinach or kale, and your choice of liquid (almond milk, coconut water, or water) to the blender. If you prefer a sweeter smoothie, add honey or maple syrup.
- Blend all ingredients on high until smooth. If the smoothie is too thick, add more liquid until you reach your desired consistency.
- Taste and adjust sweetness if necessary, adding more honey or maple syrup if desired.

What to Expect:

This smoothie delivers a powerful punch of antioxidants, which help combat oxidative stress and support cellular health. Sea buckthorn powder is rich in omega-7 fatty acids, vitamin C, and other nutrients that promote healthy skin and cardiovascular health. Acai berry powder offers antioxidants such as anthocyanins, which support heart health and improve cholesterol levels. The addition of greens and fruits not only enhances the smoothie's nutrient profile but also ensures a delicious, naturally sweet flavor. Enjoy this smoothie as a revitalizing breakfast or a nourishing snack to support your overall health and well-being.

CHAGA MUSHROOM AND CACAO HEALTH ELIXIR.

The Chaga Mushroom and Cacao Health Elixir is a sumptuous and full-bodied tonic that marries the rich, stimulating qualities of cacao with the powerful, life-enhancing antioxidants found in chaga mushrooms. Famous for its immune-boosting and restorative properties, this rejuvenating brew offers a dual load of phytonutrients and minerals, promising not only an egis to your daily routine but also a multi-faceted shroud of good taste and goodwill.

Ingredients:

- 1-2 tablespoons chaga mushroom pieces or 1 teaspoon chaga mushroom powder
- 2 cups of water
- 1 tablespoon raw cacao powder
- Optional: Honey, maple syrup, or your favorite natural sweetener to taste
- Optional: A dash of cinnamon or vanilla extract for flavor enhancement

Instructions:

- If using chaga mushroom pieces, simmer them in 2 cups of water for about 15-30 minutes. The time allows for the properties of the chaga to get well-infused into the water. Those with chaga powder should still add the water to the chaga but can skip ahead to combining it with the rest of the concoction.
- Pour the solution through a strainer into a cup, being certain to capture all the richly dark chaga blend, and without the chaga themselves. If you're applying powder, you might not need to sieve.
- Stir in 1 tablespoon of raw cacao powder until it is completely dissolved and integrated.
- Blend in honey, maple syrup, or your choice of sweetener to taste, if desired. Cinnamon or vanilla extract could be added here as flavor.
- Blend all together, making sure they are well combined. Enjoy this decoction on its own or combined with other drinks. Best enjoyed warm.

What to Expect:
Sipping Chaga Mushroom and Cacao Health Elixir can boost your immunity, promote cellular repair, reduce mental fog, and improve overall focus and concentration. This beverage is high in minerals and antioxidants. The synergy of bittersweet cacao with the earthy, autumnal flavor of chaga will warm you, heart and soul.

Turmeric, Ginger, and Black Pepper Tea for Overall Wellness.

Turmeric, Ginger, and Black Pepper Tea is a synergistic blend that combines the powerful anti-inflammatory and antioxidant properties of turmeric and ginger with the bioavailability-enhancing effects of black pepper.
Ingredients:

- 1 teaspoon turmeric powder
- 1 inch fresh ginger root, grated
- A pinch of ground black pepper
- 1 cup hot water

Instructions:

- In a cup, blend 1 teaspoon of turmeric powder, 1 inch of freshly grated ginger root, and a pinch of ground black pepper.
- Pour 1 cup of hot water over the mixture and let it steep for 10 minutes.
- Strain the tea to remove the solids before drinking.

What to Expect:
This tea offers a host of health benefits, including boosting the immune system, reducing inflammation, and aiding in digestion. The presence of black pepper enhances the absorption of curcumin from turmeric, making this tea an effective remedy for promoting overall wellness. Its warming qualities also make it a comforting beverage for any time of day.

Turmeric and Black Pepper Mix for Anti-inflammatory Benefits.

Combining turmeric powder with a pinch of black pepper creates a potent mix that leverages the anti-inflammatory properties of curcumin in turmeric, significantly enhanced by piperine in black pepper, which improves the absorption of curcumin by the body.
Ingredients:

- 1 teaspoon turmeric powder
- A pinch of black pepper

Instructions:

- Mix 1 teaspoon of turmeric powder with a pinch of black pepper thoroughly.
- Incorporate this mixture into meals, smoothies, or warm beverages. It can be added to curries, soups, or even a warm glass of milk.

What to Expect:

The regular addition of this mix to your diet can help reduce inflammation and pain associated with conditions like arthritis, muscle soreness, and various chronic diseases. The mix not only provides health benefits but also adds a warm, earthy flavor to dishes and drinks.

Chia Seed and Lemon Hydration Drink.

The Chia Seed and Lemon Hydration Drink is a refreshing and nourishing beverage that combines the hydrating power of lemon-infused water with the nutritional benefits of chia seeds. This drink is an excellent source of omega-3 fatty acids, fiber, antioxidants, and vitamins, making it perfect for boosting hydration and overall health.

Ingredients:

- 2 tablespoons chia seeds
- Juice of 1 lemon
- 2 cups water
- Optional: Honey or maple syrup to taste
- Optional: A few mint leaves for extra flavor

Instructions:

- In a pitcher or large jar, combine the juice of 1 lemon with 2 cups of water. Stir well to mix.
- Add 2 tablespoons of chia seeds to the lemon water. Stir again to ensure the seeds are well distributed.
- Let the mixture sit for about 15 to 30 minutes, allowing the chia seeds to swell and absorb the water, forming a gel-like consistency.
- Once the chia seeds have expanded, stir the drink again to break up any clumps. If desired, add honey or maple syrup to sweeten and mint leaves for additional flavor.
- Refrigerate the drink for a few hours or enjoy it immediately over ice.

What to Expect:

Drinking the Chia Seed and Lemon Hydration Drink provides a hydrating experience with added nutritional benefits. Chia seeds are rich in omega-3 fatty acids, which are essential for heart health and reducing inflammation. The lemon not only adds a refreshing taste but also supplies vitamin C, aiding in immune support and skin health. This drink is ideal for post-workout recovery, as a morning energizer, or anytime you need a hydration boost. Its unique texture and flavor make it a delightful and healthful choice for maintaining hydration and receiving essential nutrients.

Herbal Remedies for Energy and Vitality.

Ashwagandha and Licorice Root Tonic.

The Ashwagandha and Licorice Root Tonic is a rejuvenating drink that combines the adaptogenic benefits of ashwagandha with the soothing effects of licorice root. This tonic is designed to enhance energy, vitality, and resilience to stress, making it a valuable addition to your wellness routine.
Ingredients:

- 1 teaspoon ashwagandha powder
- ½ teaspoon licorice root powder
- 1 cup warm milk (dairy or plant-based) or water

Instructions:

- In a cup, mix 1 teaspoon of ashwagandha powder with ½ teaspoon of licorice root powder.
- Heat 1 cup of milk or water until warm but not boiling. Pour the warm liquid into the cup with the ashwagandha and licorice powders.
- Stir the mixture thoroughly until the powders are completely dissolved. For added sweetness and health benefits, consider adding a teaspoon of honey or maple syrup.
- Drink this tonic once daily, preferably in the evening, to maximize its stress-reducing and calming effects.

What to Expect:
Regular consumption of the Ashwagandha and Licorice Root Tonic can provide numerous health benefits, including improved energy levels and enhanced stress resilience. Ashwagandha is known for its ability to reduce cortisol levels and combat the effects of stress, while licorice root supports adrenal health and adds a naturally sweet flavor to the tonic. Together, they create a powerful blend that promotes overall vitality and well-being. This tonic is also gentle on the digestive system and can help soothe digestive discomfort, thanks to the anti-inflammatory properties of both herbs.

Maca Root and Cacao Energy Smoothie.

The Maca Root and Cacao Energy Smoothie is a delicious and energizing drink that combines the natural vitality-enhancing properties of maca root with the rich, antioxidant benefits of cacao. Paired with milk and banana for creaminess and additional nutrients, this smoothie is a perfect way to start your day or boost your energy levels naturally.

Ingredients:

- 1 teaspoon maca root powder
- 1 tablespoon raw cacao powder
- 1 cup milk of choice (almond, soy, coconut, or dairy)
- 1 ripe banana

Instructions:

- Place 1 teaspoon of maca root powder and 1 tablespoon of raw cacao powder in a blender.
- Add 1 ripe banana and 1 cup of your chosen milk to the blender.
- Blend all the ingredients on high until the mixture is smooth and creamy. If the smoothie is too thick, you can add a bit more milk or some water to reach your preferred consistency.
- Taste the smoothie and adjust the sweetness if necessary. You can add a sweetener like honey, maple syrup, or dates if you prefer it sweeter.

What to Expect:

Drinking the Maca Root and Cacao Energy Smoothie provides a natural energy boost without the jitters often associated with caffeine. Maca root is known for its ability to increase stamina and energy levels, while cacao adds mood-enhancing properties and a wealth of antioxidants. The banana not only adds natural sweetness and creaminess but also provides potassium and fiber, making this smoothie a balanced and nutritious option for an energy lift. This smoothie is ideal for breakfast, as a pre-workout drink, or anytime you need an extra boost of energy and nutrients.

GINSENG ROOT TEA FOR ENERGY AND VITALITY.

Ginseng Root Tea is a revered herbal beverage, utilized for centuries for its ability to boost energy levels and enhance overall vitality. Known for its adaptogenic properties, ginseng helps the body resist stressors and improve mental and physical performance.

Ingredients:

- 1 tablespoon sliced or whole ginseng root
- 2 cups water

Instructions:

- Place the ginseng root in a pot with 2 cups of water.
- Bring the water to a boil, then reduce the heat and simmer for 15 to 20 minutes, allowing the ginseng flavors and properties to infuse the water.
- Strain the tea into a cup, discarding the ginseng slices.

What to Expect:

Drinking Ginseng Root Tea can provide a natural energy boost without the jitters often associated with caffeine. It may improve mental clarity, enhance physical stamina, and support overall well-being. Regular consumption can help in adapting to stress and maintaining energy levels throughout the day.

Siberian Ginseng (Eleuthero) Extract for Immune and Energy.

Siberian Ginseng, also known as Eleuthero, is a herbal extract renowned for its ability to enhance energy levels and support the immune system. Taking this extract can help improve physical endurance and mental clarity while bolstering the body's defences against common illnesses.

Ingredients:

- Siberian ginseng (Eleuthero) extract (available in liquid, powder, or capsule form)

Instructions:

- Follow the dosage instructions provided on the packaging of the Siberian ginseng extract. The recommended dose can vary depending on the concentration of the extract.
- Siberian ginseng can be taken with water or juice for ease of consumption if using liquid or powder forms. Capsules can be taken with a glass of water.

What to Expect:

Regular intake of Siberian Ginseng extract can lead to increased energy, reduced fatigue, and enhanced mental performance. Its immune-boosting properties may as well help in reducing the frequency and severity of colds and other respiratory infections. It's a natural adaptogen, helping the body to manage stress more effectively.

Schisandra Berry and Goji Berry Vitality Tonic.

The Schisandra Berry and Goji Berry Vitality Tonic is a powerful concoction that combines the adaptogenic properties of schisandra berries with the nutrient-rich profile of goji berries. This tonic is designed to enhance overall vitality, well-being, and to support various aspects of health including cognitive function, energy levels, and immune system strength.

Ingredients:

- 1 tablespoon dried schisandra berries
- 1 tablespoon dried goji berries
- 1 cup hot water

Instructions:

- Place 1 tablespoon each of dried schisandra berries and dried goji berries in a cup or a tea infuser.

- Pour 1 cup of hot water over the berries and allow them to soak and steep for about 10 to 15 minutes. The longer you steep, the more potent the tonic will be.
- Strain the tonic to remove the berries, or simply remove the tea infuser if you used one.

What to Expect:

Drinking this tonic can provide a significant boost in antioxidants, which protect the body from oxidative stress and support overall health. Schisandra berries are known for their five-flavor profile and adaptogenic benefits, which help the body resist stressors of all kinds, while goji berries are celebrated for their high vitamin and mineral content, especially vitamin C and beta-carotene. Together, they create a synergistic blend that supports mental clarity, energy, immune function, and overall vitality. This tonic is a delightful way to incorporate these superfoods into your daily routine for a healthful boost.

Chia Seed and Coconut Water Hydration Mix.

The Chia Seed and Coconut Water Hydration Mix is a refreshing and hydrating beverage, perfect for replenishing fluids and nutrients, especially after physical activity or during hot weather. Chia seeds absorb several times their weight in water and release it slowly, while coconut water is rich in electrolytes, making this mix an excellent natural hydrator and energy booster.

Ingredients:

- 2 tablespoons chia seeds
- 1 cup coconut water

Instructions:

- Pour 2 tablespoons of chia seeds into 1 cup of coconut water. Stir well to combine.
- Let the mixture sit for about 10 to 15 minutes, allowing the chia seeds to swell and absorb the coconut water. Stir again to break up any clumps of chia seeds.
- Drink the mix as is, or for added flavour, consider infusing it with a squeeze of lime or lemon juice.

What to Expect:

Drinking the Chia Seed and Coconut Water Hydration Mix can significantly improve hydration and provide a sustained release of energy. Chia seeds are also a great source of omega-3 fatty acids, fiber, and protein, contributing to overall health and well-being. This mix is ideal for athletes, those leading an active lifestyle, or anyone looking to boost their hydration and nutrient intake naturally.

Chapter 2: Mental and Emotional Health.

Herbal Remedies for Stress and Anxiety.

Ashwagandha Milk for Stress.

Ashwagandha Milk combines the adaptogenic power of ashwagandha powder with the comforting warmth of milk, creating a soothing beverage ideal for reducing stress and promoting relaxation. Ashwagandha, a revered herb in Ayurvedic medicine, is known for its ability to balance the body's response to stress and improve sleep quality.

Ingredients:

- 1 teaspoon ashwagandha powder
- 1 cup milk (dairy or plant-based)

Instructions:

- Heat 1 cup of milk in a small saucepan over medium heat until it is warm but not boiling.
- Add 1 teaspoon of ashwagandha powder to the warm milk.
- Stir the mixture thoroughly to ensure the ashwagandha powder is completely dissolved. For added sweetness and flavor, you may add a touch of honey, maple syrup, or a pinch of cinnamon.
- Pour the ashwagandha milk into a cup and enjoy it warm.

What to Expect:

Drinking ashwagandha milk before bed can help soothe the nervous system, reduce stress levels, and prepare the body for a restful night's sleep. The natural compounds in ashwagandha, including withanolides, have been shown to promote relaxation and improve sleep patterns by modulating the stress response pathways in the body. The warm milk serves as a comforting base, enhancing the calming effects of the herb. This beverage is a simple and natural way to unwind at the end of the day and support overall well-being by improving sleep quality and reducing stress.

Lemon Balm Tea for Anxiety.

Lemon Balm Tea is a soothing herbal remedy made from steeping dried lemon balm leaves, a plant known for its calming properties and effectiveness in alleviating symptoms of anxiety. This gentle tea can help ease the mind, reduce stress, and promote a sense of well-being.

Ingredients:

- 1-2 teaspoons of dried lemon balm leaves
- 1 cup of boiling water

Instructions:

- Place 1-2 teaspoons of dried lemon balm leaves in a tea infuser or directly in a cup.
- Pour 1 cup of boiling water over the leaves and allow them to steep for about 10 minutes. The steeping time allows the therapeutic compounds in the lemon balm leaves to infuse into the water.
- If you used a tea infuser, remove it from the cup. If the leaves were added directly, strain the tea to remove them before drinking.
- Optional: Enhance the flavor and calming effects of the tea by adding a slice of lemon or a teaspoon of honey.

What to Expect:

Drinking Lemon Balm Tea can provide immediate relief from anxiety and stress. The compounds in lemon balm, including rosmarinic acid, have been shown to have a calming effect on the nervous system, helping to ease symptoms of anxiety such as nervousness, restlessness, and irritability. Additionally, lemon balm tea can aid in improving sleep quality, making it an excellent beverage to enjoy in the evening or anytime you need to unwind. Its pleasant, lemony flavor and aroma also contribute to the overall soothing experience. Enjoy Lemon Balm Tea as needed to help navigate through stressful moments or incorporate it into your daily routine for ongoing support of mental well-being.

Lavender Oil Bath for Relaxation.

A Lavender Oil Bath harnesses the calming and aromatic properties of lavender essential oil to create a tranquil bathing experience. This simple yet effective method is perfect for unwinding after a long day, soothing the senses, and alleviating stress.

Ingredients:

- 5-10 drops of lavender essential oil
- Warm bathwater

Instructions:

- Fill your bathtub with warm water, adjusting the temperature to your preference.
- Once the bath is drawn, add 5-10 drops of lavender essential oil directly to the water. Use your hand to gently swirl the water, helping to distribute the oil evenly.
- Step into the bath and soak for 20-30 minutes, allowing the natural properties of the lavender oil to work their magic.
- As you relax in the bath, take deep breaths to fully enjoy the soothing aroma of lavender, which is known to reduce anxiety and promote a sense of calm and well-being.

What to Expect:
Immersing yourself in a Lavender Oil Bath can provide immediate relief from stress and tension. Lavender essential oil is renowned for its ability to calm the mind, ease anxiety, and promote relaxation, making it an ideal choice for a stress-relieving bath. Additionally, the warm water can help relax muscles, further enhancing the relaxation experience. After your bath, you may find it easier to unwind and prepare for a restful night's sleep, thanks to the soothing effects of lavender. This bathing ritual can be a cherished part of your evening routine, especially on days when you need extra relaxation and stress relief.

Holy Basil (Tulsi) Tea for Stress Reduction.

Holy Basil (Tulsi) Tea is a revered herbal tea made from the leaves of the holy basil plant, known for its powerful adaptogenic properties that help the body combat stress and anxiety. This sacred herb, deeply embedded in Ayurvedic medicine, offers a natural and holistic approach to stress management and mental well-being.
Ingredients:

- 1-2 teaspoons of dried holy basil (Tulsi) leaves
- 1 cup of hot water

Instructions:

- Place 1-2 teaspoons of dried holy basil leaves in a tea infuser or directly in a cup.
- Pour 1 cup of freshly boiled water over the leaves and allow them to steep for about 10 minutes. This duration ensures that the water absorbs the full spectrum of the herb's therapeutic properties.
- If you used a tea infuser, remove it from the cup. If the leaves were added directly, strain the tea to remove them before drinking.
- Optional: You can add a natural sweetener like honey or a slice of lemon to enhance the flavor of the tea.

What to Expect:
Drinking Holy Basil (Tulsi) Tea can significantly reduce stress and anxiety levels, promoting a sense of calm and relaxation. Holy basil is known for its adaptogenic effects, which help balance cortisol levels, improve mood, and enhance mental clarity. Its subtle, minty flavor is both refreshing and soothing, making it an ideal beverage for moments when you need to de-stress or before meditation. Regular consumption can also support immune health, metabolic function, and overall vitality. Tulsi tea offers a comforting, therapeutic experience that nurtures the body, mind, and spirit.

RHODIOLA ROSEA EXTRACT FOR STRESS RELIEF.

Rhodiola Rosea Extract is a natural supplement derived from the roots of the Rhodiola rosea plant, known for its adaptogenic properties that help the body adapt to and resist physical, chemical, and environmental stress. This powerful herb has been used for centuries in traditional medicine to increase energy, stamina, strength, and mental capacity.

How to Use:

- Opt for a high-quality, commercially prepared Rhodiola Rosea extract. Ensure it specifies the percentage of active compounds, such as rosavins and salidrosides, which are critical for its stress-relief properties.
- Follow the dosing instructions provided on the product label. The typical dosage ranges, but it's essential to start with the lower end of the recommended dose to assess your tolerance.
- Rhodiola can be taken in various forms, including capsules, tablets, or liquid extracts. Choose the form that best suits your preference and lifestyle.

What to Expect:

Incorporating Rhodiola Rosea Extract into your daily regimen can offer significant benefits for stress relief and overall well-being. Users often report an increase in energy, endurance, strength, and mental performance shortly after beginning supplementation. Rhodiola is particularly beneficial during periods of high stress or fatigue, as it can help improve your body's stress response, reduce anxiety, and elevate mood levels. Additionally, Rhodiola has been shown to support cognitive functions, such as memory and attention, and may aid in reducing symptoms of depression. It's a natural way to enhance your resilience to stress without the side effects commonly associated with pharmaceuticals. As with any supplement, it's advisable to consult with a healthcare professional before starting, especially if you have underlying health conditions or are taking other medications.

CATNIP AND CHAMOMILE RELAXATION TEA.

Catnip and Chamomile Relaxation Tea is a calming herbal blend that combines the soothing properties of chamomile with the relaxing effects of catnip. This tea is perfect for unwinding after a long day, promoting relaxation, and preparing the body for a restful night's sleep.

Ingredients:

- 1 teaspoon dried catnip leaves
- 1 teaspoon dried chamomile flowers
- 1 cup hot water

Instructions:

- Mix 1 teaspoon of dried catnip leaves and 1 teaspoon of dried chamomile flowers in a tea infuser or directly in a cup.
- Pour 1 cup of boiling water over the herbal blend and allow it to steep for about 10 minutes. The steeping time allows the therapeutic properties of the herbs to infuse into the water, creating a potent relaxation tea.
- If using a tea infuser, remove it from the cup. If the herbs were added directly, strain the tea to remove the leaves and flowers before drinking.
- Optional: Enhance the tea's natural flavors and benefits by adding a touch of honey, lemon, or mint according to your preference.

What to Expect:

Drinking Catnip and Chamomile Relaxation Tea can help soothe the nervous system, reduce feelings of stress and anxiety, and facilitate a sense of calm. Chamomile is widely regarded for its gentle sedative effects, making it a popular choice for promoting sleep. Catnip, while known for stimulating cats, has the opposite effect on humans, offering mild sedative properties that can enhance relaxation. Together, these herbs create a synergistic blend that supports relaxation and mental well-being. This tea is an excellent choice for anyone seeking a natural way to unwind and destress, especially before bedtime, to encourage deep and restorative sleep.

Kava Kava Root Brew for Anxiety.

Kava Kava Root Brew is a traditional beverage made from the dried roots of the kava plant, known for its potent anxiety-reducing properties. Consumed for centuries in the Pacific Islands for its calming effects, kava kava offers a natural way to ease anxiety and promote relaxation. However, it's important to use kava with caution due to concerns about its potential impact on liver health.

Ingredients:

- 2-3 tablespoons of dried kava kava root
- 2 cups of water

Instructions:

- Place 2-3 tablespoons of dried kava kava root into a bowl or strainer bag designed for brewing kava.
- Warm 2 cups of water until it is hot but not boiling. The optimal temperature enhances the extraction of kavalactones, the active compounds in kava.
- Pour the warm water over the kava kava root and let it steep for 10-15 minutes. If using a bowl, knead and squeeze the root in the water

to help release its active ingredients. If in a strainer bag, gently massage the bag in the water.

- Strain the mixture to remove the solid particles. The resulting brew will have a muddy appearance and a distinctive earthy taste.
- Consume the kava kava brew slowly over the course of 30 minutes to an hour.

What to Expect:

Drinking Kava Kava Root Brew can provide significant relief from anxiety and stress, promoting a sense of calm and relaxation without impairing cognitive function. Users often experience a noticeable reduction in anxiety, improved mood, and a feeling of well-being. Kava's effects can vary from person to person, and it may take some time to find the right dosage for your needs. Due to concerns about liver toxicity, it's recommended to use kava sparingly and not as a daily supplement. Always consult with a healthcare provider before adding kava to your regimen, especially if you have liver issues or take medications that affect the liver. Note that kava is not recommended for pregnant or breastfeeding women.

Ashwagandha Root Powder Mix for Stress Reduction.

The Ashwagandha Root Powder Mix is a traditional remedy known for its stress-reducing and sleep-improving properties. Ashwagandha, a powerful adaptogen, helps the body manage stress more effectively, promoting relaxation and a sense of calm. Mixed with warm milk or water, this drink is ideal for unwinding before bedtime, leading to a more restful night's sleep.

Ingredients:

- 1 teaspoon ashwagandha root powder
- 1 cup milk (dairy or plant-based) or water

Instructions:

- Heat the milk or water until it is warm but not boiling. Warmth is key to maximizing the solubility and effectiveness of the ashwagandha powder.
- Add 1 teaspoon of ashwagandha root powder to the warm milk or water. Stir thoroughly until the powder is completely dissolved. For added taste and benefits, consider incorporating a natural sweetener like honey or a dash of cinnamon.
- Consume the Ashwagandha Root Powder Mix approximately 30 minutes before bedtime to allow its calming effects to take place.

What to Expect:

Regular consumption of the Ashwagandha Root Powder Mix can lead to noticeable reductions in stress levels and improvements in sleep quality. Ashwagandha works by regulating the stress response system, reducing cortisol levels, and promoting a balanced mood. This can result in decreased anxiety, improved concentration, and a more restful night's sleep. Additionally, ashwagandha's anti-inflammatory and antioxidant properties contribute to overall well-being. However, it's important to use ashwagandha cautiously and consult with a healthcare professional before starting, especially for those with thyroid conditions, autoimmune diseases, or who are pregnant or breastfeeding, due to its potent effects.

Scullcap and Hops Tea for Anxiety Relief.

Scullcap and Hops Tea is a natural herbal blend designed to calm anxiety and ease nervous tension. Both scullcap and hops are renowned for their sedative properties, making this tea an excellent choice for those seeking natural remedies to promote relaxation and mental well-being.

Ingredients:

- 1 teaspoon dried scullcap herb
- 1 teaspoon dried hops
- 1 cup hot water

Instructions:

- Combine 1 teaspoon of dried scullcap herb with 1 teaspoon of dried hops in a tea infuser or tea bag.
- Place the infuser or tea bag in a cup and pour 1 cup of boiling water over it.
- Allow the herbs to steep for about 10 minutes. Steeping for this duration ensures the active compounds are effectively extracted into the water, maximizing the tea's therapeutic potential.
- Remove the infuser or tea bag from the cup. Optionally, you can sweeten the tea with honey or add a slice of lemon to enhance its flavor.

What to Expect:

Drinking Scullcap and Hops Tea can provide significant relief from anxiety and nervous tension. Scullcap is known for its ability to soothe the nervous system, offering relief from occasional stress and anxiety. Hops, commonly used in brewing beer, also possess natural sedative effects that can enhance sleep quality and promote relaxation. Together, these herbs create a powerful synergy that can help calm the mind and prepare the body for rest, making this tea especially beneficial in the evening or during times of heightened stress. However, it's important to note that while scullcap and hops are generally safe for most people, it's wise to consult with a healthcare provider before incorporating them into your routine, especially if you are pregnant, nursing, or taking medications.

PASSIONFLOWER AND VALERIAN ROOT TEA FOR STRESS RELIEF.

Passionflower and Valerian Root Tea is a soothing herbal remedy crafted to alleviate stress and anxiety. This blend harnesses the calming properties of passionflower, known for its ability to reduce nervous tension, and valerian root, widely recognized for its sedative qualities and effectiveness in promoting relaxation and sleep.

Ingredients:

- 1 teaspoon dried passionflower
- 1 teaspoon dried valerian root
- 1 cup hot water

Instructions:

- Combine 1 teaspoon of dried passionflower with 1 teaspoon of dried valerian root in a tea infuser or directly in a cup.
- Pour 1 cup of boiling water over the herbal blend, ensuring the herbs are fully submerged.
- Allow the tea to steep for 10 to 15 minutes, granting the hot water ample time to extract the therapeutic compounds from the herbs.
- If using a tea infuser, remove it from the cup. If the herbs were added directly, strain the tea to remove the solid pieces before drinking.
- Optional: You may add a natural sweetener like honey or a slice of lemon to enhance the flavor of the tea.

What to Expect:

Drinking Passionflower and Valerian Root Tea can provide significant relief from stress and anxiety, promoting a sense of calm and relaxation. This tea is particularly beneficial in the evening or before bedtime, as it can help prepare the body and mind for a restful night's sleep. The effects of valerian root and passionflower have been studied for their impact on improving sleep quality and reducing the time it takes to fall asleep. While this tea is a natural and effective way to manage stress and anxiety, it's important to use these herbs responsibly, especially valerian root, due to its potent sedative effects. As with any herbal remedy, consulting with a healthcare provider before incorporating it into your routine is advisable, especially if you are pregnant, nursing, or taking other medications.

RHODIOLA ROSEA CAPSULES FOR ADAPTOGENIC SUPPORT.

Rhodiola Rosea Capsules are a convenient and effective way to incorporate the adaptogenic benefits of Rhodiola rosea into your daily routine. Known for its ability to enhance the body's resistance to stress, Rhodiola rosea is a powerful herb that has been used for centuries to combat fatigue, improve mental performance, and support overall well-being.

How to Use:

- Select high-quality Rhodiola rosea capsules from a reputable supplier, ensuring the product specifies the percentage of active compounds such as rosavins and salidroside.
- Follow the manufacturer's recommended dosage on the product label. Dosages may vary, but they typically range from 100 to 400 mg per day, taken in the morning or early afternoon to avoid potential interference with sleep.
- Begin with the lower end of the recommended dose to assess your tolerance and gradually increase as needed.

What to Expect:
Taking Rhodiola Rosea Capsules can lead to noticeable improvements in your ability to handle stress, both mentally and physically. Users often report increased energy levels, enhanced mental clarity, and improved mood. The adaptogenic properties of Rhodiola rosea help balance the stress-response system in the body, reducing the impact of stress hormones and enhancing resilience to stressors. Additionally, Rhodiola may contribute to improved exercise performance and recovery by supporting physical endurance and reducing fatigue. It's a natural way to support your body and mind during demanding times, promoting adaptability, and well-being. As with any dietary supplement, it's prudent to consult with a healthcare professional before starting Rhodiola rosea, especially if you have underlying health conditions or are taking other medications, to ensure it is appropriate for your health needs.

Lemon Balm and Rosemary Tea for Stress Relief.

Lemon Balm and Rosemary Tea is a fragrant and soothing herbal beverage, blending the calming properties of lemon balm with the uplifting and cognitive-enhancing effects of rosemary. This tea is perfect for those seeking natural ways to alleviate stress, improve mood, and enhance mental clarity.
Ingredients:

- 1 teaspoon dried lemon balm leaves
- 1 teaspoon dried rosemary leaves
- 1 cup hot water

Instructions:

- Combine 1 teaspoon of dried lemon balm leaves with 1 teaspoon of dried rosemary leaves in a tea infuser or directly in a cup.
- Pour 1 cup of boiling water over the herbs and allow them to steep for about 10 minutes. This steeping time allows the herbs to release their full spectrum of flavors and therapeutic properties.
- Remove the tea infuser or strain the tea to remove the herbs before drinking.

- Optional: Enhance the tea with a slice of lemon or a teaspoon of honey for added flavor and benefits.

What to Expect:
Drinking Lemon Balm and Rosemary Tea can have a soothing effect on the nervous system, helping to reduce feelings of stress and anxiety. Lemon balm is well-known for its ability to ease stress and promote a sense of calm, while rosemary has been associated with improved mood and cognitive function, including better concentration and memory. The combination of these two herbs creates a tea that not only helps to relax the mind and body but also stimulates mental clarity and focus. Enjoy this tea during moments of stress or when you need a mental boost. Its refreshing flavor and aroma make it a delightful choice for any time of the day.

HOPS AND LAVENDER SLEEP PILLOW FOR ANXIETY.

Creating a Hops and Lavender Sleep Pillow involves blending dried hops and lavender flowers, known for their calming and sleep-inducing properties. This natural remedy is perfect for those seeking a non-intrusive way to soothe anxiety and promote restful sleep. The aromatic compounds in both hops and lavender have been used traditionally to reduce stress, alleviate insomnia, and improve sleep quality.

Ingredients:

- ½ cup dried hops
- ½ cup dried lavender flowers
- A small cloth pillow or sachet bag

Instructions:

- In a bowl, mix together ½ cup of dried hops and ½ cup of dried lavender flowers until well combined.
- Fill a small cloth pillow or sachet bag with the hops and lavender blend. If using a pillow, sew it shut or use a drawstring closure. For a sachet bag, simply tie the bag securely.
- Place the sleep pillow near your sleeping area, under your regular pillow, or on a bedside table. The goal is to have the pillow close enough that you can inhale the calming scents as you sleep.

What to Expect:
Using a Hops and Lavender Sleep Pillow can help create a tranquil environment conducive to sleep. The scent of lavender is widely recognized for its ability to relax the mind, reduce anxiety, and induce sleep, while hops contribute sedative qualities that can deepen sleep and improve sleep duration. Together, these herbs can help calm nervous tension and make it easier to fall asleep and stay asleep through the night. This natural approach to enhancing sleep quality is gentle and can be particularly beneficial for those

who prefer not to rely on sleep medications. Enjoy the soothing aroma as you drift off to sleep, and wake feeling more rested and less anxious.

HOLY BASIL (TULSI) AND CHAMOMILE TEA.

Holy Basil (Tulsi) and Chamomile Tea is a calming herbal beverage that combines the stress-reducing properties of holy basil with the soothing effects of chamomile. This tea is an ideal choice for those looking to alleviate stress, calm anxiety, and promote a sense of serenity and well-being.
Ingredients:

- 1 teaspoon dried holy basil (Tulsi) leaves
- 1 teaspoon dried chamomile flowers
- 1 cup hot water

Instructions:

- Mix 1 teaspoon of dried holy basil leaves with 1 teaspoon of dried chamomile flowers in a tea infuser or directly in a cup.
- Pour 1 cup of boiling water over the herbal mixture, ensuring the herbs are fully submerged.
- Allow the tea to steep for about 10 minutes, giving the water ample time to extract the beneficial compounds from the herbs.
- If using a tea infuser, remove it from the cup. If the herbs were added directly, strain the tea to remove the herbs before drinking.
- Optional: You may add a natural sweetener like honey or a slice of lemon to enhance the flavor of the tea.

What to Expect:
Drinking Holy Basil (Tulsi) and Chamomile Tea can offer immediate relief from stress and anxiety. Holy basil, revered in Ayurvedic medicine as an adaptogen, helps the body adapt to stress and promotes mental balance. Chamomile is well-known for its calming effects, especially in reducing anxiety and facilitating a good night's sleep. The combination of these two herbs in a single tea provides a powerful tool for managing daily stress and improving overall mood. Enjoy this tea in the evening to unwind before bed or anytime during the day when you need a moment of calm. The gentle, floral flavor and aromatic blend make it a delightful and therapeutic addition to your stress management routine.

PASSIONFLOWER AND LEMON BALM NIGHTTIME TEA.

Passionflower and Lemon Balm Nighttime Tea is a soothing herbal infusion designed to promote relaxation and enhance sleep quality. By blending the calming effects of passionflower, known for its ability to ease insomnia and anxiety, with the stress-reducing properties of lemon balm, this tea serves as an ideal nighttime beverage for those seeking a natural way to unwind and encourage restful sleep.

Ingredients:

- 1 teaspoon dried passionflower
- 1 teaspoon dried lemon balm
- 1 cup hot water

Instructions:

- Combine 1 teaspoon of dried passionflower with 1 teaspoon of dried lemon balm in a tea infuser or directly in a cup.
- Pour 1 cup of boiling water over the herbal blend and allow it to steep for 10 to 15 minutes. The longer steeping time ensures a strong infusion, maximizing the herbs' sedative and calming effects.
- Remove the tea infuser or strain the tea to remove the loose herbs before drinking.
- Optional: For added flavor or sweetness, consider adding a teaspoon of honey or a few drops of lemon juice to the tea.

What to Expect:

Drinking Passionflower and Lemon Balm Nighttime Tea before bed can significantly aid in relaxation and help prepare the mind and body for sleep. Passionflower is particularly effective in reducing anxiety and improving sleep quality, making it easier to fall asleep and stay asleep throughout the night. Lemon balm complements passionflower by reducing stress and promoting a sense of calm. Together, these herbs create a potent combination that can alleviate restlessness and insomnia, leading to a more peaceful and restorative night's sleep. This tea is a natural and gentle option for those looking to enhance their nighttime routine and improve overall sleep health.

ASHWAGANDHA AND HOLY BASIL ADRENAL SUPPORT TONIC.

The Ashwagandha and Holy Basil Adrenal Support Tonic is a powerful drink designed to combat stress and alleviate symptoms of adrenal fatigue. By combining ashwagandha, known for its adaptogenic properties, with holy basil (tulsi), revered for its stress-relieving effects, this tonic offers a holistic approach to supporting adrenal health and enhancing overall vitality.

Ingredients:

- 1 teaspoon ashwagandha powder
- 1 teaspoon holy basil (tulsi) powder
- 1 cup warm milk (dairy or plant-based) or water

Instructions:

- Mix 1 teaspoon of ashwagandha powder with 1 teaspoon of holy basil powder in a cup.

- Heat 1 cup of milk or water until warm but not boiling. Pour the warm liquid into the cup with the ashwagandha and holy basil powders.
- Stir the mixture thoroughly until the powders are completely dissolved. If desired, sweeten with honey or maple syrup to taste.
- Drink the tonic once daily, preferably in the morning or early afternoon, to maximize its stress-relieving and adrenal-supportive benefits.

What to Expect:
Regular consumption of the Ashwagandha and Holy Basil Adrenal Support Tonic can help reduce physical and mental stress, thereby supporting the adrenal glands' function. Ashwagandha assists in regulating cortisol levels, enhancing the body's resilience to stress, while holy basil promotes mental clarity and energy. This combination can lead to improved energy levels, reduced anxiety, and a more balanced mood. Additionally, the tonic can aid in improving sleep quality and overall well-being. It's a natural and effective way to support your body's stress response system and maintain optimal health. As with any supplement, it's wise to consult with a healthcare provider before starting, especially if you have existing health conditions or are taking medications.

DAMIANA LEAF TEA FOR ANXIETY AND RELAXATION.

Damiana Leaf Tea is a herbal tea made from the leaves of the damiana plant, renowned for its mild sedative effects that can help ease anxiety and promote relaxation. Traditionally used for its mood-enhancing properties, damiana is a great choice for those seeking a natural way to unwind and alleviate stress.
Ingredients:

- 1-2 teaspoons dried damiana leaves
- 1 cup hot water

Instructions:

- Place 1-2 teaspoons of dried damiana leaves in a tea infuser or directly in a cup.
- Pour 1 cup of boiling water over the damiana leaves, ensuring they are fully immersed.
- Allow the leaves to steep for 10 to 15 minutes, allowing the water to extract the active compounds from the leaves fully.
- If using a tea infuser, remove it from the cup. If the leaves were added directly, strain the tea to remove the leaves before drinking.
- Optional: Enhance the flavor of the tea with honey, lemon, or mint according to your preference.

What to Expect:

Drinking Damiana Leaf Tea can provide a soothing effect, helping to reduce feelings of anxiety and stress. The tea may promote a sense of well-being and relaxation, making it ideal for consumption in the evening or during moments of high stress. Damiana is also thought to have aphrodisiac properties, although this is more anecdotal than scientifically proven. As with any herbal remedy, it's important to start with a small amount to ensure your body's tolerance and consult with a healthcare provider if you're pregnant, nursing, or taking medication, as damiana can interact with certain substances. Enjoy the calming benefits of Damiana Leaf Tea as part of your daily routine to support overall mental health and relaxation.

LEMON VERBENA AND PASSIONFLOWER RELAXING TEA.

Lemon Verbena and Passionflower Relaxing Tea is an aromatic and soothing herbal blend designed to reduce stress and promote relaxation. This tea combines the calming properties of passionflower, known for its ability to ease anxiety and improve sleep, with the refreshing and mood-enhancing qualities of lemon verbena. Together, they create a delicious and therapeutic beverage perfect for unwinding after a long day.

Ingredients:

- 1 teaspoon dried lemon verbena leaves
- 1 teaspoon dried passionflower
- 1 cup hot water

Instructions:

- Mix 1 teaspoon of dried lemon verbena leaves with 1 teaspoon of dried passionflower in a tea infuser or directly in a cup.
- Pour 1 cup of boiling water over the herbs, allowing them to steep for about 10 minutes. This duration lets the water fully absorb the herbs' flavors and medicinal properties.
- Remove the tea infuser or strain the tea to remove the loose herbs before drinking.
- Optional: Add a touch of honey, stevia, or lemon slice to enhance the flavor of the tea without compromising its relaxing effects.

What to Expect:

Drinking Lemon Verbena and Passionflower Relaxing Tea can help soothe the nervous system, reduce feelings of stress, and prepare the body and mind for a restful night's sleep. Passionflower is particularly effective for those experiencing anxiety or insomnia, as it promotes deeper sleep and relaxation. Lemon verbena adds a light, citrusy flavor that uplifts the mood while also aiding in digestion. This tea is an excellent choice for the evening or any time you need to relax and de-stress. Its natural ingredients work synergistically to provide a calming effect, making it a gentle, effective way to support your overall well-being.

WITHANIA (ASHWAGANDHA) ROOT NIGHTTIME MILK.

Withania Root Nighttime Milk, commonly known as Ashwagandha Milk, is a traditional Ayurvedic remedy used to alleviate stress and promote restful sleep. Ashwagandha, also known as Withania somnifera, is a powerful adaptogen that helps balance the body's stress hormones, making it perfect for a soothing nighttime beverage.

Ingredients:

- 1 teaspoon ashwagandha (withania) root powder
- 1 cup milk (can be dairy or a plant-based alternative like almond, coconut, or oat milk)
- 1 teaspoon honey, or to taste (optional)
- A pinch of cinnamon or nutmeg for flavor enhancement (optional)

Instructions:

- Gently heat 1 cup of milk in a small saucepan over medium heat. Avoid bringing it to a boil to preserve the milk's nutritional properties and prevent scalding.
- Once the milk is warm, add 1 teaspoon of ashwagandha root powder. Stir well to ensure the powder is fully dissolved in the milk.
- Simmer the mixture for a few minutes, allowing the ashwagandha to infuse into the milk. Stir occasionally to prevent sticking and ensure even distribution of the herb.
- Remove from heat and add 1 teaspoon of honey for sweetness, if desired. You can also sprinkle a pinch of cinnamon or nutmeg to enhance the flavor.
- Stir the mixture well, then pour it into a cup.

What to Expect:

Drinking Withania (Ashwagandha) Root Nighttime Milk before bed can significantly reduce stress levels and promote a more restful sleep. Ashwagandha's adaptogenic properties help to regulate cortisol levels, reducing the effects of stress on the body. The addition of honey not only sweetens the drink but also has natural relaxing properties that can enhance the sleep-inducing effects of the milk. Cinnamon or nutmeg adds a comforting warmth and aroma to the beverage, making it even more soothing. This nighttime milk is a holistic way to unwind at the end of the day, setting the stage for a peaceful night's sleep and improved overall well-being.

ST. JOHN'S WORT AND LEMON BALM TEA FOR MOOD SUPPORT.

St. John's Wort and Lemon Balm Tea is a therapeutic herbal blend crafted to support mood and alleviate symptoms of mild depression and anxiety. St. John's Wort is well-known for its antidepressant properties, while lemon

balm brings calming effects to the nervous system, making this tea an excellent choice for those seeking natural remedies to enhance emotional well-being.
Ingredients:

- 1 teaspoon dried St. John's Wort
- 1 teaspoon dried lemon balm leaves
- 1 cup hot water

Instructions:

- Combine 1 teaspoon of dried St. John's Wort with 1 teaspoon of dried lemon balm leaves in a tea infuser or directly in a cup.
- Pour 1 cup of boiling water over the herbal mixture, ensuring that the herbs are fully submerged.
- Allow the herbs to steep for about 10 minutes. This steeping time allows the therapeutic compounds to be released into the water.
- Remove the tea infuser or strain the tea to remove the loose herbs before drinking.
- Optional: Add a natural sweetener like honey or a slice of lemon to enhance the flavor if desired.

What to Expect:
Drinking St. John's Wort and Lemon Balm Tea can provide mood-enhancing benefits and help alleviate symptoms of mild depression and anxiety. The combination of these two herbs can promote a sense of calm, reduce stress levels, and improve overall emotional balance. St. John's Wort is particularly effective for mild to moderate depression, while lemon balm aids in relaxation and stress relief. Enjoy this tea during times of emotional unrest or daily as part of your routine to support mental health. However, it's important to note that St. John's Wort can interact with certain medications, including antidepressants and birth control pills. Consult with a healthcare professional before adding St. John's Wort to your regimen, especially if you are currently taking any medications.

RHODIOLA ROSEA ROOT EXTRACT FOR STRESS REDUCTION.

Rhodiola Rosea Root Extract is a natural supplement derived from the Rhodiola rosea plant, famed for its adaptogenic properties that help the body resist and adapt to stress, fatigue, and anxiety. This powerful herb is utilized to enhance mental clarity, energy levels, and overall resilience against stress.
How to Use:

- Opt for a high-quality, commercially prepared Rhodiola Rosea extract, ensuring it specifies the active ingredients like rosavins and salidroside, which contribute to its efficacy.
- Follow the manufacturer's instructions regarding dosage. Typically, the dosage ranges from 100 to 600 mg per day, depending on the

extract's concentration and the individual's response to the supplement.
- Rhodiola can be taken in various forms, including capsules, tablets, or liquid extracts. Select the form that best fits your lifestyle and preference.

What to Expect:
Incorporating Rhodiola Rosea Root Extract into your daily routine can significantly aid in reducing stress and enhancing mental performance. Users often report an improvement in energy levels, mood, and focus shortly after beginning supplementation. Rhodiola works by stimulating the body's stress response system, helping to increase stamina and reduce fatigue in stressful situations. It's particularly beneficial during periods of high mental and physical stress, as well as for combating fatigue and improving cognitive functions. As with any supplement, it's wise to start with a low dose to assess your body's reaction and consult with a healthcare professional, especially if you have existing health conditions or are taking other medications, to ensure its suitability for your health regimen.

Ashwagandha Root and Holy Basil Tea for Stress Relief.

Ashwagandha Root and Holy Basil (Tulsi) Tea is a powerful herbal infusion designed to provide relief from stress and anxiety. This tea combines the adaptogenic benefits of ashwagandha root, known for its ability to balance the body's stress hormones, with the calming properties of holy basil, revered for its spiritual and medicinal significance in Ayurvedic medicine. Together, they create a soothing beverage that supports mental well-being and resilience.

Ingredients:
- 1 teaspoon dried ashwagandha root
- 1 teaspoon dried holy basil (tulsi) leaves
- 1 cup hot water

Instructions:
- Combine 1 teaspoon of dried ashwagandha root with 1 teaspoon of dried holy basil leaves in a tea infuser or directly in a cup.
- Pour 1 cup of boiling water over the herbs, ensuring they are fully immersed.
- Allow the tea to steep for about 10 to 15 minutes, allowing the herbs to release their beneficial compounds into the water.
- Remove the tea infuser or strain the tea to remove the loose herbs before drinking.
- Optional: Enhance the tea with natural sweeteners like honey or add a slice of lemon for additional flavor and benefits.

What to Expect:
Drinking Ashwagandha Root and Holy Basil Tea can significantly reduce stress levels and alleviate anxiety. Ashwagandha's adaptogenic properties help mitigate the body's stress response, promoting a sense of calm and helping to manage cortisol levels. Holy basil complements ashwagandha by enhancing mental clarity and providing a sense of peace. This combination not only aids in reducing stress and anxiety but also supports overall vitality and immune health. The tea has a grounding, earthy flavor, making it a comforting choice for relaxation and stress management. Incorporate this tea into your evening routine or enjoy it during moments of high stress to foster tranquility and well-being.

Blue Vervain and Lavender Stress-Relief Tea.

Blue Vervain and Lavender Stress-Relief Tea is a calming herbal concoction designed to alleviate stress, tension, and promote a sense of tranquility. Blue vervain, with its natural soothing properties, synergizes with the calming aroma of lavender to create a tea that not only relaxes the body but also the mind.

Ingredients:

- 1 teaspoon dried blue vervain
- 1 teaspoon dried lavender flowers
- 1 cup hot water

Instructions:

- Combine 1 teaspoon of dried blue vervain with 1 teaspoon of dried lavender flowers in a tea infuser or directly in a cup.
- Pour 1 cup of boiling water over the herb mixture, ensuring that the herbs are fully immersed.
- Allow the tea to steep for about 10 to 15 minutes, allowing ample time for the herbs to release their beneficial compounds.
- Remove the tea infuser or strain the tea to remove the loose herbs before drinking.
- Optional: You may add a natural sweetener like honey or a slice of lemon to enhance the flavor of the tea.

What to Expect:
Drinking Blue Vervain and Lavender Stress-Relief Tea can help reduce feelings of stress and tension, promoting a serene state of mind. Blue vervain is known for its ability to ease nervous tension, while lavender's aromatic properties have been widely recognized for their relaxing effects. This tea is perfect for unwinding after a long day, helping to soothe anxiety and prepare the body for a restful night's sleep. The floral and slightly earthy flavor of this tea makes it a delightful choice for those seeking natural remedies to support mental well-being and relaxation.

KAVA KAVA ROOT BREW FOR RELAXATION.

Kava Kava Root Brew is a traditional drink known for its potent relaxing and anxiety-reducing properties. Made from the root of the kava plant, this brew has been used for centuries in Pacific Island cultures to promote relaxation, socialization, and relieve stress. However, it's important to approach kava with caution due to concerns about its potential effects on liver health.
Ingredients:

- 2-4 tablespoons dried kava kava root
- 2 cups of water

Instructions:

- Place 2-4 tablespoons of dried kava kava root into a strainer bag or cheesecloth.
- In a bowl, add the kava kava root to 2 cups of warm (not hot) water. The traditional method involves kneading and squeezing the bag in the water for about 10-15 minutes to extract the kavalactones, which are the active compounds in kava.
- Continue to massage and squeeze the bag in the water until it becomes milky and opaque.
- Once done, remove the strainer bag or cheesecloth, squeezing out as much liquid as possible.
- Serve the brew in a cup. It can be consumed as is or diluted further with water to taste.

What to Expect:
Kava Kava Root Brew can produce a sense of relaxation and euphoria, reducing anxiety and stress without impairing cognitive function. It's known for its muscle-relaxing and sedative effects, making it a popular choice for those seeking natural relief from tension and insomnia. However, due to concerns about liver toxicity, it's crucial to use kava sparingly and to be mindful of any health advisories or restrictions regarding its consumption. It is also advised to consult with a healthcare provider before integrating kava into your routine, especially if you have liver issues, are pregnant, nursing, or taking medications. Enjoy kava kava root brew responsibly and in moderation to experience its calming benefits while minimizing potential risks.

OATSTRAW AND LAVENDER TEA FOR NERVOUS SYSTEM SUPPORT.

Oatstraw and Lavender Tea is a gentle, soothing blend designed to calm the nervous system and promote a sense of well-being. Oatstraw, the green stalks of the oat plant, is rich in vitamins and minerals that support nervous system health, while lavender flowers offer calming and relaxing properties. This tea is ideal for those looking to reduce stress, anxiety, and promote relaxation.

Ingredients:

- 1 teaspoon dried oatstraw
- 1 teaspoon dried lavender flowers
- 1 cup hot water

Instructions:

- Combine 1 teaspoon of dried oatstraw with 1 teaspoon of dried lavender flowers in a tea infuser or directly in a cup.
- Pour 1 cup of boiling water over the herbs, ensuring they are fully submerged.
- Allow the tea to steep for about 10 to 15 minutes. The longer steeping time allows the herbs to release their beneficial compounds, maximizing the tea's calming effects.
- Remove the tea infuser or strain the tea to remove the loose herbs before drinking.
- Optional: Add a natural sweetener like honey or a slice of lemon to enhance the flavor of the tea.

What to Expect:

Drinking Oatstraw and Lavender Tea can provide immediate and lasting benefits for the nervous system. Oatstraw is known for its ability to nourish and strengthen nerves, making it beneficial for those dealing with stress, exhaustion, or anxiety. Lavender adds a layer of relaxation, helping to soothe the mind and promote a peaceful state. This combination makes the tea a perfect choice for evening consumption to wind down before bed or anytime you need to calm a frazzled nervous system. The tea's mild, earthy flavor, complemented by the floral notes of lavender, creates a delightful sensory experience that enhances its therapeutic effects.

Herbal Remedies for Mental Clarity and Focus.

Rosemary Tea for Mental Alertness.

Rosemary Tea is an aromatic and invigorating herbal beverage known for its ability to enhance mental clarity, focus, and alertness. Made from the leaves of the rosemary plant, this tea leverages rosemary's natural compounds that have been linked to improved cognitive function and memory retention. It's an excellent choice for those seeking a natural boost to their mental performance.

Ingredients:

- 1 teaspoon fresh or dried rosemary leaves
- 1 cup hot water

Instructions:

- Place 1 teaspoon of fresh or dried rosemary leaves in a tea infuser or directly in a cup.
- Pour 1 cup of boiling water over the rosemary leaves, ensuring they are fully immersed.
- Allow the rosemary to steep for about 5 to 10 minutes, depending on your taste preference and desired strength. The longer it steeps, the more potent the flavor and effects.
- Remove the tea infuser or strain the tea to remove the rosemary leaves before drinking.
- Optional: Enhance the tea with a slice of lemon or a teaspoon of honey, which can complement rosemary's robust flavor.

What to Expect:
Drinking Rosemary Tea can provide a noticeable increase in mental alertness and cognitive function. Rosemary contains compounds such as 1,8-cineole, which have been shown to have positive effects on memory performance and brain function. This tea is perfect for mornings, study sessions, or any time you need a mental boost without the jittery side effects of caffeine. Its refreshing and distinctive flavor is both uplifting and soothing, making it a delightful beverage for enhancing mental clarity and concentration. Enjoy Rosemary Tea as a part of your daily routine to support your cognitive health and performance.

Ginkgo Biloba Leaf Infusion for Improved Concentration.

Ginkgo Biloba Leaf Infusion is a traditional herbal remedy known for its powerful effects on cognitive function and memory enhancement. Ginkgo biloba, one of the oldest living tree species, contains flavonoids and terpenoids, antioxidants that improve blood flow to the brain and protect neurons, supporting overall brain health and concentration.
Ingredients:

- 1-2 teaspoons dried ginkgo biloba leaves
- 1 cup hot water

Instructions:

- Place 1-2 teaspoons of dried ginkgo biloba leaves in a tea infuser or directly in a cup.
- Pour 1 cup of boiling water over the ginkgo biloba leaves, ensuring they are fully immersed.
- Allow the leaves to infuse in the hot water for about 10 minutes. The steeping time allows the beneficial compounds of the leaves to be released into the water.
- Remove the tea infuser or strain the tea to remove the leaves before drinking.

- Optional: Add a natural sweetener or a slice of lemon to enhance the flavor of the infusion.

What to Expect:

Drinking Ginkgo Biloba Leaf Infusion can lead to an improvement in cognitive functions, including enhanced concentration, memory, and mental clarity. Many users report feeling more alert and focused after consuming the tea, making it an excellent beverage for study sessions, work, or any activity that requires sustained mental effort. Additionally, ginkgo biloba has been associated with supporting brain health over time, potentially slowing the cognitive decline related to aging. Enjoy this herbal infusion as part of your daily routine to support cognitive health and improve concentration. However, it's important to consult with a healthcare provider before adding ginkgo biloba to your regimen, especially if you are taking medications, due to its blood-thinning properties.

Sleep Aid and Herbal Remedies for Sleep Disorders.

Valerian Root Infusion for Insomnia.

Valerian Root Infusion is a natural remedy known for its sedative qualities, making it an effective treatment for insomnia and other sleep disorders. By steeping dried valerian root in hot water, you can create a potent herbal tea that promotes relaxation and improves sleep quality.

Ingredients:

- 1 teaspoon dried valerian root
- 1 cup hot water

Instructions:

- Place 1 teaspoon of dried valerian root in a tea infuser or directly in a cup.
- Pour 1 cup of boiling water over the valerian root, ensuring it is fully submerged.
- Allow the valerian root to steep for about 10 minutes. This steeping time allows the valerian root to release its active compounds, which contribute to its sleep-promoting effects.
- Remove the tea infuser or strain the tea to remove the valerian root before drinking.
- Optional: If the taste is too strong, you can add a natural sweetener like honey or mix with a more flavorful herbal tea to improve the taste.

What to Expect:

Drinking Valerian Root Infusion before bed can help calm the nervous system, reduce anxiety, and facilitate a deeper, more restful sleep. Valerian root contains several compounds that have been shown to enhance GABA (gamma-aminobutyric acid) levels in the brain, which helps regulate nerve impulses and has a calming effect. Due to its potent effects, it's recommended to consume valerian root infusion sparingly and not rely on it as a long-term solution without consulting a healthcare provider. Some people may experience mild side effects such as dizziness or grogginess, so it's advisable to see how your body responds before continuing regular use. Incorporate Valerian Root Infusion into your nighttime routine to improve sleep quality and overcome insomnia naturally.

Passionflower Nighttime Tea.

Passionflower Nighttime Tea is a natural beverage crafted from dried passionflower, a herb celebrated for its sleep-inducing properties. By infusing passionflower in boiling water, this tea becomes an effective aid for those seeking to improve their sleep quality and find relaxation before bedtime.
Ingredients:

- 1 teaspoon dried passionflower
- 1 cup boiling water

Instructions:

- Place 1 teaspoon of dried passionflower in a tea infuser or directly in a cup.
- Pour 1 cup of boiling water over the dried passionflower, ensuring it's fully submerged.
- Allow the tea to steep for about 15 minutes. This duration allows the water to fully extract the sleep-promoting compounds from the passionflower.
- Remove the tea infuser or strain the tea to remove the loose herbs before drinking.
- Optional: For added flavor or sweetness, you can add honey or a slice of lemon to the tea.

What to Expect:
Drinking Passionflower Nighttime Tea before bed can significantly contribute to a peaceful and restful night's sleep. Passionflower is known for its calming effects on the nervous system, helping to ease anxiety and insomnia by increasing levels of GABA in the brain, which helps reduce brain activity and promote relaxation. This herbal tea is especially beneficial for those who experience difficulty falling asleep or staying asleep throughout the night. Its gentle sedative effect can help you drift off to sleep more easily and enjoy a deeper, more restorative sleep. Enjoy this soothing beverage as part of your nightly routine to embrace its tranquility-promoting benefits.

Hops Pillow for Deep Sleep.

A Hops Pillow, filled with dried hops flowers, is a traditional remedy utilized for its sleep-inducing properties. The subtle aroma released by the hops is known to enhance sleep quality and promote a state of deep relaxation. This natural approach is perfect for those seeking a gentle aid to improve their sleep experience.

Ingredients:

- Dried hops flowers
- A small pillowcase or fabric pouch

Instructions:

- Fill a small pillowcase or fabric pouch with dried hops flowers. The amount of hops needed will depend on the size of your pillow or pouch but aim for enough to fill the pillow while allowing it to remain pliable.
- Sew the opening shut or use a drawstring closure if your pillowcase or pouch is designed with one. Ensure the hops are securely contained within the pillow.
- Place the hops pillow near your head or under your regular pillow at night. The proximity will allow you to inhale the relaxing aroma as you sleep.
- Optional: For added relaxation benefits, you can combine the hops with other calming herbs such as lavender or chamomile. Just mix these in with the hops flowers before filling your pillow.

What to Expect:

Using a Hops Pillow can significantly contribute to achieving a deeper, more restful sleep. Hops contain naturally occurring compounds that have sedative effects, which can help to reduce sleep latency (the time it takes to fall asleep) and improve overall sleep quality. The calming aroma of hops is subtle and should not be overwhelming, making it a suitable sleep aid for nightly use. Over time, you may find that your sleep patterns improve and that you feel more rested upon waking. This simple, natural solution can be a valuable addition to your bedtime routine, especially if you prefer non-ingestible methods of enhancing sleep quality.

Magnolia Bark Tea for Sleep Disturbances.

Magnolia Bark Tea is a traditional herbal remedy made from the bark of the magnolia tree, known for its ability to promote restful sleep and alleviate sleep disturbances. The bioactive compounds in magnolia bark, such as magnolol and honokiol, have sedative properties that can help calm the mind and prepare the body for sleep.

Ingredients:

- 1-2 teaspoons dried magnolia bark
- 1 cup boiling water

Instructions:

- Place 1-2 teaspoons of dried magnolia bark in a tea infuser or directly in a cup.
- Pour 1 cup of boiling water over the magnolia bark, ensuring it is fully immersed.
- Allow the bark to steep for about 10-15 minutes, allowing enough time for the therapeutic compounds to infuse into the water.
- Remove the tea infuser or strain the tea to remove the bark pieces before drinking.
- Optional: Add a natural sweetener like honey or a slice of lemon to enhance the flavor of the tea, if desired.

What to Expect:

Drinking Magnolia Bark Tea before bedtime can significantly improve the quality of your sleep. The natural compounds in magnolia bark have been shown to reduce the time it takes to fall asleep and increase the duration of deep sleep. This tea is particularly beneficial for those who experience insomnia or other sleep disturbances, helping to relax the body and mind, and reduce anxiety that can interfere with sleep. While magnolia bark is generally safe for most people, it's potent and should be used with caution. It's recommended to start with a lower dose to assess your tolerance and avoid potential drowsiness in the morning. As with any herbal remedy, consult with a healthcare provider before incorporating magnolia bark tea into your nighttime routine, especially if you are pregnant, nursing, or taking medications.

HOPS AND VALERIAN ROOT PILLOW FOR INSOMNIA.

The Hops and Valerian Root Pillow is a natural sleep aid that combines the sedative effects of hops with the calming properties of valerian root. This unique blend is designed to support deep sleep and alleviate insomnia by promoting relaxation and easing the mind. Placing this herbal pillow near the head at night can significantly improve sleep quality without the need for pharmaceutical sleep aids.

Ingredients:

- ½ cup dried hops
- ½ cup dried valerian root
- A small, breathable fabric pillowcase or sachet bag

Instructions:

- In a bowl, thoroughly mix ½ cup of dried hops with ½ cup of dried valerian root.

- Fill a small, breathable fabric pillowcase or sachet bag with the herb mixture. If using a pillowcase, sew it shut or tie it securely to prevent the herbs from spilling out.
- Place the filled pillow or sachet near your head or under your regular pillow at night.

What to Expect:
Using a Hops and Valerian Root Pillow can help ease the transition into sleep by calming the nervous system and reducing anxiety. Hops contain compounds that have a mild sedative effect, which can be beneficial for those who have difficulty falling asleep. Valerian root is known for its ability to improve sleep quality and reduce nighttime awakenings. Together, these herbs create a synergistic effect that supports restful sleep.
This natural remedy is especially useful for individuals looking for a non-invasive method to improve their sleep patterns and combat insomnia. The aroma of the herbs can vary, with valerian root having a particularly strong scent, but many find the overall effect to be soothing and conducive to sleep. As with any herbal treatment, it's important to monitor your body's response, and consult with a healthcare provider if you have any concerns or are taking other sleep medications.

Lavender and Chamomile Sleep Sachet.

The Lavender and Chamomile Sleep Sachet is a natural sleep aid crafted from a blend of dried lavender and chamomile, two herbs renowned for their calming and sleep-inducing properties. This sachet is designed to promote restful sleep by creating a soothing aroma environment that relaxes the mind and body, making it easier to fall asleep and enjoy a deeper sleep cycle.
Ingredients:

- ½ cup dried lavender flowers
- ½ cup dried chamomile flowers
- A small, breathable fabric sachet or pouch

Instructions:

- In a bowl, mix together ½ cup of dried lavender flowers with ½ cup of dried chamomile flowers until well combined.
- Fill a small, breathable fabric sachet or pouch with the lavender and chamomile blend. Secure the sachet closed to prevent the herbs from spilling out.
- Place the filled sachet under your pillow or near your head on the bedstand before going to sleep.

What to Expect:
Using the Lavender and Chamomile Sleep Sachet can significantly enhance the quality of your sleep. Lavender is well-known for its ability to decrease

anxiety and induce a state of calm, while chamomile is often used for its gentle sedative effects. The combined aroma of these herbs can help soothe the nervous system, reduce sleep disturbances, and make it easier to fall asleep and stay asleep throughout the night. The scent of lavender and chamomile is also known to reduce stress levels and create a tranquil atmosphere conducive to relaxation and sleep. This simple, natural approach to improving sleep is gentle and can be particularly beneficial for those seeking alternatives to sleep medications. Enjoy the subtle, calming fragrances of lavender and chamomile as you drift off to a restful night's sleep.

CHERRY AND CHAMOMILE SLEEPY TIME TEA.

Cherry and Chamomile Sleepy Time Tea is a delightful and effective natural remedy designed to promote restful sleep. This unique blend combines the natural sleep-inducing properties of cherries, known for their melatonin content, with the calming effects of chamomile flowers. Together, they create a soothing tea that helps prepare the body and mind for a peaceful night's sleep.

Ingredients:

- 1 tablespoon dried cherries, chopped
- 1 tablespoon dried chamomile flowers
- 1 cup hot water

Instructions:

- In a tea infuser or directly in a cup, combine 1 tablespoon of chopped dried cherries with 1 tablespoon of dried chamomile flowers.
- Pour 1 cup of boiling water over the cherry and chamomile blend, ensuring that the ingredients are fully submerged.
- Allow the mixture to steep for about 10 minutes. The steeping time allows the water to extract the beneficial compounds from the cherries and chamomile, creating a potent brew.
- Remove the tea infuser or strain the tea to remove the solid ingredients before drinking.
- Optional: Add a natural sweetener like honey or a slice of lemon to enhance the tea's flavor.

What to Expect:

Drinking Cherry and Chamomile Sleepy Time Tea before bedtime can significantly improve the quality of your sleep. The natural melatonin in cherries helps regulate the sleep-wake cycle, while chamomile's calming properties reduce anxiety and promote relaxation. This combination not only makes it easier to fall asleep but also contributes to a deeper and more restful sleep. The tea has a subtle, fruity flavor with the soothing aroma of chamomile, making it a perfect nighttime beverage. Enjoy this tea as part of your evening routine to unwind and prepare for a night of peaceful sleep.

LEMON VERBENA AND MAGNOLIA BARK SLEEP AID.

Lemon Verbena and Magnolia Bark Sleep Aid is a soothing herbal tea crafted to support restful sleep and promote relaxation. By blending the refreshing and calming properties of lemon verbena with the sleep-enhancing effects of magnolia bark, this tea serves as a natural remedy for those seeking to improve their sleep quality without relying on pharmaceutical sleep aids.
Ingredients:

- 1 teaspoon dried lemon verbena leaves
- 1 teaspoon dried magnolia bark
- 1 cup hot water

Instructions:

- Combine 1 teaspoon of dried lemon verbena leaves with 1 teaspoon of dried magnolia bark in a tea infuser or directly in a cup.
- Pour 1 cup of boiling water over the herbal mixture, making sure the ingredients are fully immersed.
- Allow the tea to steep for about 10 to 15 minutes, providing ample time for the therapeutic properties of lemon verbena and magnolia bark to infuse into the water.
- Remove the tea infuser or strain the tea to remove the solid ingredients before drinking.
- Optional: For added flavor or sweetness, consider adding honey or a slice of lemon to the tea.

What to Expect:
Drinking Lemon Verbena and Magnolia Bark Sleep Aid before bedtime can significantly contribute to a tranquil and restorative night's sleep. Lemon verbena is known for its ability to ease stress and promote a sense of calm, while magnolia bark contains compounds that have been shown to reduce anxiety and improve sleep quality by increasing GABA activity in the brain, a neurotransmitter that promotes relaxation. This herbal tea blend offers a gentle yet effective way to unwind at the end of the day, helping you to fall asleep more easily and enjoy a deeper, more restful sleep. Enjoy this calming beverage as part of your nightly routine to embrace its sleep-supportive benefits.

CHERRY JUICE AND CHAMOMILE SLEEP AID.

Cherry Juice and Chamomile Sleep Aid is a natural beverage designed to enhance sleep quality and promote relaxation. Combining the melatonin-rich benefits of cherry juice with the calming properties of chamomile tea, this sleep aid is an effective and delicious way to prepare your body and mind for restful sleep.

Ingredients:

- ½ cup cherry juice (preferably tart cherry juice for its higher melatonin content)
- 1 cup freshly brewed chamomile tea

Instructions:

- Brew 1 cup of chamomile tea by steeping 1-2 teaspoons of dried chamomile flowers or a chamomile tea bag in boiling water for about 5-10 minutes.
- Remove the chamomile flowers or tea bag, ensuring the tea is strong and well-infused.
- In a mug or glass, mix ½ cup of cherry juice with the freshly brewed chamomile tea.
- Stir the mixture well to combine the cherry juice and chamomile tea evenly.
- Optional: Adjust the flavor to your liking by adding a natural sweetener like honey or a slice of lemon. You can also adjust the ratio of cherry juice to chamomile tea based on your taste preferences.

What to Expect:

Drinking Cherry Juice and Chamomile Sleep Aid in the evening can help improve your sleep quality. Tart cherry juice is a natural source of melatonin, the hormone that regulates the sleep-wake cycle, while chamomile tea is known for its gentle sedative effects that promote relaxation and reduce anxiety. This combination works synergistically to help you unwind, fall asleep more easily, and achieve a deeper, more restful night's sleep. Enjoy this beverage about an hour before bedtime as part of your nightly routine to maximize its sleep-promoting benefits.

LINDEN FLOWER AND CHAMOMILE BEDTIME TEA.

Linden Flower and Chamomile Bedtime Tea is a soothing herbal blend designed to promote a restful night's sleep. This tea combines the relaxing effects of chamomile with the tranquil properties of linden flowers, creating a perfect beverage for unwinding before bed.

Ingredients:

- 1 teaspoon dried linden flowers
- 1 teaspoon dried chamomile flowers
- 1 cup hot water

Instructions:

- Combine 1 teaspoon of dried linden flowers with 1 teaspoon of dried chamomile flowers in a tea infuser or directly in a cup.

- Pour 1 cup of boiling water over the herbal mixture, ensuring the herbs are fully immersed.
- Allow the tea to steep for about 10 to 15 minutes. This duration allows the therapeutic properties of linden and chamomile to infuse into the water, creating a potent brew for relaxation.
- Remove the tea infuser or strain the tea to remove the loose herbs before drinking.
- Optional: You may add a natural sweetener like honey or a slice of lemon to enhance the tea's flavor.

What to Expect:

Drinking Linden Flower and Chamomile Bedtime Tea before bed can help calm the mind, ease anxiety, and facilitate a deep and restful sleep. Linden flowers are known for their mild sedative properties, which can help relieve tension and promote relaxation. Chamomile is widely regarded for its ability to improve sleep quality and reduce stress. Together, these herbs offer a gentle yet effective way to unwind at the end of the day, preparing your body and mind for a peaceful night's sleep. The tea has a pleasant, floral taste with subtle sweet and earthy notes, making it a delightful part of your nighttime routine. Enjoy this calming beverage to support your sleep and overall well-being.

LAVENDER AND MUGWORT DREAM PILLOW.

A Lavender and Mugwort Dream Pillow combines the relaxing aroma of lavender with the dream-enhancing properties of mugwort. This herbal pillow is designed to be placed near the head during sleep, providing a night of restful sleep and vivid dreams. The soothing scent of lavender promotes relaxation and stress relief, while mugwort is traditionally used for its ability to stimulate dreams and enhance dream recall.

Ingredients:

- ½ cup dried lavender flowers
- ½ cup dried mugwort
- A small, breathable fabric pillowcase or pouch

Instructions:

- In a bowl, mix together ½ cup of dried lavender flowers with ½ cup of dried mugwort until well combined.
- Fill a small, breathable fabric pillowcase or pouch with the lavender and mugwort blend. If using a pillowcase, sew it shut or use a drawstring closure to ensure the herbs stay inside.
- Place the dream pillow near your head or under your regular pillow when you go to sleep.

What to Expect:

Using a Lavender and Mugwort Dream Pillow can enhance the quality of your sleep and the vividness of your dreams. The lavender provides a calming and soothing effect, helping to reduce anxiety and promote deep sleep. Mugwort, on the other hand, is known for its ability to encourage vivid and memorable dreams, making it a popular herb among those who practice dream work or seek more lucid dreaming experiences. The combination of these two herbs in a dream pillow offers a natural way to support restful sleep and explore the rich tapestry of your dreams. Enjoy the gentle, aromatic benefits of this dream pillow as part of your nightly routine to encourage relaxation and dream exploration.

LAVENDER AND CATNIP SLEEP TEA.

Lavender and Catnip Sleep Tea is a calming herbal infusion crafted to promote restful sleep and relaxation. Lavender, known for its soothing aroma and stress-relieving properties, pairs beautifully with catnip, a herb celebrated for its mild sedative effects on humans. This blend is perfect for those seeking a natural way to unwind and encourage a deep, restorative sleep.

Ingredients:

- 1 teaspoon dried lavender flowers
- 1 teaspoon dried catnip leaves
- 1 cup hot water

Instructions:

- Combine 1 teaspoon of dried lavender flowers with 1 teaspoon of dried catnip leaves in a tea infuser or directly in a cup.
- Pour 1 cup of boiling water over the herbs, making sure they are fully immersed.
- Allow the mixture to steep for about 10 minutes, giving the water ample time to absorb the herbs' beneficial properties.
- Remove the tea infuser or strain the tea to remove the loose herbs before drinking.
- Optional: Enhance the tea's natural flavors with a touch of honey or a slice of lemon.

What to Expect:

Drinking Lavender and Catnip Sleep Tea before bedtime can significantly improve the quality of your sleep. The lavender contributes a calming effect that helps reduce stress and anxiety, making it easier to fall asleep. Catnip complements lavender by promoting relaxation and drowsiness, further aiding in the transition to sleep. This herbal tea has a delightful, floral taste with subtle minty notes from the catnip, creating a comforting bedtime ritual.

Enjoy this tea as part of your evening routine to support a night of peaceful, uninterrupted sleep.

Poppy Seed and Honey Sleep Elixir.

The Poppy Seed and Honey Sleep Elixir is a natural concoction designed to aid sleep and promote relaxation. Poppy seeds contain small amounts of opium alkaloids which, while not strong enough to induce significant psychoactive effects, can contribute to a sense of calm and well-being. When combined with the natural soothing properties of honey, this elixir becomes a gentle remedy for sleeplessness.

Ingredients:

- 1 tablespoon crushed poppy seeds
- 2 tablespoons honey

Instructions:

- Crush 1 tablespoon of poppy seeds using a mortar and pestle or a spice grinder, ensuring they are finely ground.
- Mix the crushed poppy seeds with 2 tablespoons of honey in a small bowl until well combined.
- Consume a small amount of the mixture, about 1 teaspoon, before bed.

What to Expect:

Consuming the Poppy Seed and Honey Sleep Elixir before bedtime can help soothe the mind and body, making it easier to fall asleep. The calming effects of poppy seeds, coupled with the natural sweetness and comforting properties of honey, work together to promote relaxation and support a restful night's sleep. This elixir is particularly beneficial for those who have difficulty winding down at the end of the day or experience mild insomnia. The taste is pleasantly sweet, with a nutty flavor from the poppy seeds. As with any natural remedy, it's important to use this elixir in moderation and consult with a healthcare provider if you have any concerns or are taking other medications, especially those that affect sleep or mood.

Cherry Juice and Magnolia Bark Sleep Aid.

The Cherry Juice and Magnolia Bark Sleep Aid is a natural beverage crafted to support healthy sleep patterns and promote relaxation. Combining the melatonin-rich properties of cherry juice, particularly tart cherry juice, with the sleep-enhancing effects of magnolia bark extract, this sleep aid is designed for those seeking a natural remedy to improve sleep quality and duration.

Ingredients:

- ½ cup tart cherry juice

- 1 teaspoon magnolia bark extract
- 1 cup water (optional, to dilute if desired)

Instructions:

- In a glass, mix ½ cup of tart cherry juice with 1 teaspoon of magnolia bark extract. Stir well to ensure the magnolia bark extract is fully integrated into the cherry juice.
- If the taste is too strong or if you prefer a lighter beverage, dilute the mixture with 1 cup of water. Adjust the amount of water according to your taste preference.
- Drink this mixture in the evening, about 1-2 hours before bedtime, to maximize its sleep-promoting benefits.

What to Expect:

Drinking the Cherry Juice and Magnolia Bark Sleep Aid in the evening can help regulate your sleep-wake cycle, thanks to the natural melatonin content in cherry juice. Melatonin is a hormone that plays a crucial role in signaling the body to prepare for sleep. Magnolia bark extract, on the other hand, has compounds that may reduce anxiety and improve the quality of sleep by acting on GABA receptors in the brain, which are involved in promoting relaxation. This combination makes for a powerful sleep aid that not only helps you fall asleep more easily but also contributes to a deeper and more restful night's sleep. Enjoy this simple, natural remedy to support your sleep health and overall well-being.

Passionflower and Hop Sleep Capsules.

Passionflower and Hop Sleep Capsules are a natural dietary supplement designed to improve sleep quality and promote relaxation. This blend combines the sedative properties of hops with the calming effects of passionflower, both of which have been traditionally used to support sleep and alleviate anxiety. Encapsulating these herbs provides a convenient and effective way to consume them, especially for those seeking a natural alternative to improve their sleep patterns.

Ingredients:

- Dried passionflower
- Dried hops
- Empty capsules (available at health food stores or online)

Instructions:

- In a grinder, blend equal parts of dried passionflower and dried hops until you achieve a fine powder. The ratio can be adjusted based on your specific needs or preferences.
- Once ground into a fine powder, carefully fill empty capsules with the mixture using a capsule machine or a small spoon. Follow the

instructions provided with your capsules or capsule machine for best results.
- Store the filled capsules in a cool, dry place until ready to use.

Dosage:
- Take one or two capsules approximately 30-60 minutes before bedtime, or as directed by a healthcare professional. It's important to start with a lower dose to assess your body's response before increasing the dosage if needed.

What to Expect:
Taking Passionflower and Hop Sleep Capsules before bedtime can help calm the mind, ease anxiety, and promote a restful night's sleep. Passionflower is known for its ability to increase GABA levels in the brain, a neurotransmitter that promotes relaxation. Hops contain compounds that have sedative effects, further supporting sleep. This combination can be particularly beneficial for individuals experiencing insomnia, restlessness, or those who have difficulty maintaining sleep throughout the night. As with any herbal supplement, it's wise to consult with a healthcare provider before beginning use, especially if you are pregnant, nursing, or taking other medications, to ensure safety and appropriateness for your health needs.

VALERIAN ROOT AND HOPS CAPSULES FOR INSOMNIA.

Valerian Root and Hops Capsules are a potent herbal remedy designed to aid sleep and combat insomnia. This combination utilizes the sedative properties of valerian root along with the calming effects of hops to create a natural supplement that promotes relaxation and improves sleep quality.

Ingredients:
- Dried valerian root, powdered
- Dried hops, powdered
- Empty capsules (suitable for dietary supplements)

Instructions:
- Blend equal parts of powdered valerian root and powdered hops until you achieve a uniform mixture. The exact ratio can be adjusted based on your preference or the advice of a healthcare professional.
- Using a capsule filling machine or a small spoon and a steady hand, carefully fill the empty capsules with the valerian and hops mixture. Ensure each capsule is filled consistently for even dosages.
- Seal the capsules if necessary, depending on the type of empty capsules used.
- Store the filled capsules in a cool, dry place, away from direct sunlight.

Dosage:

- Take one or two capsules about 30-60 minutes before bedtime, or as recommended by a healthcare provider. It's important to start with the lower dosage to see how your body responds before adjusting.

What to Expect:
Valerian Root and Hops Capsules can significantly improve sleep onset and quality for those struggling with insomnia or sleep disturbances. Valerian root works by increasing GABA levels in the brain, which helps reduce anxiety and promote relaxation. Hops complement valerian by providing mild sedative effects, making it easier to fall asleep and stay asleep throughout the night. Together, they offer a powerful, natural approach to improving sleep without the hangover effect often associated with over-the-counter sleep aids. As with any supplement, it's advisable to consult with a healthcare provider before starting, especially if you are pregnant, nursing, or have any medical conditions, to ensure this remedy is suitable for your specific health needs.

CHAMOMILE AND PASSIONFLOWER TEA FOR RESTFUL SLEEP.

Chamomile and Passionflower Tea is a calming herbal infusion aimed at promoting restful sleep. This blend leverages the soothing properties of chamomile, known for its ability to relax the body and mind, with the sedative qualities of passionflower, a herb often used to treat insomnia and anxiety. Together, they create a potent natural remedy for improving sleep quality.

Ingredients:
- 1 teaspoon dried chamomile flowers
- 1 teaspoon dried passionflower
- 1 cup hot water

Instructions:
- Combine 1 teaspoon of dried chamomile flowers with 1 teaspoon of dried passionflower in a tea infuser or directly in a cup.
- Pour 1 cup of boiling water over the herbs, ensuring they are fully submerged.
- Allow the mixture to steep for about 10 minutes, giving the water ample time to absorb the beneficial properties of the herbs.
- Remove the tea infuser or strain the tea to remove the loose herbs before drinking.
- Optional: Add a natural sweetener like honey or a slice of lemon to enhance the flavor of the tea.

What to Expect:
Drinking Chamomile and Passionflower Tea before bedtime can significantly enhance the quality of your sleep. Chamomile's gentle calming effect helps

to soothe the nervous system, easing stress and preparing the body for sleep. Passionflower increases levels of GABA in the brain, a neurotransmitter that promotes relaxation. This combination not only aids in falling asleep more quickly but also contributes to a deeper and more uninterrupted sleep cycle. The tea has a floral, slightly sweet taste that is both comforting and enjoyable. Incorporate this tea into your nightly routine to naturally support restful sleep and wake up feeling refreshed.

Lemon Balm and Rose Petal Calming Tea.

Lemon Balm and Rose Petal Calming Tea is a delicate and aromatic herbal infusion designed to calm the mind, soothe the spirit, and provide a moment of peaceful relaxation. Lemon balm, with its mild sedative properties, pairs beautifully with the gentle floral notes of rose petals, creating a cup of tea that not only delights the senses but also promotes a sense of well-being and tranquility.

Ingredients:

- 1 tablespoon dried lemon balm leaves
- 1 tablespoon dried rose petals
- 1 cup hot water

Instructions:

- Combine 1 tablespoon of dried lemon balm leaves with 1 tablespoon of dried rose petals in a tea infuser or directly in a cup.
- Pour 1 cup of boiling water over the herbal blend, covering the leaves and petals completely.
- Allow the tea to infuse for 5 to 10 minutes, depending on your preference for strength. The longer it steeps, the more pronounced the flavors and therapeutic properties will become.
- If you've used a tea infuser, remove it from the cup. If the herbs were added directly, strain the tea into another cup to remove the leaves and petals.
- Optionally, you can sweeten the tea with a teaspoon of honey or enjoy it as is to fully appreciate the natural flavors.

What to Expect:

Drinking Lemon Balm and Rose Petal Calming Tea can help reduce stress and anxiety, promote relaxation, and support a good night's sleep. The soothing properties of lemon balm, combined with the comforting essence of rose petals, make this tea a perfect choice for unwinding after a long day or whenever you need a peaceful moment to yourself. This tea is not just a beverage but a gentle remedy that nurtures both body and soul, inviting calm and serenity into your daily routine.

CHAPTER 3: DIGESTIVE AND DETOXIFICATION SYSTEMS.

DIGESTIVE HEALTH REMEDIES.

ALOE VERA JUICE FOR DIGESTIVE HEALTH.

Aloe Vera Juice is a soothing and nourishing drink known for its ability to support digestive health. Extracted from the aloe vera plant, this juice contains enzymes, vitamins, minerals, and anti-inflammatory compounds that help soothe the digestive tract, promote gut healing, and enhance nutrient absorption.

Ingredients:

- Pure aloe vera juice (readily available in health food stores or online)

Instructions:

- Purchase pure, food-grade aloe vera juice, ensuring it is suitable for internal use. Check the product label for any additional ingredients and recommended dosages.
- Follow the recommended dosage on the product label, which is typically about 2 to 8 ounces per day. You can consume the aloe vera juice directly or dilute it with water or another juice to improve the taste.
- For best results, drink aloe vera juice on an empty stomach in the morning to maximize its digestive health benefits.

What to Expect:

Regular consumption of Aloe Vera Juice can offer various benefits for digestive health, including soothing irritation and inflammation in the gut, aiding in the healing of the intestinal lining, and promoting regular bowel movements. It may also help in reducing symptoms of digestive disorders such as irritable bowel syndrome (IBS) and acid reflux. Additionally, aloe vera juice can support overall hydration and provide a gentle detoxification effect on the body. As with any supplement, it's important to start with a small dose to assess your body's response and consult with a healthcare provider if you have any medical conditions or concerns.

DANDELION ROOT DETOX TEA.

Dandelion Root Detox Tea is known for its detoxifying properties, targeting liver health by cleansing and rejuvenating this vital organ. It's rich in antioxidants and compounds that support digestion and liver function.

Ingredients:

- 1 tablespoon dried dandelion root

- 2 cups water

Instructions:

- Boil 2 cups of water and add 1 tablespoon of dried dandelion root. Reduce heat and simmer for 15 minutes.
- Strain the tea into a cup. Optionally, add lemon or honey for flavor.

What to Expect:

This tea supports liver detoxification, promoting toxin elimination and digestive health. It may lead to increased energy and reduced digestive discomfort. Enjoy as part of a balanced diet for optimal benefits.

Licorice Root Tea for Digestive Health.

Licorice Root Tea is celebrated for its soothing effects on gastrointestinal health, aiding in the relief of digestive issues through its anti-inflammatory and soothing properties.

Ingredients:

- 1 tablespoon dried licorice root
- 1 cup hot water

Instructions:

- Place 1 tablespoon of dried licorice root in a cup.
- Pour 1 cup of hot water over the licorice root and let it steep for 10 minutes.
- Strain the tea into another cup to remove the licorice root.

What to Expect:

Drinking Licorice Root Tea may ease digestive discomfort, such as heartburn and indigestion, by promoting a healthy gastrointestinal tract. Its sweet, natural flavor makes it a pleasant, therapeutic drink. Enjoy regularly to support digestive health.

Lemon Balm and Mint Digestive Tea.

Lemon Balm and Mint Digestive Tea is a soothing and flavorful herbal beverage that combines the calming properties of lemon balm with the refreshing and digestive aid of mint. This tea is perfect for relieving digestive discomfort while also promoting relaxation and a sense of well-being.

Ingredients:

- 1 tablespoon dried lemon balm leaves
- 1 tablespoon dried mint leaves
- 1 cup hot water

Instructions:

- Mix 1 tablespoon each of dried lemon balm leaves and dried mint leaves in a tea infuser or directly in a cup.

- Pour 1 cup of boiling water over the herbs, allowing them to steep for about 5 to 10 minutes, depending on your preference for strength.
- If you've used a tea infuser, remove it from the cup. If the herbs were added directly, strain the tea to remove them before drinking.

What to Expect:
Drinking Lemon Balm and Mint Digestive Tea can help ease digestive issues such as bloating, gas, and indigestion due to the soothing properties of both herbs. Lemon balm is known for its ability to reduce anxiety and promote a sense of calm, while mint helps to relax the muscles of the digestive tract, further aiding in the relief of discomfort. This tea is ideal for enjoying after meals or anytime you need a moment of calm and relief from digestive distress.

PEPPERMINT TEA FOR INDIGESTION.

Peppermint Tea is a refreshing and therapeutic drink, widely acclaimed for its ability to ease indigestion and soothe gastrointestinal discomfort. The active ingredient in peppermint, menthol, has antispasmodic properties that relax the muscles of the digestive tract, making it an excellent natural remedy for bloating, gas, and other digestive issues.
Ingredients:

- 1 teaspoon dried peppermint leaves
- 1 cup boiling water

Instructions:

- Boil 1 cup of water and then remove it from heat.
- Place 1 teaspoon of dried peppermint leaves in a tea infuser or directly into the cup.
- Pour the boiling water over the peppermint leaves, ensuring they are fully submerged.
- Allow the tea to steep for about 10 minutes. This steeping time allows the peppermint to release its essential oils and active compounds.
- After steeping, remove the tea infuser or strain the tea to remove the leaves.
- Optional: You can add a natural sweetener like honey if desired, but many find the natural flavor of peppermint tea to be pleasantly sweet and refreshing on its own.

What to Expect:
Drinking Peppermint Tea after meals can provide quick relief from indigestion symptoms. You may experience a cooling sensation and overall soothing effect in your stomach and intestines, which helps to alleviate discomfort associated with indigestion, including bloating and gas.

Peppermint tea is also beneficial for easing nausea and improving overall digestion. Enjoy this tea as needed, particularly after large meals or when experiencing digestive discomfort, to harness its digestive health benefits. However, individuals with GERD (gastroesophageal reflux disease) or certain other conditions may find that peppermint exacerbates their symptoms, so it's wise to consult with a healthcare provider if you have ongoing digestive health issues.

SENNA LEAF AND FENNEL SEED LAXATIVE BLEND.

The Senna Leaf and Fennel Seed Laxative Blend combines the potent natural laxative properties of senna leaves with the digestive benefits of fennel seeds. This herbal tea is designed to relieve occasional constipation and promote digestive health, offering a gentle yet effective solution.
Ingredients:

- 1 teaspoon dried senna leaves
- 1 teaspoon fennel seeds
- 1 cup hot water

Instructions:

- Mix 1 teaspoon of dried senna leaves with 1 teaspoon of fennel seeds in a tea infuser or directly in a cup.
- Pour 1 cup of boiling water over the senna and fennel blend, allowing it to steep for 5 to 10 minutes. The steeping time should be adjusted according to personal tolerance and the desired strength, as senna is a powerful laxative.
- If you've used a tea infuser, remove it from the cup. If the leaves and seeds were added directly, strain the tea into another cup to remove them.

What to Expect:
Senna works by stimulating the muscles of the colon to promote bowel movements, while fennel seeds can help reduce gas and bloating associated with constipation. This blend should be consumed preferably before bedtime, allowing it to work overnight. Effects typically occur within 6 to 12 hours after consumption. It's important to stay hydrated and use this tea only as needed for occasional constipation relief, not as a long-term solution.

SENNA LEAF AND ANISE SEED GENTLE LAXATIVE TEA.

Senna Leaf and Anise Seed Gentle Laxative Tea is a natural remedy designed to relieve occasional constipation and promote digestive health. The senna leaf acts as a powerful laxative, stimulating bowel movements, while anise seeds offer a soothing effect on the digestive tract, reducing gas and bloating.
Ingredients:

- 1 teaspoon dried senna leaves
- 1 teaspoon anise seeds
- 1 cup hot water

Instructions:

- Mix 1 teaspoon of dried senna leaves with 1 teaspoon of anise seeds in a tea infuser or directly in a cup.
- Pour 1 cup of boiling water over the senna and anise, allowing them to steep for about 5 to 10 minutes. Adjust the steeping time based on personal sensitivity and the desired effect, as senna is very potent.
- If using a tea infuser, remove it from the cup. If the herbs were added directly, strain the tea to remove them before drinking.

What to Expect:

This tea should be consumed occasionally and responsibly due to the potent effects of senna, which typically induce a bowel movement within 6 to 12 hours after consumption. Anise seeds not only add a sweet, licorice-like flavor to the tea but also help to mitigate any potential cramping that may occur due to senna's action. This combination offers a gentle yet effective solution for those experiencing temporary constipation, promoting a smoother digestive process.

Cinnamon Infusion for Blood Sugar Control.

Cinnamon Infusion is a natural remedy known for its ability to help regulate blood sugar levels, thanks to the active compounds in cinnamon that mimic insulin and improve insulin sensitivity.

Ingredients:

- 2 cinnamon sticks
- 1 cup hot water

Instructions:

- Place 2 cinnamon sticks in a cup.
- Pour 1 cup of hot water over the cinnamon sticks and let them steep for 10 minutes.
- Remove the cinnamon sticks before drinking.

What to Expect:

Consuming Cinnamon Infusion can aid in managing blood sugar levels, making it beneficial for those monitoring their glucose levels or those with insulin resistance. Its warming, sweet flavor also makes it an enjoyable drink, suitable for daily consumption as part of a balanced diet.

CINNAMON AND HONEY MIX FOR BLOOD SUGAR CONTROL.

The Cinnamon and Honey Mix combines the blood sugar-regulating properties of cinnamon with the natural sweetness of honey, offering a tasty way to help manage blood sugar levels.

Ingredients:

- 1 teaspoon cinnamon powder
- 2 teaspoons honey

Instructions:

- In a small bowl, mix 1 teaspoon of cinnamon powder with 2 teaspoons of honey until they form a consistent blend.
- Consume this mixture regularly, about half a teaspoon to one teaspoon daily, either directly or by adding it to warm water, tea, or spread over toast.

What to Expect:

Regular intake of the Cinnamon and Honey Mix can aid in the regulation of blood sugar levels, thanks to the natural compounds in cinnamon that improve insulin sensitivity. Honey provides a healthier sweetening option that, in moderation, can contribute to a balanced diet, especially for those monitoring their blood sugar.

GINGER ROOT DECOCTION FOR NAUSEA.

Ginger Root Decoction is a potent natural remedy known for its effectiveness in alleviating nausea. Ginger, with its powerful bioactive compounds such as gingerol, acts as an anti-emetic, helping to soothe the stomach and reduce feelings of nausea. This simple yet effective decoction can be particularly beneficial for motion sickness, morning sickness, or nausea resulting from medical treatments.

Ingredients:

- A 2-inch piece of fresh ginger root
- 2 cups of water

Instructions:

- Thoroughly wash the fresh ginger root and slice it into thin pieces to maximize the surface area exposed to the water.
- In a small pot, combine the sliced ginger with 2 cups of water.
- Bring the water to a simmer over medium heat, then reduce the heat to maintain a gentle simmer.
- Allow the ginger to simmer for about 15 minutes. This slow cooking process helps to extract the beneficial compounds from the ginger into the water.
- After simmering, strain the decoction to remove the ginger slices, leaving a clear liquid.

- Sip the ginger decoction slowly to alleviate nausea. It can be consumed warm or cooled, depending on your preference.

What to Expect:
Drinking Ginger Root Decoction can provide rapid relief from nausea thanks to ginger's natural anti-emetic properties. You may feel a warming sensation in your stomach, followed by a gradual reduction in nausea. The decoction can be especially comforting and effective when consumed at the first sign of stomach upset. Ginger is also known for its anti-inflammatory effects, which can contribute to overall digestive health. This remedy is safe for most people, including pregnant women dealing with morning sickness (though it's always wise to consult with a healthcare provider if you're pregnant). Enjoy this natural, soothing treatment as needed to combat nausea and promote a sense of well-being.

FENNEL SEED INFUSION FOR BLOATING.

Fennel Seed Infusion is a natural and effective remedy known for its ability to relieve bloating, gas, and digestive discomfort. Fennel seeds contain compounds that relax the muscles in the gastrointestinal tract, helping to release trapped gas and reduce bloating. This herbal infusion can be a soothing option for those experiencing digestive issues.

Ingredients:

- 1 tablespoon fennel seeds
- 1 cup boiling water

Instructions:

- Crush 1 tablespoon of fennel seeds using a mortar and pestle or the back of a spoon to release their volatile oils and enhance their digestive benefits.
- Place the crushed fennel seeds in a tea infuser or directly in a cup.
- Pour 1 cup of boiling water over the crushed fennel seeds.
- Allow the mixture to steep for about 10 minutes. This steeping time lets the fennel seeds release their active compounds into the water.
- If you used a tea infuser, remove it from the cup. If the seeds were added directly, strain the infusion to remove the seeds before drinking.
- Drink the fennel seed infusion warm for the best results in relieving bloating and gas.

What to Expect:
Drinking a warm cup of Fennel Seed Infusion can offer quick relief from bloating and gas. You may notice a reduction in digestive discomfort shortly after consuming the infusion. Fennel seeds have a mild, licorice-like flavor that makes this remedy not only effective but also enjoyable to drink. This

herbal infusion can be consumed after meals or anytime you are experiencing bloating and digestive issues. It's a gentle, natural way to support digestive health and comfort.

CHAMOMILE TEA FOR DIGESTIVE COMFORT.

Chamomile Tea is a timeless herbal remedy renowned for its gentle, soothing properties, particularly in aiding digestive comfort. Made from the dried flowers of the chamomile plant, this tea is a natural way to ease digestive discomfort, including bloating, cramping, and gas, while promoting overall relaxation.

Ingredients:

- 1-2 teaspoons dried chamomile flowers
- 1 cup hot water

Instructions:

- Place 1-2 teaspoons of dried chamomile flowers in a tea infuser or directly in a cup.
- Pour 1 cup of boiling water over the chamomile flowers, ensuring they are fully submerged.
- Allow the chamomile to steep for about 10 minutes, which allows ample time for the water to extract the soothing compounds from the chamomile flowers.
- Remove the tea infuser or strain the tea to remove the loose flowers before drinking.
- Optional: You can add a natural sweetener like honey or a slice of lemon to enhance the flavor of the tea.

What to Expect:

Drinking Chamomile Tea can provide immediate relief from digestive discomfort. Chamomile's natural anti-inflammatory and antispasmodic properties help to relax the muscles of the digestive tract, easing cramps, bloating, and gas. Additionally, chamomile tea can help reduce stress and anxiety, which are often contributing factors to digestive issues. Its mild, floral flavor and aroma contribute to its calming effect, making it a perfect beverage for winding down in the evening or anytime you need to soothe digestive discomfort. Incorporate Chamomile Tea into your routine as a natural and effective solution for promoting digestive health and overall well-being.

SLIPPERY ELM BARK GRUEL FOR GASTRIC ULCERS.

Slippery Elm Bark Gruel is a traditional remedy known for its soothing properties, particularly effective in treating and providing relief for gastric ulcers. Slippery elm bark contains mucilage, a gel-like substance that coats and protects the mucous membranes of the gastrointestinal tract, helping to heal ulcers and reduce inflammation.

Ingredients:

- 1-2 tablespoons slippery elm powder
- 1 cup water

Instructions:

- In a small saucepan, mix 1-2 tablespoons of slippery elm powder with 1 cup of water. The amount of slippery elm powder can be adjusted depending on the desired thickness of the gruel.
- Stir the mixture well to ensure the powder is fully dissolved in the water.
- Heat the mixture over low heat, stirring constantly, until it thickens into a gruel. This usually takes about 3-5 minutes.
- Once the gruel has reached the desired consistency, remove it from the heat and let it cool to a safe temperature for consumption.

What to Expect:

Consuming Slippery Elm Bark Gruel can provide immediate relief for the discomfort associated with gastric ulcers. The mucilage forms a protective layer over ulcers and inflamed areas in the stomach and intestines, promoting healing and preventing irritation from stomach acids. This remedy can also be beneficial for other digestive issues such as acid reflux, gastritis, and irritable bowel syndrome (IBS) due to its soothing and anti-inflammatory properties. Slippery elm gruel has a mild, slightly sweet taste and can be consumed 2-3 times daily or as needed for relief. It's important to consult with a healthcare provider before using slippery elm, especially if you have chronic digestive issues or are taking medication, to ensure it is appropriate for your specific health needs.

Slippery Elm and Marshmallow Root Tea for Gut Health.

Slippery Elm and Marshmallow Root Tea is a gentle, soothing tea blend designed to support gut health and promote digestive comfort. Both slippery elm bark and marshmallow root contain high amounts of mucilage, a gelatinous substance that coats and protects the lining of the digestive tract, easing inflammation, and providing relief from various digestive issues.

Ingredients:

- 1 teaspoon slippery elm bark powder
- 1 teaspoon marshmallow root (dried or powdered)
- 1 cup hot water

Instructions:

- Mix 1 teaspoon of slippery elm bark powder with 1 teaspoon of dried or powdered marshmallow root in a tea infuser or directly in a cup.

- Pour 1 cup of boiling water over the herbal mixture, ensuring the herbs are fully immersed.
- Allow the tea to steep for about 10 minutes. This steeping time allows the herbs to release their mucilage and other beneficial compounds into the water.
- Remove the tea infuser or strain the tea to remove the loose herbs before drinking.
- Optional: Add a natural sweetener like honey to enhance the flavor of the tea, if desired.

What to Expect:
Drinking Slippery Elm and Marshmallow Root Tea can offer significant relief for those experiencing digestive discomfort, including symptoms associated with conditions like irritable bowel syndrome (IBS), acid reflux, and gastritis. The mucilage from both slippery elm and marshmallow root forms a soothing film over the mucous membranes, which can help heal and prevent irritation in the digestive tract. Additionally, this tea can aid in reducing inflammation and soothing sore throats. Its natural, mild flavor makes it a pleasant remedy to consume. Enjoy this tea 2-3 times a day, especially before meals or at bedtime, to maximize its digestive health benefits. Always consult with a healthcare provider before incorporating new herbal remedies into your routine, especially if you have existing health conditions or are taking medications.

DANDELION AND BURDOCK ROOT TEA FOR LIVER DETOX.

Dandelion and Burdock Root Tea is a potent herbal blend designed to support liver detoxification and promote overall liver health. Both dandelion and burdock root are revered in herbal medicine for their cleansing properties and ability to stimulate liver function, making this tea an excellent choice for those looking to naturally enhance their body's detoxification processes.

Ingredients:

- 1 tablespoon dandelion root
- 1 tablespoon burdock root
- 4 cups of water

Instructions:

- Combine 1 tablespoon of dandelion root and 1 tablespoon of burdock root in a medium saucepan.
- Add 4 cups of water to the saucepan and bring the mixture to a boil.
- Once boiling, reduce the heat and allow the mixture to simmer for about 15 minutes. This simmering process helps to extract the beneficial compounds from the roots, infusing the water with their detoxifying properties.

- After simmering, strain the tea to remove the roots, pouring the liquid into a teapot or directly into cups.
- Optional: Adjust the flavor to your liking with natural sweeteners such as honey or lemon, though many prefer to drink the tea unsweetened to maximize its detoxifying benefits.

What to Expect:
Drinking Dandelion and Burdock Root Tea can help stimulate liver function and enhance the body's natural detoxification pathways. Dandelion root acts as a diuretic, supporting the elimination of toxins through increased urine production, while burdock root is known for its blood-purifying properties. Together, these herbs can improve digestion, reduce inflammation, and support overall liver health. This tea is best enjoyed regularly as part of a healthy diet and lifestyle to maximize its detoxifying effects. As with any detox regimen, it's wise to consult with a healthcare provider, especially if you have existing health conditions or are taking medications, to ensure that this herbal tea is suitable for you.

PEPPERMINT AND CARAWAY SEED DIGESTIVE BLEND.

The Peppermint and Caraway Seed Digestive Blend is a natural herbal tea designed to aid digestion and relieve digestive discomforts such as bloating, gas, and indigestion. Peppermint is renowned for its soothing effect on the gastrointestinal tract, while caraway seeds have been used traditionally to treat digestive issues and improve gut health.
Ingredients:

- 1 teaspoon dried peppermint leaves
- 1 teaspoon caraway seeds
- 1 cup hot water

Instructions:

- Mix 1 teaspoon of dried peppermint leaves with 1 teaspoon of caraway seeds in a tea infuser or directly in a cup.
- Pour 1 cup of boiling water over the peppermint and caraway blend, making sure the ingredients are fully submerged.
- Allow the mixture to steep for about 10 minutes. This duration allows the water to extract the active compounds from the peppermint and caraway, creating a potent digestive aid.
- Remove the tea infuser or strain the tea to remove the seeds and leaves before drinking.
- Optional: You may add a natural sweetener like honey to enhance the flavor of the tea, although it's typically enjoyed without sweeteners to maximize its digestive benefits.

What to Expect:

Drinking the Peppermint and Caraway Seed Digestive Blend after meals can significantly aid in digestion and provide relief from common digestive discomforts. Peppermint's natural antispasmodic properties help relax the muscles of the digestive tract, reducing cramps and bloating. Caraway seeds, on the other hand, can help alleviate gas and indigestion, promoting overall digestive health. This blend offers a refreshing and slightly spicy flavor, making it a delightful way to end a meal and support your digestive system. Enjoy this tea regularly to harness its full digestive health benefits.

MILK THISTLE SEED TEA FOR LIVER SUPPORT.

Milk Thistle Seed Tea is a herbal tea known for its liver-supporting properties. Made from the seeds of the milk thistle plant, which contain silymarin, a group of compounds said to have antioxidant and anti-inflammatory effects that protect the liver. This tea is beneficial for those looking to support liver function, detoxify the liver, and aid in the liver's recovery from damage caused by toxins, alcohol, or diseases.

Ingredients:

- 1 tablespoon crushed milk thistle seeds
- 1 cup boiling water

Instructions:

- Crush 1 tablespoon of milk thistle seeds using a mortar and pestle or a spice grinder to release their active compounds.
- Place the crushed seeds in a tea infuser or directly in a cup.
- Pour 1 cup of boiling water over the crushed seeds, ensuring they are fully immersed.
- Allow the tea to steep for about 10-15 minutes, allowing the silymarin and other beneficial compounds to infuse into the water.
- If you used a tea infuser, remove it from the cup. If the seeds were added directly, strain the tea to remove the seeds before drinking.
- Optional: You can add honey or lemon to taste, but many prefer it plain to fully enjoy the benefits.

What to Expect:

Drinking Milk Thistle Seed Tea can support liver health by promoting the regeneration of liver cells and protecting the liver from toxins. Silymarin, the active compound in milk thistle, acts as an antioxidant that reduces free radical production and oxidative stress, which are linked to liver disease. This tea may be particularly beneficial for those who have liver conditions, are recovering from liver damage, or wish to support their liver health due to lifestyle factors. Milk thistle tea has a slightly bitter, earthy taste, which is typical of liver-supportive herbs. Incorporate this tea into your daily routine to harness its liver-protective benefits. As with any herbal remedy, consulting with a healthcare provider is advisable, especially if you have a liver condition or are taking medication, to ensure it is appropriate for your health needs.

GINGER AND LEMON BALM TEA FOR NAUSEA.

Ginger and Lemon Balm Tea is a comforting herbal infusion designed to alleviate nausea and promote digestive health. Ginger, with its potent anti-nausea properties, pairs excellently with the calming effects of lemon balm, making this tea an effective natural remedy for soothing stomach upset, motion sickness, and nausea of various origins.

Ingredients:

- 1 inch fresh ginger root, thinly sliced or grated
- 1 teaspoon dried lemon balm leaves
- 1 cup boiling water

Instructions:

- Prepare the fresh ginger by thinly slicing or grating a 1-inch piece. This process helps to release the ginger's active compounds.
- In a tea infuser or directly in a cup, combine the prepared ginger with 1 teaspoon of dried lemon balm leaves.
- Pour 1 cup of boiling water over the ginger and lemon balm mixture, ensuring the ingredients are fully submerged.
- Allow the tea to steep for about 10 minutes. Steeping time can be adjusted based on your preference for strength and flavor intensity.
- Remove the tea infuser or strain the tea to remove the ginger pieces and lemon balm leaves before drinking.
- Optional: Enhance the flavor of the tea with a squeeze of lemon juice or a teaspoon of honey, which can also provide additional soothing benefits.

What to Expect:

Sipping Ginger and Lemon Balm Tea can provide quick relief from nausea and promote a sense of digestive well-being. The active compounds in ginger, such as gingerol, have been shown to effectively reduce nausea and prevent vomiting. Lemon balm complements ginger by promoting relaxation and reducing stress, which can further alleviate stomach discomfort. This tea has a warming, slightly spicy flavor from the ginger, balanced by the subtle, citrusy notes of lemon balm, making it both therapeutic and enjoyable to drink. Enjoy this tea as needed, especially before or after meals, during travel, or whenever nausea arises, to harness its anti-nausea and digestive soothing benefits.

ARTICHOKE LEAF TEA FOR LIVER HEALTH.

Artichoke Leaf Tea is a healthful infusion known for its beneficial effects on liver function and bile production. Made from the leaves of the artichoke plant, this tea contains cynarin and silymarin, compounds that have antioxidant and liver-protective properties. Drinking artichoke leaf tea is an excellent way to support digestive health, improve bile flow, and enhance the liver's detoxification processes.

Ingredients:

- 1-2 teaspoons dried artichoke leaves
- 1 cup boiling water

Instructions:

- Place 1-2 teaspoons of dried artichoke leaves in a tea infuser or directly in a cup.
- Pour 1 cup of boiling water over the artichoke leaves, making sure they are fully submerged.
- Allow the tea to steep for about 10-15 minutes, which allows ample time for the active compounds to be released into the water.
- Remove the tea infuser or strain the tea to remove the loose leaves before drinking.
- Optional: If you find the taste to be slightly bitter, you can add a natural sweetener like honey or a slice of lemon to enhance the flavor.

What to Expect:

Drinking Artichoke Leaf Tea can provide several benefits for liver health and digestion. The cynarin in artichoke leaves helps to stimulate bile production, which is essential for digesting fats and the detoxification of the liver. Silymarin acts as an antioxidant, protecting liver cells from damage and supporting liver regeneration. Regular consumption of this tea may also help lower blood lipid levels, contributing to cardiovascular health. The tea has a slightly bitter, earthy taste, characteristic of many liver-supportive herbs. Incorporating Artichoke Leaf Tea into your daily routine can be a simple and natural way to support your liver's health and overall well-being.

YELLOW DOCK ROOT TEA FOR DIGESTIVE SUPPORT.

Yellow Dock Root Tea is a traditional herbal remedy known for its ability to aid digestion and support liver function. Made from the root of the yellow dock plant, this tea contains compounds that act as mild laxatives and detoxifiers, making it beneficial for improving bowel movements and cleansing the liver.

Ingredients:

- 1 teaspoon dried yellow dock root
- 1 cup water

Instructions:

- In a small saucepan, combine 1 teaspoon of dried yellow dock root with 1 cup of water.
- Bring the mixture to a boil, then reduce the heat and allow it to simmer for about 15 minutes. Simmering helps to extract the beneficial compounds from the yellow dock root into the water.
- After simmering, strain the tea to remove the root pieces, leaving a clear liquid.
- The tea can be consumed warm or allowed to cool down to a comfortable temperature before drinking.

What to Expect:
Drinking Yellow Dock Root Tea can provide significant digestive support. It may help relieve constipation by stimulating bowel movements and enhancing liver function by promoting the elimination of toxins from the body. Yellow dock root is also known for its ability to increase bile production, which further aids in digestion and nutrient absorption. However, due to its laxative effect, it's important to start with a small amount to see how your body responds. Regular consumption should be approached with caution, and it's wise to consult with a healthcare provider before incorporating yellow dock root tea into your regimen, especially if you have a history of kidney stones or if you're pregnant or nursing, as the oxalates in yellow dock can contribute to kidney stone formation in susceptible individuals. Enjoy this tea as part of a holistic approach to digestive health and detoxification.

Barberry Bark Decoction for Gallbladder Health.

Barberry Bark Decoction is a potent herbal remedy known for its positive effects on gallbladder and liver health. Derived from the bark of the barberry plant, this decoction contains berberine, a compound with antimicrobial, anti-inflammatory, and bile-stimulating properties. It is especially beneficial for stimulating bile flow and supporting the liver's detoxifying functions, making it an effective natural treatment for gallbladder issues.
Ingredients:

- 1-2 teaspoons dried barberry bark
- 1 cup water

Instructions:

- Place 1-2 teaspoons of dried barberry bark into a small saucepan.
- Add 1 cup of water to the saucepan and bring the mixture to a boil.
- Once boiling, reduce the heat to a simmer and cover the saucepan. Allow the barberry bark to simmer for about 15-20 minutes. This

process will extract the berberine and other beneficial compounds from the bark into the water.
- After simmering, remove the saucepan from the heat and strain the decoction to remove the pieces of bark, leaving a clear liquid.
- The decoction can be consumed warm, or you can let it cool to a comfortable drinking temperature.

What to Expect:
Drinking Barberry Bark Decoction can offer support for gallbladder and liver health by promoting the flow of bile, which is crucial for digestion and the elimination of toxins from the body. The berberine in barberry has been shown to help in the treatment of gallstones, liver diseases, and other digestive disorders. Additionally, its antimicrobial and anti-inflammatory properties can contribute to overall health and wellness. It is important to note that barberry bark is potent, and its use should be approached with caution. Always start with a small dose to assess your body's reaction, and consult with a healthcare provider before using barberry, especially if you are pregnant, nursing, or have health conditions related to blood pressure or blood sugar. Regular use of this decoction should be part of a balanced approach to digestive and gallbladder health.

PEPPERMINT AND LICORICE TEA FOR INDIGESTION.

Peppermint and Licorice Tea is a soothing herbal blend designed to ease indigestion and soothe stomach discomfort. Peppermint leaves offer natural antispasmodic properties that relax the digestive tract muscles, while licorice root supports the health of the stomach lining and may ease the symptoms of acid reflux and heartburn. This tea combines the refreshing flavor of peppermint with the sweet, comforting taste of licorice, making it a pleasant remedy for digestive woes.

Ingredients:
- 1 teaspoon dried peppermint leaves
- 1 teaspoon chopped licorice root
- 1 cup boiling water

Instructions:
- Combine 1 teaspoon of dried peppermint leaves with 1 teaspoon of chopped licorice root in a tea infuser or directly in a cup.
- Pour 1 cup of boiling water over the peppermint and licorice mixture, ensuring the ingredients are fully immersed.
- Allow the tea to steep for about 10 minutes. This duration allows the water to extract the beneficial compounds from the herbs effectively.
- Remove the tea infuser or strain the tea to remove the loose herbs before drinking.

- Optional: Adjust the flavor according to your preference. You can add a natural sweetener like honey, although the licorice root naturally imparts a sweet taste to the tea.

What to Expect:

Drinking Peppermint and Licorice Tea can provide quick relief from indigestion and stomach discomfort. The peppermint in the tea helps to relieve symptoms like bloating, gas, and cramps by relaxing the digestive system muscles. Licorice root has soothing properties that protect the stomach lining and may help reduce the discomfort associated with acid reflux. This tea is best consumed after meals or at the first sign of digestive upset. However, individuals with high blood pressure should consume licorice root sparingly, as it can affect blood pressure levels when consumed in large quantities over an extended period. Enjoy this comforting and effective herbal tea to support your digestive health.

Triphala Powder for Digestive Regularity.

Triphala Powder is a traditional Ayurvedic blend made from the dried fruits of three plants: Amalaki (Emblica officinalis), Bibhitaki (Terminalia bellirica), and Haritaki (Terminalia chebula). This potent combination is revered for its ability to promote digestive regularity, support detoxification, and rejuvenate the entire digestive system. Triphala is known for its gentle laxative effect, antioxidant properties, and balancing effect on the three doshas (body energies): Vata, Pitta, and Kapha.

Ingredients:

- ½ to 1 teaspoon Triphala powder
- 1 cup warm water

Instructions:

- Add ½ to 1 teaspoon of Triphala powder to 1 cup of warm water. The amount of Triphala can be adjusted based on your individual tolerance and needs.
- Stir the mixture well until the Triphala powder is completely dissolved in the water.
- Drink this mixture before bed, allowing its cleansing and balancing effects to work overnight.
- For best results, consume Triphala on an empty stomach, either a few hours after dinner or right before bedtime.

What to Expect:

Regular consumption of Triphala Powder mixed in warm water can lead to improved digestive regularity and a gentle detoxifying effect on the body. It may help alleviate constipation, reduce bloating, and promote a healthy and balanced digestive tract. Triphala's antioxidant components also contribute to overall health by combating oxidative stress and supporting immune function. As a rejuvenative, Triphala can aid in nourishing the body and promoting vitality. The taste of Triphala is somewhat bitter and astringent, which can be unusual at first but is often considered refreshing once accustomed to it. If you are new to Triphala, start with a smaller dose to assess your body's response, as its potency can vary among individuals. Always consult with a healthcare provider or an Ayurvedic practitioner before adding new herbal supplements to your routine, especially if you have existing health conditions or are taking medications.

ANGELICA AND PEPPERMINT DIGESTIVE TONIC.

Angelica and Peppermint Digestive Tonic is a herbal blend designed to aid digestion and soothe stomach discomfort. Angelica root, known for its carminative and digestive properties, works in harmony with the soothing and antispasmodic effects of peppermint leaves. This tonic is ideal for relieving symptoms of indigestion, bloating, and gas, promoting a healthy digestive process.

Ingredients:

- 1 teaspoon dried angelica root
- 1 teaspoon dried peppermint leaves
- 1 cup boiling water

Instructions:

- Combine 1 teaspoon of dried angelica root with 1 teaspoon of dried peppermint leaves in a tea infuser or directly in a cup.
- Pour 1 cup of boiling water over the herbal mixture, ensuring that the herbs are fully submerged.
- Cover and allow the mixture to steep for about 10 minutes. Covering the cup helps to retain the essential oils and active compounds within the water.
- After steeping, remove the tea infuser or strain the tea to remove the loose herbs.
- Optional: If desired, you can sweeten the tonic with honey or add a slice of lemon for additional flavor.

What to Expect:

Drinking the Angelica and Peppermint Digestive Tonic can offer immediate relief from digestive discomfort. Angelica root enhances digestive health by stimulating bile production and improving gut motility, while peppermint leaves soothe the stomach lining and reduce muscle spasms in the gastrointestinal tract. This combination not only helps to alleviate symptoms like bloating and gas but also promotes a more efficient digestion process. The tonic has a refreshing and slightly spicy flavor, making it a pleasant remedy to enjoy after meals or whenever digestive issues arise. Regular consumption can contribute to overall digestive wellness and comfort. However, it's important to note that angelica root may interact with certain medications and conditions, so consulting with a healthcare provider before incorporating it into your routine is advisable.

FENNEL AND GINGER DIGESTIVE AID.

Fennel and Ginger Digestive Aid is a warming herbal tea that combines the carminative properties of fennel seeds with the soothing effects of fresh ginger. This blend is perfect for alleviating digestive discomfort, reducing bloating, and promoting overall digestive health. Both fennel and ginger are renowned for their ability to ease gas, support digestion, and soothe the stomach.

Ingredients:

- 1 teaspoon fennel seeds
- 1-inch piece of fresh ginger, thinly sliced
- 1 cup boiling water

Instructions:

- Crush 1 teaspoon of fennel seeds lightly to release their essential oils. Slice a 1-inch piece of fresh ginger into thin slices.
- Place the crushed fennel seeds and ginger slices in a tea infuser or directly into a cup.
- Pour 1 cup of boiling water over the fennel and ginger. Ensure the ingredients are fully submerged in the water.
- Cover and allow the mixture to steep for about 10 minutes. Covering the cup during steeping helps to preserve the volatile oils and active compounds in the tea.
- Remove the tea infuser or strain the tea to remove the fennel seeds and ginger slices before drinking.
- Optional: You may add a teaspoon of honey or a slice of lemon to the tea for added flavor.

What to Expect:

Drinking Fennel and Ginger Digestive Aid can provide soothing relief from various digestive issues, including bloating, gas, and indigestion. Fennel seeds are known for their ability to relax the muscles of the gastrointestinal tract, reducing cramping and gas, while ginger has anti-inflammatory properties that can soothe the stomach lining and aid in digestion. The combination of these two powerful digestive herbs results in a tea that not only helps to alleviate discomfort but also promotes a healthy and efficient digestive process. The tea has a refreshing and slightly spicy taste, making it an enjoyable remedy to consume after meals or whenever digestive discomfort arises. Enjoy this natural and gentle digestive aid to support your digestive health.

Meadowsweet Infusion for Acid Reflux.

Meadowsweet Infusion is a gentle, herbal remedy known for its ability to soothe acid reflux and protect the digestive lining. Meadowsweet, with its natural anti-inflammatory and antacid properties, offers a soothing effect on the stomach and esophagus, making it an excellent choice for those suffering from discomfort due to acid reflux.

Ingredients:

- 1-2 teaspoons dried meadowsweet flowers
- 1 cup boiling water

Instructions:

- Place 1-2 teaspoons of dried meadowsweet flowers in a tea infuser or directly in a cup.
- Pour 1 cup of boiling water over the meadowsweet flowers, ensuring they are fully immersed.
- Cover and allow the flowers to steep for about 10 minutes. Covering the cup helps to retain the essential oils and beneficial compounds in the tea.
- Remove the tea infuser or strain the tea to remove the flowers before drinking.
- Optional: The tea has a naturally sweet and pleasant flavor, but you can add honey or a slice of lemon for additional taste if desired.

What to Expect:

Drinking Meadowsweet Infusion can provide relief from the symptoms of acid reflux, such as heartburn, indigestion, and discomfort in the stomach or esophagus. Meadowsweet contains salicylic acid, which contributes to its anti-inflammatory and pain-relieving effects, and it also offers protective properties for the mucous membranes of the digestive tract. This herbal tea not only helps to neutralize excess stomach acid but also promotes the healing of the digestive lining. Enjoy this soothing infusion up to three times a day, especially after meals or when experiencing acid reflux symptoms, to harness its full benefits. However, individuals with salicylate sensitivity or those taking blood-thinning medications should consult with a healthcare provider before incorporating meadowsweet into their routine, due to its natural salicylic acid content.

Cardamom and Ginger Digestive Chai.

Cardamom and Ginger Digestive Chai is a flavorful and therapeutic beverage that combines the digestive benefits of cardamom and ginger with the rich, aromatic spices typical of chai. This tea is designed to aid digestion, soothe the stomach, and provide a warming, comforting experience. Enjoy it as a delightful way to end a meal or as a soothing drink to ease digestive discomfort.

Ingredients:

- ½ teaspoon ground cardamom
- ½ inch fresh ginger, grated or thinly sliced
- ¼ teaspoon ground cinnamon
- ¼ teaspoon ground cloves
- ¼ teaspoon ground black pepper
- 1 cup water
- 1 cup milk (dairy or plant-based)
- 1-2 teaspoons honey, or to taste
- 1 black tea bag or 1 teaspoon loose black tea (optional)

Instructions:

- In a small saucepan, combine the ground cardamom, grated ginger, ground cinnamon, ground cloves, and ground black pepper with 1 cup of water. If you're adding black tea, include it in this step.
- Bring the mixture to a boil, then reduce the heat and simmer for 5-10 minutes to allow the spices to infuse their flavors into the water.
- Add 1 cup of milk to the saucepan and return to a simmer. Be careful not to let the mixture boil over.
- Once the chai is hot and the flavors have melded together, remove it from the heat. If you used a tea bag, remove it now.
- Strain the chai to remove the solid spices and ginger pieces.
- Stir in 1-2 teaspoons of honey, adjusting to taste.
- Serve the chai warm in your favorite mug.

What to Expect:

Drinking Cardamom and Ginger Digestive Chai offers a warming and soothing effect on the digestive system. Cardamom and ginger are known for their carminative properties, which help reduce bloating, gas, and indigestion. The additional spices not only add depth and complexity to the flavor but also contribute their own digestive benefits. Cinnamon, for example, can help regulate blood sugar levels, while cloves and black pepper stimulate digestion. This chai is a comforting, tasty beverage that supports digestive health and can be enjoyed throughout the day, especially after meals. Enjoy the rich flavors and digestive benefits of this homemade chai as a natural and delicious way to support your digestive well-being.

ARTICHOKE AND MINT DIGESTIVE TEA.

Artichoke and Mint Digestive Tea is a herbal infusion designed to support digestion and offer relief from digestive discomforts such as bloating and indigestion. Artichoke leaves are known for their liver-supporting properties and ability to stimulate bile production, which is essential for fat digestion and detoxification. Mint adds a refreshing flavor to the tea and has antispasmodic properties that can soothe the stomach and alleviate symptoms of irritable bowel syndrome (IBS).

Ingredients:

- 1 teaspoon dried artichoke leaves
- 1 teaspoon dried mint leaves
- 1 cup boiling water

Instructions:

- Combine 1 teaspoon of dried artichoke leaves with 1 teaspoon of dried mint leaves in a tea infuser or directly in a cup.
- Pour 1 cup of boiling water over the herbal mixture, ensuring the leaves are fully submerged.
- Allow the tea to steep for about 10 minutes. This steeping time allows the water to extract the active compounds from the herbs, maximizing their digestive benefits.
- Remove the tea infuser or strain the tea to remove the loose leaves before drinking.
- Optional: You may add a teaspoon of honey or a slice of lemon to enhance the flavor of the tea, although it's also delightful on its own.

What to Expect:

Drinking Artichoke and Mint Digestive Tea after meals can help improve digestion and relieve digestive discomfort. The artichoke leaves in the tea promote bile flow, aiding in the digestion of fats and supporting liver health. Mint leaves help to relax the muscles of the digestive tract, reducing symptoms of bloating, gas, and abdominal pain. This tea offers a refreshing and slightly bitter taste that is both soothing and beneficial for digestive health. Incorporating this tea into your daily routine, especially after heavy or fatty meals, can support your digestive system and enhance overall well-being.

SLIPPERY ELM AND MARSHMALLOW ROOT SOOTHING GRUEL.

Slippery Elm and Marshmallow Root Soothing Gruel is a gentle, nutritious concoction designed to calm and protect the digestive tract. Both slippery elm bark and marshmallow root are rich in mucilage, a type of soluble fiber that becomes gel-like when mixed with water. This mucilage coats the lining of the digestive system, providing relief from irritation, inflammation, and various digestive issues. This gruel is particularly beneficial for those suffering from conditions like acid reflux, gastritis, ulcers, and irritable bowel syndrome (IBS).

Ingredients:

- 2 tablespoons slippery elm bark powder
- 2 tablespoons marshmallow root powder
- 2 cups water

Instructions:

- In a small saucepan, combine 2 tablespoons of slippery elm bark powder with 2 tablespoons of marshmallow root powder.
- Gradually add 2 cups of water to the powders, stirring constantly to ensure a smooth, lump-free mixture.
- Place the saucepan over low heat and cook the mixture, stirring continuously, until it thickens into a gruel. This may take about 5-10 minutes.
- Once the gruel has reached the desired consistency, remove it from heat and allow it to cool to a safe temperature for consumption.
- Optional: You can add a natural sweetener like honey or maple syrup to enhance the taste, or a pinch of cinnamon for additional flavor.

What to Expect:

Consuming Slippery Elm and Marshmallow Root Soothing Gruel can provide immediate relief for the digestive tract. The mucilage forms a protective layer that can help heal and prevent further irritation of the mucous membranes. This gruel is not only soothing but also nutritious, as slippery elm bark is known for its vitamins, minerals, and antioxidants. Marshmallow root further enhances the soothing effect with its own healing properties. This remedy is mild and safe for most people, including children and adults with sensitive digestive systems. Enjoy this gruel 1-2 times daily, especially before meals or at bedtime, to support digestive health and comfort.

GINGER AND PEPPERMINT DIGESTIVE AID CAPSULES.

Ginger and Peppermint Digestive Aid Capsules are a natural and convenient way to support digestive health and alleviate discomfort such as bloating, gas, and indigestion. Ginger is renowned for its ability to ease nausea and promote gastric motility, while peppermint relaxes the digestive tract muscles, offering relief from symptoms of IBS and other digestive issues. These capsules combine the benefits of both herbs, making them a potent digestive aid.

Ingredients:

- Powdered ginger
- Powdered peppermint leaves
- Empty capsules

Instructions:

- In a bowl, mix equal parts of powdered ginger and powdered peppermint leaves. The exact amounts will depend on how many capsules you wish to make. A good starting ratio is 1 tablespoon of each powder for a small batch.
- Carefully open the empty capsules (they typically come in two pieces) and fill each half with the ginger and peppermint powder mixture. If you have a capsule filling machine, follow the manufacturer's instructions for filling the capsules.
- Once filled, carefully close the capsules by pressing the two halves together.
- Store the filled capsules in a cool, dry place, ideally in a container that blocks out light to preserve the potency of the herbs.

Dosage:

- Take one or two capsules after meals, or as needed to relieve digestive discomfort. Begin with the lower dosage to assess your body's response.

What to Expect:

Taking Ginger and Peppermint Digestive Aid Capsules after meals can help facilitate digestion and relieve discomfort associated with indigestion, bloating, and gas. You may notice a reduction in symptoms such as nausea and abdominal cramping. These capsules offer a convenient and discreet way to harness the digestive benefits of ginger and peppermint, especially when you are on the go or do not have time to prepare herbal tea. As with any dietary supplement, it's wise to consult with a healthcare provider before starting, especially if you are pregnant, nursing, or have any existing health conditions or concerns.

CHAMOMILE AND LICORICE TEA FOR STOMACH COMFORT.

Chamomile and Licorice Tea is a soothing herbal infusion designed to provide relief and comfort to the digestive tract. Chamomile, with its natural calming properties, helps to ease discomfort, reduce inflammation, and relax the muscles of the digestive system. Licorice root complements chamomile by coating and protecting the mucous membranes of the stomach and intestines, offering relief from acidity and gastritis.

Ingredients:

- 1 teaspoon dried chamomile flowers
- 1 teaspoon chopped licorice root
- 1 cup boiling water

Instructions:

- Combine 1 teaspoon of dried chamomile flowers with 1 teaspoon of chopped licorice root in a tea infuser or directly in a cup.
- Pour 1 cup of boiling water over the chamomile and licorice mixture, ensuring that the herbs are fully immersed.
- Allow the tea to steep for about 10 minutes. This steeping time allows the herbs to release their beneficial compounds into the water.
- Remove the tea infuser or strain the tea to remove the loose herbs before drinking.
- Optional: If desired, you can sweeten the tea with honey or add a slice of lemon for additional flavor.

What to Expect:

Drinking Chamomile and Licorice Tea can provide significant relief from digestive discomfort. You may experience a reduction in symptoms such as bloating, gas, and indigestion shortly after consuming the tea. The chamomile in the tea promotes relaxation and aids in reducing stress, which can often exacerbate digestive issues. Licorice root is known for its ability to soothe and protect the gastrointestinal lining, making it particularly beneficial for those with acid reflux or gastritis. Enjoy this tea after meals or anytime you need digestive support. The natural sweetness of licorice and the gentle flavor of chamomile make this tea not only therapeutic but also enjoyable to drink. Regular consumption can contribute to overall digestive wellness and comfort.

Ginger and Fennel Seed Anti-Nausea Blend.

Ginger and Fennel Seed Anti-Nausea Blend is a natural herbal tea designed to relieve nausea and digestive discomfort. This blend harnesses the potent anti-nausea effects of ginger, a well-known natural remedy for stomach upset, with the carminative properties of fennel seeds, which aid in relieving gas, bloating, and digestive spasms. Together, they create a powerful tea that can help soothe the stomach and improve digestion.

Ingredients:

- 1-inch piece of fresh ginger, thinly sliced
- 1 teaspoon fennel seeds
- 1 cup boiling water

Instructions:

- Prepare the fresh ginger by thinly slicing a 1-inch piece. This increases the surface area, allowing more of its active compounds to infuse into the water.
- In a tea infuser or directly in a cup, combine the sliced ginger with 1 teaspoon of fennel seeds.

- Pour 1 cup of boiling water over the ginger and fennel seeds, making sure they are fully submerged.
- Allow the mixture to steep for about 10 minutes. Covering the cup during this time can help trap the essential oils and increase the potency of the tea.
- After steeping, remove the tea infuser or strain the tea to remove the ginger slices and fennel seeds before drinking.
- Optional: If you prefer, you can add a small amount of honey or lemon to taste, although the natural flavors are often pleasant and soothing on their own.

What to Expect:

Drinking the Ginger and Fennel Seed Anti-Nausea Blend can provide quick relief from nausea and digestive discomfort. Ginger's active compounds, such as gingerol, have been shown to effectively reduce feelings of nausea and prevent vomiting. Fennel seeds add a sweet, licorice-like flavor to the tea and can help relax the digestive tract, reducing gas and bloating. This tea is ideal for consumption before or after meals, during bouts of nausea, or anytime you need digestive support. Its warming and slightly spicy flavor makes it a comforting choice, especially during cold weather or when you need an extra digestive aid. Enjoy this natural and soothing blend to help maintain digestive comfort and health.

HERBAL REMEDIES FOR LIVER HEALTH.

DANDELION TEA FOR LIVER DETOX.

Dandelion Tea combines the detoxifying benefits of both dandelion root and leaves, aiding in liver health by promoting the removal of toxins and supporting liver function.

Ingredients:

- 1 tablespoon dried dandelion root
- 1 tablespoon dried dandelion leaves
- 2 cups water

Instructions:

- Combine 1 tablespoon each of dried dandelion root and leaves in a pot with 2 cups of water.
- Bring to a boil, then reduce heat and simmer for 15 minutes.
- Strain the tea into a cup, discarding the solids.

What to Expect:

Drinking Dandelion Tea for Liver Detox can enhance liver function and aid in the detoxification process. It may also support digestive health and provide a boost in energy and wellness. Its natural diuretic properties help in flushing out toxins more efficiently

Milk Thistle Seed Decoction.

Milk Thistle Seed Decoction is a traditional herbal remedy known for its liver-supporting benefits. Milk thistle contains silymarin, a group of compounds believed to have antioxidant, anti-inflammatory, and detoxifying properties. This decoction is particularly beneficial for those looking to support liver function, detoxify the liver, and protect it from damage caused by toxins, alcohol, and other harmful substances.

Ingredients:

- 1 tablespoon milk thistle seeds
- 2 cups water

Instructions:

- Crush the milk thistle seeds lightly to enhance the extraction of silymarin and other beneficial compounds. You can use a mortar and pestle or a spice grinder for this purpose.
- Add the crushed milk thistle seeds to a pot with 2 cups of water.
- Bring the mixture to a boil, then reduce the heat and simmer gently for about 20 minutes. This prolonged simmering allows for the maximum extraction of silymarin from the seeds into the water.
- After simmering, strain the decoction to remove the milk thistle seeds, leaving a clear liquid.
- The decoction can be consumed warm or allowed to cool down to a comfortable temperature before drinking.

What to Expect:

Drinking Milk Thistle Seed Decoction can provide several benefits for liver health. You may notice improved digestion and a general feeling of well-being as your liver function improves. Milk thistle's antioxidant properties can also help protect liver cells from damage and may support the liver's natural repair and regeneration processes. This decoction has a slightly bitter, earthy taste, which is characteristic of many liver-supportive herbs. For those new to milk thistle, starting with a small amount and gradually increasing to a full dose can help the body adjust to its effects. It's recommended to consult with a healthcare provider before starting any new herbal remedy, especially if you have existing health conditions or are taking medications, to ensure it is appropriate for your health needs. Incorporating Milk Thistle Seed Decoction into your routine can be a powerful way to support and maintain liver health.

Milk Thistle Seed Extract for Liver Health.

Milk Thistle Seed Extract is widely recognized for its liver-protective qualities, bolstering liver health through its potent antioxidant and anti-inflammatory properties.

Ingredients:

- Commercially prepared milk thistle extract (Follow the manufacturer's recommended dosage, usually found on the packaging.)

Instructions:

- Purchase a high-quality, commercially prepared milk thistle seed extract from a reputable source.
- Follow the recommended dosage instructions on the product label. This typically involves taking the extract with a glass of water.
- Consistency is key. Take the extract regularly as directed for best results.

What to Expect:

Milk Thistle Seed Extract supports the liver in various ways, including promoting regeneration of damaged liver tissue, protecting against toxins, and supporting overall liver function. Users may notice improvements in liver enzyme levels, a reduction in inflammation, and enhanced detoxification processes. It's a supportive supplement for those focusing on liver health maintenance or recovery.

Dandelion and Peppermint Liver Detox Tea.

Dandelion and Peppermint Liver Detox Tea is a refreshing and therapeutic herbal blend that supports liver health and detoxification. Combining the diuretic and liver-supportive properties of dandelion root with the soothing and digestive benefits of peppermint leaves, this tea is an ideal choice for those looking to enhance liver function and overall wellness.

Ingredients:

- 1 teaspoon dried dandelion root
- 1 teaspoon dried peppermint leaves
- 1 cup hot water

Instructions:

- Mix 1 teaspoon of dried dandelion root with 1 teaspoon of dried peppermint leaves in a tea infuser or directly in a cup.
- Pour 1 cup of boiling water over the dandelion root and peppermint leaves, allowing them to steep for about 10 minutes. The longer steeping time allows for the full extraction of the beneficial compounds from the herbs.

- If you've used a tea infuser, remove it from the cup. If the herbs were added directly, strain the tea to remove the leaves and roots before drinking.

What to Expect:
Drinking Dandelion and Peppermint Liver Detox Tea can help support the body's natural detoxification processes, specifically aiding in liver function. Dandelion root acts as a natural liver tonic, promoting the elimination of toxins, while peppermint leaves soothe the digestive system and reduce symptoms of bloating and discomfort. This tea is not only beneficial for liver health but also promotes hydration and digestion, making it a wholesome addition to your daily routine for maintaining optimal health.

DANDELION ROOT AND BURDOCK TEA.

Dandelion Root and Burdock Tea is a powerful herbal infusion aimed at promoting liver and kidney health. Both dandelion root and burdock root are celebrated for their detoxifying properties and their ability to support the natural cleansing processes of the liver and kidneys. This tea blend is not only beneficial for detoxification but also supports overall digestive health and blood purification.

Ingredients:

- 1 teaspoon dried dandelion root
- 1 teaspoon dried burdock root
- 1 cup boiling water

Instructions:

- Combine 1 teaspoon of dried dandelion root with 1 teaspoon of dried burdock root in a tea infuser or directly in a heat-resistant cup.
- Pour 1 cup of boiling water over the roots, making sure they are fully submerged.
- Cover and allow the tea to steep for about 10-15 minutes. Covering the tea while it steeps helps to retain the volatile oils and beneficial compounds in the water.
- After steeping, remove the tea infuser or strain the tea to remove the loose roots before drinking.
- Optional: If desired, you can sweeten the tea with honey or enhance its flavor with a slice of lemon.

What to Expect:
Drinking Dandelion Root and Burdock Tea can offer several health benefits, particularly for the liver and kidneys. You may notice improved digestion and a gentle diuretic effect, which aids in the elimination of toxins through increased urine production. The tea can also stimulate bile flow, further supporting liver function and the digestion of fats. Dandelion and burdock

have a slightly bitter taste, which is characteristic of many liver-supportive herbs and can stimulate digestive enzymes. This tea is ideal for those looking to naturally support their body's detoxification processes and can be enjoyed regularly as part of a healthy diet and lifestyle. Regular consumption can contribute to improved liver and kidney function and overall well-being.

Dandelion and Lemon Detox Tea.

Dandelion and Lemon Detox Tea is a simple yet powerful herbal beverage that combines the liver-supportive properties of dandelion leaves with the detoxifying benefits of lemon. This tea is ideal for those looking to support their liver's natural detoxification processes and enhance overall wellness.
Ingredients:

- 1 tablespoon fresh or dried dandelion leaves
- 1 slice of lemon
- 1 cup hot water

Instructions:

- Place 1 tablespoon of fresh or dried dandelion leaves in a tea infuser or directly in a cup.
- Add a slice of lemon to the cup.
- Pour 1 cup of hot water over the dandelion leaves and lemon slice, allowing them to steep for about 5 to 10 minutes.
- If you used a tea infuser, remove it from the cup. If the leaves were added directly, strain the tea to remove them and the lemon slice before drinking.

What to Expect:
Drinking Dandelion and Lemon Detox Tea can aid in liver detoxification, helping to flush out toxins and improve liver function. Dandelion leaves are rich in vitamins and minerals that support detoxification and kidney function, while lemon adds a vitamin C boost and aids in digestion. This tea is a refreshing and effective way to support your body's natural detox processes, promote hydration, and maintain a healthy liver.

Schisandra Berry Tea for Liver Health and Stress Reduction.

Schisandra Berry Tea, made from the dried berries of the Schisandra chinensis plant, is a traditional remedy known for its liver-protective properties and ability to reduce stress. This adaptogenic tea helps balance the body's stress response while supporting overall liver function.
Ingredients:

- 1 tablespoon dried schisandra berries
- 1 cup hot water

Instructions:

- Place 1 tablespoon of dried schisandra berries in a cup.
- Pour 1 cup of hot water over the berries and let them steep for 10 to 15 minutes.
- Strain the tea to remove the berries. If desired, the berries can be steeped a second time to extract more flavor and nutrients.

What to Expect:
Drinking Schisandra Berry Tea can contribute to improved liver health by supporting the organ's detoxifying processes. Additionally, its adaptogenic qualities can help reduce physical and mental stress, enhancing overall vitality and well-being. The tea has a unique flavor profile, often described as having five tastes: sweet, sour, salty, bitter, and pungent, making it a distinctive herbal beverage experience.

Dandelion Green and Mint Refreshing Tea.

Dandelion Green and Mint Refreshing Tea is a delightful herbal beverage that combines the liver-supportive benefits of dandelion greens with the cooling and soothing properties of mint leaves. This tea is ideal for those looking to support their liver health while enjoying a naturally refreshing and uplifting drink.
Ingredients:

- A handful of fresh dandelion greens (or 1 tablespoon dried dandelion leaves)
- A handful of fresh mint leaves (or 1 tablespoon dried mint leaves)
- 1 cup hot water

Instructions:

- Roughly chop the fresh dandelion greens and mint leaves to release their flavors. If you're using dried leaves, measure out 1 tablespoon of each.
- Place the chopped greens and leaves or the dried herbs in a tea infuser or directly in a cup.
- Pour 1 cup of boiling water over the dandelion and mint, allowing them to steep for about 5 to 10 minutes, depending on how strong you like your tea.
- If you've used a tea infuser, remove it from the cup. If the herbs were added directly, strain the tea into another cup to remove the leaves.

What to Expect:
Drinking Dandelion Green and Mint Refreshing Tea can provide a gentle liver detoxification boost, thanks to the diuretic properties of dandelion, which help to flush toxins from the liver and kidneys. Mint contributes a cooling and soothing effect, aiding in digestion and offering a refreshing taste. This combination makes for a perfect spring or summer drink,

supporting hydration, liver health, and overall well-being with its nutrient-rich composition. It's also a great alternative to caffeinated beverages for a midday pick-me-up.

Lemon and Ginger Detoxifying Water.

Lemon and Ginger Detoxifying Water is a refreshing and simple way to boost your hydration and support your body's natural detoxification processes. This infused water combines the digestive benefits of ginger with the cleansing properties of lemon, making it an ideal drink to consume throughout the day for maintaining hydration and enhancing overall health.
Ingredients:

- 1 lemon, thinly sliced
- 1-inch piece of ginger, thinly sliced or grated
- 1 liter of water

Instructions:

- Add the thinly sliced lemon and ginger to a pitcher or large water bottle.
- Fill the pitcher or bottle with 1 liter of water.
- Let the water infuse for at least 1 hour in the refrigerator, allowing the flavors and nutrients to meld. For a stronger infusion, you can let it sit overnight.
- Drink the Lemon and Ginger Detoxifying Water throughout the day.

What to Expect:

Drinking this infused water can aid in digestion, help to detoxify the liver, and support the immune system thanks to the vitamin C from the lemon and the anti-inflammatory properties of ginger. Additionally, staying well-hydrated is essential for all bodily functions, including detoxification and elimination of wastes. This detoxifying water is not only beneficial for your health but also offers a more flavorful and enjoyable way to increase your daily water intake.

Stinging Nettle and Lemon Spring Detox Tea.

Stinging Nettle and Lemon Spring Detox Tea is a revitalizing herbal beverage that combines the cleansing properties of stinging nettle leaves with the detoxifying benefits of lemon. This tea is perfect for a springtime detox or any time you wish to refresh and purify your body.
Ingredients:

- 1 tablespoon dried stinging nettle leaves
- 1 slice of lemon
- 1 cup hot water

Instructions:

- Place 1 tablespoon of dried stinging nettle leaves in a tea infuser or directly in a cup.
- Add a slice of lemon to the cup.
- Pour 1 cup of hot water over the nettle leaves and lemon slice, allowing them to steep for 10 to 15 minutes.
- Remove the tea infuser or strain the tea to remove the leaves and lemon slice before drinking.

What to Expect:

Drinking Stinging Nettle and Lemon Spring Detox Tea can help detoxify the body, support kidney function, and reduce inflammation. Stinging nettle is rich in nutrients and has been traditionally used to cleanse the blood and remove toxins. Lemon adds a refreshing taste and boosts the detoxifying effects with its vitamin C and antioxidants. This tea is a gentle way to support overall health and vitality, making it a great addition to your daily wellness routine.

Nettle Tea for Allergy Relief.

Nettle Tea is known for its natural antihistamine properties, making it an effective remedy for alleviating allergy symptoms such as sneezing, itching, and nasal congestion.

Ingredients:

- 1 tablespoon dried nettle leaves
- 1 cup hot water

Instructions:

- Place 1 tablespoon of dried nettle leaves in a cup.
- Pour 1 cup of hot water over the nettle leaves and let it steep for 15 minutes.
- Strain the tea into another cup to remove the nettle leaves.

What to Expect:

Regular consumption of Nettle Tea may provide relief from allergy symptoms by naturally reducing histamine production. Its anti-inflammatory benefits can help ease seasonal or environmental allergy reactions, offering a soothing, natural solution.

Chlorella and Spirulina Detox Smoothie.

The Chlorella and Spirulina Detox Smoothie is a powerful blend that combines the detoxifying and nutrient-rich properties of chlorella and spirulina with the natural sweetness and vitamins of fruits. This smoothie is an excellent way to support your body's detoxification processes while also providing a significant boost in essential nutrients.

Ingredients:

- 1 teaspoon chlorella powder
- 1 teaspoon spirulina powder
- 1 banana (for sweetness and creaminess)
- ½ cup of mixed berries (such as blueberries, strawberries, or raspberries for antioxidants)
- 1 cup spinach (for additional vitamins and minerals)
- 1 cup almond milk or water (for blending)
- Optional: 1 tablespoon honey or maple syrup for added sweetness

Instructions:

- Add 1 teaspoon each of chlorella and spirulina powders to a blender.
- Add the banana, mixed berries, spinach, and your choice of almond milk or water to the blender. If you prefer a sweeter taste, add honey or maple syrup.
- Blend all ingredients until smooth and creamy. Adjust the amount of liquid to achieve your desired smoothie consistency.
- Taste and adjust sweetness if necessary by adding more honey or maple syrup.

What to Expect:
This detox smoothie is designed to aid in the body's natural detoxification process, thanks to the chelating properties of chlorella and the nutrient density of spirulina. The added fruits and spinach provide a wealth of vitamins, minerals, and antioxidants, contributing to overall health and vitality. Taking this smoothie can help improve energy levels, support immune function, and promote healthy skin, making it a nutritious and delicious addition to your wellness routine.

Chlorella and Spirulina Powder for Detoxification.

Blending chlorella and spirulina powder into a smoothie creates a powerful detoxifying and nutrient-rich drink. Both chlorella and spirulina are renowned for their high concentrations of vitamins, minerals, and antioxidants, offering support for detoxification processes and overall nutrient intake.

Ingredients:

- 1 teaspoon chlorella powder
- 1 teaspoon spirulina powder
- 1 cup of your preferred liquid (water, almond milk, coconut water)
- Optional: fruits (banana, berries, apple) and vegetables (spinach, kale) for added flavor and nutrients

Instructions:

- Add 1 teaspoon each of chlorella and spirulina powder to a blender.
- Pour in 1 cup of your chosen liquid. Add any optional fruits and vegetables for enhanced taste and additional vitamins.

- Blend until smooth and fully combined.

What to Expect:
This smoothie supports the body's natural detoxification mechanisms, helping to remove toxins and heavy metals. The high levels of chlorophyll in chlorella and the nutrient density of spirulina boost energy, immune function, and overall health. Consuming this smoothie regularly can contribute to improved wellness and vitality.

HERBAL REMEDIES FOR KIDNEY HEALTH.

NETTLE AND HORSETAIL KIDNEY SUPPORT TEA.

Nettle and Horsetail Kidney Support Tea is a herbal infusion specifically designed to enhance kidney health and support urinary tract function. Both nettle and horsetail are renowned for their diuretic properties, helping to flush toxins from the body and improve urinary flow. This tea blend is beneficial for those looking to naturally support their kidney function and promote overall urinary health.
Ingredients:

- 1 teaspoon dried nettle leaves
- 1 teaspoon dried horsetail
- 1 cup boiling water

Instructions:

- Combine 1 teaspoon of dried nettle leaves with 1 teaspoon of dried horsetail in a tea infuser or directly in a heat-resistant cup.
- Pour 1 cup of boiling water over the herbs, ensuring they are fully immersed.
- Cover and allow the tea to steep for about 10-15 minutes. The cover helps to retain essential oils and active compounds within the tea.
- After steeping, remove the tea infuser or strain the tea to remove the loose herbs.
- Optional: The tea has a natural, earthy flavor, but you can add honey or a slice of lemon for additional taste if desired.

What to Expect:
Drinking Nettle and Horsetail Kidney Support Tea can provide several benefits for kidney and urinary tract health. The diuretic effect of both herbs aids in flushing out toxins and excess fluids from the body, which can help prevent urinary tract infections and support kidney function. Nettle is also rich in nutrients that are beneficial for overall health, while horsetail can help strengthen the urinary tract tissues. This tea can be enjoyed regularly to support the body's natural detoxification processes and promote healthy kidney and urinary tract function. However, it's important to consume

diuretic teas in moderation and stay hydrated by drinking plenty of water throughout the day. As with any herbal remedy, consulting with a healthcare provider is advisable, especially if you have existing health conditions or are taking medications.

HERBAL REMEDIES FOR URINARY TRACT HEALTH.

CORN SILK TEA FOR URINARY COMFORT.

Corn Silk Tea is a gentle, traditional remedy used to soothe urinary tract discomfort. Made from the silky threads found under the husk of a corn cob, corn silk contains compounds that are beneficial for urinary health, including anti-inflammatory and diuretic properties. This tea is particularly helpful for those experiencing irritation or inflammation of the bladder and urinary tract.
Ingredients:

- 1-2 tablespoons dried corn silk
- 1 cup boiling water

Instructions:

- Place 1-2 tablespoons of dried corn silk in a tea infuser or directly in a cup.
- Pour 1 cup of boiling water over the corn silk, ensuring it is fully submerged.
- Allow the corn silk to steep for about 10-15 minutes, covering the cup to preserve the natural compounds in the steam.
- After steeping, remove the tea infuser or strain the tea to remove the loose corn silk before drinking.
- Optional: The tea has a mild, slightly sweet flavor, but you can add honey or lemon to enhance its taste if desired.

What to Expect:
Drinking Corn Silk Tea can offer relief from urinary tract discomfort, such as pain or irritation during urination. Its diuretic effect helps to flush out toxins and can reduce bloating by eliminating excess water from the body. Additionally, corn silk's anti-inflammatory properties may help soothe the lining of the urinary tract, providing comfort and support for urinary health. This tea can be consumed 2-3 times a day, especially when experiencing symptoms of urinary discomfort, to help promote a sense of relief and well-being. Always ensure to stay hydrated by drinking plenty of water in addition to herbal teas like corn silk tea. As with any herbal remedy, it's wise to consult with a healthcare provider before incorporating corn silk tea into your health regimen, particularly if you have pre-existing conditions or are taking medications.

BEARBERRY (UVA URSI) TEA FOR URINARY TRACT INFECTIONS.

Bearberry (Uva Ursi) Tea is a potent herbal remedy traditionally used to support urinary tract health and combat urinary tract infections (UTIs). The active compound in bearberry leaves, arbutin, is converted into hydroquinone in the body, which has antiseptic and antibacterial properties. This makes bearberry tea an effective natural option for flushing out bacteria from the urinary tract. However, due to its potency and the presence of tannins, bearberry tea is recommended for short-term use only.

Ingredients:

- 1 teaspoon dried bearberry (uva ursi) leaves
- 1 cup boiling water

Instructions:

- Place 1 teaspoon of dried bearberry leaves in a tea infuser or directly in a cup.
- Pour 1 cup of boiling water over the bearberry leaves, ensuring they are fully submerged.
- Cover and allow the leaves to steep for about 10-15 minutes. Covering the cup helps to retain the therapeutic compounds in the tea.
- After steeping, remove the tea infuser or strain the tea to remove the loose leaves before drinking.
- Optional: Bearberry tea has a strong, slightly bitter flavor, so it's generally not sweetened. However, if necessary for taste, a small amount of honey can be added.

What to Expect:

Drinking Bearberry (Uva Ursi) Tea can provide support for urinary tract health, especially during a UTI. The tea's antibacterial properties can help reduce bacteria levels in the urinary tract, alleviating symptoms such as pain, burning, and urgency. It is important to note that bearberry tea should be used with caution and for a short duration (typically not exceeding one week) due to potential side effects from prolonged use, such as liver damage or interference with nutrient absorption. Bearberry is not recommended for pregnant or nursing women, children, or individuals with kidney disease. Always consult with a healthcare provider before starting any new herbal remedy, especially if you have existing health conditions or are taking medications. Drinking plenty of water and seeking medical advice for UTIs is also crucial, as they can lead to more serious conditions if not properly treated.

Cranberry and Dandelion Tea for UTI Prevention.

Cranberry and Dandelion Tea is a healthful blend designed to support urinary tract health and prevent urinary tract infections (UTIs). Cranberries are well-known for their ability to prevent bacteria from adhering to the urinary tract walls, while dandelion leaves act as a natural diuretic, promoting the flushing of toxins and bacteria from the system. This combination makes for a powerful tea that not only supports urinary health but also provides a rich source of vitamins and antioxidants.

Ingredients:

- 1 tablespoon dried cranberries
- 1 teaspoon dried dandelion leaves
- 1 cup boiling water

Instructions:

- Roughly chop the dried cranberries to increase the surface area for infusion.
- Combine the chopped dried cranberries with dried dandelion leaves in a tea infuser or directly in a heat-resistant cup.
- Pour 1 cup of boiling water over the cranberry and dandelion mixture, ensuring the ingredients are fully immersed.
- Allow the mixture to steep for about 10-15 minutes. Covering the cup during steeping can help retain the essential oils and active compounds within the tea.
- After steeping, remove the tea infuser or strain the tea to remove the cranberry pieces and dandelion leaves.
- Optional: You may add a natural sweetener like honey or a slice of lemon to enhance the flavor of the tea.

What to Expect:

Drinking Cranberry and Dandelion Tea can provide several benefits for urinary tract health, including aiding in the prevention of UTIs. The diuretic properties of dandelion help increase urine production, facilitating the removal of toxins and potentially harmful bacteria from the urinary tract. Cranberries contain proanthocyanidins (PACs) that can prevent bacteria from adhering to the urinary tract walls, reducing the risk of infection. This tea offers a tart and slightly bitter flavor, which can be moderated with natural sweeteners if desired. Enjoy this tea regularly, especially if you are prone to UTIs or wish to support overall urinary tract health. However, it's important to note that while cranberry and dandelion tea can help prevent UTIs, it should not replace medical treatment for existing infections. Always consult with a healthcare provider for guidance if you suspect a UTI or have ongoing urinary tract issues.

Juniper Berry and Uva Ursi Diuretic Blend.

Juniper Berry and Uva Ursi Diuretic Blend is a powerful herbal tea designed to naturally promote diuresis and support urinary tract health. This combination harnesses the diuretic properties of juniper berries, known for stimulating kidney function and flushing out toxins, with the antiseptic benefits of uva ursi leaves, which can help cleanse the urinary tract and prevent infections. This tea is particularly beneficial for those looking to support their kidney and bladder health.

Ingredients:

- 1 teaspoon dried juniper berries
- 1 teaspoon dried uva ursi leaves
- 1 cup boiling water

Instructions:

- Crush the dried juniper berries slightly to release their essential oils.
- Combine the crushed juniper berries with dried uva ursi leaves in a tea infuser or directly in a heat-resistant cup.
- Pour 1 cup of boiling water over the herbal mixture, making sure the ingredients are fully immersed.
- Cover and allow the mixture to steep for about 10-15 minutes. Covering the cup helps to preserve the volatile oils and active compounds in the tea.
- After steeping, remove the tea infuser or strain the tea to remove the herbs before drinking.
- Optional: The flavor of this blend can be strong and somewhat bitter. If desired, you can add a natural sweetener like honey to soften the taste.

What to Expect:

Drinking Juniper Berry and Uva Ursi Diuretic Blend can increase urine production, helping to flush out excess fluids and toxins from the body. This can be particularly helpful for reducing bloating and supporting the body's natural detoxification processes. The antiseptic properties of uva ursi can also aid in preventing urinary tract infections by reducing bacteria in the urinary tract. It's important to use this tea responsibly, as excessive consumption of juniper berries can be irritating to the kidneys. Also, due to the potent effects of both herbs, this tea should be consumed for short periods and not used continuously. Pregnant and nursing women, as well as individuals with kidney disease, should avoid this tea. Always consult with a healthcare provider before adding new herbal remedies to your regimen, especially if you have existing health conditions or are on medication.

BEARBERRY TEA FOR BLADDER INFECTIONS.

Bearberry Tea, made from the leaves of the bearberry plant (also known as uva ursi), is a traditional herbal remedy used to help treat urinary tract and bladder infections. The active compound in bearberry leaves, arbutin, is metabolized into hydroquinone in the body, which possesses antimicrobial properties that can help fight bacterial infections in the urinary tract.
Ingredients:

- 1-2 teaspoons dried bearberry (uva ursi) leaves
- 1 cup boiling water

Instructions:

- Place 1-2 teaspoons of dried bearberry leaves in a tea infuser or directly in a cup.
- Pour 1 cup of boiling water over the bearberry leaves, ensuring they are fully submerged.
- Cover and allow the leaves to steep for about 10-15 minutes. Covering the cup during steeping helps to maintain the essential oils and active compounds in the tea.
- After steeping, remove the tea infuser or strain the tea to remove the loose leaves.
- Optional: Bearberry tea has a naturally strong and somewhat bitter taste. If desired, you can add a small amount of honey to improve its palatability, although it's typically consumed plain for its medicinal benefits.

What to Expect:
Drinking Bearberry Tea can offer relief for symptoms associated with urinary tract and bladder infections, such as pain during urination, urgency, and frequency. The antimicrobial action of the converted hydroquinone helps to reduce bacterial growth, aiding in the treatment of the infection. It's important to note that bearberry tea should be used under the guidance of a healthcare provider, as excessive consumption can lead to potential side effects, including liver damage. Additionally, bearberry tea is not recommended for long-term use, pregnant or nursing women, or individuals with kidney disorders. For best results in treating UTIs, it's also crucial to maintain adequate hydration by drinking plenty of water and to seek professional medical advice to ensure appropriate treatment.

CLEAVERS AND DANDELION DIURETIC INFUSION.

Cleavers and Dandelion Diuretic Infusion is a natural herbal tea designed to support urinary tract health through its diuretic properties. Cleavers (Galium aparine) is known for its ability to flush toxins from the lymphatic system and kidneys, while dandelion leaves are celebrated for their diuretic effects that promote kidney function and reduce water retention. This combination not only aids in detoxifying the body but also supports the health of the urinary tract.

Ingredients:

- 1 teaspoon dried cleavers
- 1 teaspoon dried dandelion leaves
- 1 cup boiling water

Instructions:

- Combine 1 teaspoon of dried cleavers with 1 teaspoon of dried dandelion leaves in a tea infuser or directly in a heat-resistant cup.
- Pour 1 cup of boiling water over the herbal blend, ensuring the herbs are fully immersed.
- Cover and allow the infusion to steep for about 10-15 minutes. Covering the cup during steeping helps to preserve the volatile oils and beneficial compounds of the herbs.
- After steeping, remove the tea infuser or strain the tea to remove the loose herbs.
- Optional: The tea has a natural, earthy flavor. If desired, you can add honey or a slice of lemon to enhance its taste.

What to Expect:

Drinking Cleavers and Dandelion Diuretic Infusion can provide significant benefits for urinary tract health. The natural diuretic properties of both cleavers and dandelion can increase urine production, helping to flush out excess fluids and toxins from the body. This process supports kidney function and may help in preventing urinary tract infections by maintaining a healthy flow of urine. Additionally, this infusion can aid in reducing bloating and water retention. Enjoy this tea regularly, especially if you are looking for a natural way to support urinary and kidney health. However, it's important to consume diuretic teas in moderation and maintain adequate hydration by drinking plenty of water throughout the day. As with any herbal remedy, consulting with a healthcare provider before starting regular use is advisable, especially for those with existing health conditions or those taking medications.

Buchu and Uva Ursi Tea for Bladder Infections.

Buchu and Uva Ursi Tea is a potent herbal remedy specifically formulated to alleviate bladder infections and support urinary tract health. Both buchu and uva ursi leaves have been traditionally used for their strong antiseptic and diuretic properties. Buchu contains compounds that can help disinfect the urinary tract, while uva ursi (bearberry) is valued for its arbutin content, which metabolizes into hydroquinone, a compound with antimicrobial

properties. Together, they form a powerful blend that can help flush out bacteria from the bladder, providing relief from infections.
Ingredients:

- 1 teaspoon dried buchu leaves
- 1 teaspoon dried uva ursi leaves
- 1 cup boiling water

Instructions:

- Combine 1 teaspoon of dried buchu leaves with 1 teaspoon of dried uva ursi leaves in a tea infuser or directly in a heat-resistant cup.
- Pour 1 cup of boiling water over the herbal mixture, ensuring the leaves are fully submerged.
- Cover and allow the tea to steep for about 10-15 minutes. Covering the cup during steeping helps to preserve the essential oils and active compounds within the tea.
- After steeping, remove the tea infuser or strain the tea to remove the loose leaves.
- Optional: The taste of this tea can be quite strong and somewhat bitter due to the potent nature of the herbs. If desired, you can add a small amount of honey to improve its palatability.

What to Expect:
Drinking Buchu and Uva Ursi Tea can offer relief from the symptoms of bladder infections, such as urgency, frequency, and pain during urination. The tea's diuretic effect encourages the flushing of bacteria and toxins from the urinary system. For best results, consume the tea 2-3 times daily while experiencing symptoms. However, due to the potent effects of both herbs, this tea should be used with caution and for short periods, typically not exceeding one week. It is not recommended for pregnant or nursing women, children, or individuals with kidney disease. As with any remedy for bladder infections, it's crucial to consult with a healthcare provider to ensure appropriate treatment, especially since bladder infections can lead to more serious conditions if not properly addressed. Stay hydrated by drinking plenty of water in addition to this herbal tea to help flush bacteria from the urinary tract.

JUNIPER BERRY AND PARSLEY SEED DIURETIC BLEND.

The Juniper Berry and Parsley Seed Diuretic Blend is a natural herbal tea formulated to support urinary tract function through its diuretic properties. Juniper berries are well-known for their ability to stimulate kidney function and increase urine output, helping to flush out toxins from the body. Parsley seeds, similarly, are recognized for their diuretic effects and their role in promoting kidney health and urinary tract function. Together, these ingredients create a potent blend that can aid in reducing water retention and supporting the body's natural detoxification processes.

Ingredients:

- 1 teaspoon crushed juniper berries
- 1 teaspoon parsley seeds
- 1 cup boiling water

Instructions:

- Crush 1 teaspoon of juniper berries to release their volatile oils. Combine the crushed berries with 1 teaspoon of parsley seeds in a tea infuser or directly in a heat-resistant cup.
- Pour 1 cup of boiling water over the juniper berries and parsley seeds, ensuring they are fully submerged.
- Cover and allow the mixture to steep for about 10-15 minutes. The cover helps to preserve the essential oils and active compounds, maximizing the tea's diuretic effect.
- After steeping, remove the tea infuser or strain the tea to remove the solids before drinking.
- Optional: The flavor of this blend can be quite strong and a bit bitter. If needed, you can add a small amount of honey or a slice of lemon to enhance the taste.

What to Expect:

Drinking the Juniper Berry and Parsley Seed Diuretic Blend can help support urinary tract function by increasing urine production, which aids in flushing out excess fluids and toxins. This can be particularly beneficial for those experiencing water retention or seeking to support their kidney and urinary tract health. It's important to use this tea with caution, as both juniper berries and parsley seeds are potent diuretics. Excessive consumption can lead to dehydration and electrolyte imbalances. It is also not recommended for pregnant women, nursing mothers, or individuals with kidney disorders. As with any diuretic, ensure to stay well-hydrated by drinking plenty of water throughout the day. Consult with a healthcare provider before incorporating this blend into your routine, especially if you have existing health conditions or are taking medications.

COUCH GRASS AND CORN SILK TEA FOR UTI RELIEF.

Couch Grass and Corn Silk Tea is a natural herbal infusion designed to support urinary tract health and provide relief from the symptoms of urinary tract infections (UTIs). Couch grass offers antibacterial and diuretic properties that can help flush out bacteria from the urinary tract, while corn silk is known for its soothing effect on the urinary system, reducing inflammation and irritation. Together, these herbs create a tea that can aid in the relief of UTI symptoms and promote overall urinary health.

Ingredients:

- 1 teaspoon dried couch grass (Elytrigia repens)
- 1 teaspoon dried corn silk
- 1 cup boiling water

Instructions:

- Combine 1 teaspoon of dried couch grass with 1 teaspoon of dried corn silk in a tea infuser or directly in a heat-resistant cup.
- Pour 1 cup of boiling water over the herbal mixture, ensuring that the herbs are fully submerged.
- Cover and allow the tea to steep for about 10-15 minutes. Covering the cup during steeping helps to maintain the essential oils and active compounds within the tea.
- After steeping, remove the tea infuser or strain the tea to remove the loose herbs before drinking.
- Optional: The tea has a mild, slightly sweet flavor from the corn silk. If desired, you can add honey or lemon to taste, although many find it pleasant to drink as is.

What to Expect:

Drinking Couch Grass and Corn Silk Tea can offer supportive relief for those experiencing UTI symptoms, such as urgency, frequency, and pain during urination. The diuretic properties of both couch grass and corn silk help increase urine production, aiding in the flushing out of bacteria and toxins. Additionally, the soothing properties of corn silk can help reduce inflammation and discomfort associated with UTIs. This tea can be consumed 2-3 times a day while symptoms persist. However, it's important to note that while this herbal tea can provide symptomatic relief, it should not replace medical treatment for UTIs. If symptoms persist or worsen, it is crucial to seek professional medical advice. Always ensure to stay well-hydrated by drinking plenty of water in addition to this herbal tea to help clear the infection more effectively. As with any herbal remedy, consulting with a healthcare provider before starting regular use is advisable, especially for those with existing health conditions or those taking medications.

Cranberry and D-Mannose Drink for Bladder Health.

The Cranberry and D-Mannose Drink is a synergistic blend specifically formulated to enhance bladder health and aid in the prevention of urinary tract infections (UTIs). This combination utilizes the unique properties of cranberries and D-Mannose to create a protective barrier against UTI-causing bacteria. Cranberries are renowned for their ability to prevent bacterial adhesion to the urinary tract walls, while D-Mannose acts as a natural sugar that bacteria preferentially bind to, allowing them to be flushed out of the system more easily.

Ingredients:

- ½ cup pure cranberry juice (unsweetened)
- 1 teaspoon D-Mannose powder
- 1 cup water (optional, for dilution)

Instructions:

- Combine ½ cup of pure, unsweetened cranberry juice with 1 teaspoon of D-Mannose powder in a glass. Stir thoroughly until the D-Mannose is fully dissolved.
- If desired, dilute the mixture with 1 cup of water to adjust the taste and concentration of the cranberry juice to your preference.
- Consume this drink once or twice daily, particularly if you are at risk of urinary tract infections or as part of a preventive approach to maintaining urinary tract health.

What to Expect:

Regularly consuming the Cranberry and D-Mannose Drink can significantly contribute to urinary tract health by creating an environment that is less conducive to bacterial infections. The drink's proactive approach to UTI prevention is especially beneficial for those with a history of recurrent infections. The cranberry component reduces bacterial adhesion, effectively lowering the risk of infection, while D-Mannose helps eliminate bacteria from the urinary tract. This preventive measure is a natural and effective strategy for maintaining urinary health, complementing hydration and proper urinary hygiene practices. However, it's essential to seek medical advice for active UTI symptoms or if infections frequently recur, as this drink is most effective as part of a comprehensive approach to urinary tract care.

Goldenrod and Birch Leaf Diuretic Tea.

Goldenrod and Birch Leaf Diuretic Tea is a natural herbal infusion crafted to support urinary tract health through its diuretic properties. Goldenrod is traditionally used for its ability to support kidney and urinary tract function, while birch leaves are known for their cleansing properties, aiding in the elimination of water retention and flushing toxins from the urinary system. This blend offers a gentle yet effective means of promoting urinary health.

Ingredients:

- 1 teaspoon dried goldenrod
- 1 teaspoon dried birch leaves
- 1 cup boiling water

Instructions:

- Combine 1 teaspoon of dried goldenrod with 1 teaspoon of dried birch leaves in a tea infuser or directly in a heat-resistant cup.
- Pour 1 cup of boiling water over the herbs, making sure they are fully immersed.
- Allow the tea to steep for about 10-15 minutes. Covering the cup during steeping can help preserve the essential oils and beneficial compounds of the herbs.
- After steeping, remove the tea infuser or strain the tea to remove the loose herbs.
- Optional: The tea has a naturally mild and earthy flavor. If desired, you can add honey or lemon to taste.

What to Expect:
Drinking Goldenrod and Birch Leaf Diuretic Tea can provide several benefits for urinary tract health. The natural diuretic effect of both goldenrod and birch helps increase urine production, facilitating the removal of waste and excess fluids from the body. This process can aid in reducing bloating and supporting kidney function by helping to clear the urinary tract of toxins. Additionally, this tea may help in preventing urinary tract infections by maintaining a healthy flow of urine. Enjoy this tea regularly, especially if you are looking to support your urinary tract and kidney health. However, it's important to use diuretic teas responsibly, as excessive diuresis can lead to dehydration and electrolyte imbalances. Ensure to stay well-hydrated by drinking plenty of water throughout the day. As with any herbal remedy, consulting with a healthcare provider before starting regular use is advisable, especially for those with existing health conditions or those taking medications.

Cucumber and Parsley Kidney Flush Drink.

The Cucumber and Parsley Kidney Flush Drink is a refreshing and detoxifying beverage designed to cleanse and support kidney function. Cucumbers, with their high water content and kidney-friendly nutrients, along with parsley, known for its diuretic properties and rich antioxidant content, make for a powerful combination to help flush toxins from the kidneys and improve urinary tract health.

Ingredients:
- 1 medium cucumber
- A handful of fresh parsley
- 2 cups of water

Instructions:
- Wash the cucumber thoroughly and chop it into chunks. There's no need to peel it unless it's waxed.
- Wash the parsley thoroughly to remove any dirt or residue.

- In a blender, combine the cucumber chunks, fresh parsley, and 2 cups of water.
- Blend the mixture until smooth. If you prefer a thinner consistency, you can add more water to taste.
- Optional: For added flavor and detoxifying benefits, you can squeeze in the juice of half a lemon.

What to Expect:
Drinking the Cucumber and Parsley Kidney Flush Drink can provide a gentle yet effective way to support kidney health and promote the natural detoxification process. The high water content of cucumber helps to hydrate the body and flush out toxins, while parsley serves as a natural diuretic, increasing urine output to help cleanse the kidneys. This drink is not only beneficial for kidney health but also supports overall hydration and can contribute to clearer skin. Enjoy this kidney flush drink regularly, especially in the morning to kickstart your day, or anytime you wish to support your body's natural detoxification systems. It's important to maintain a balanced diet and proper hydration for optimal health. As always, consult with a healthcare provider if you have existing kidney issues or are on medication, to ensure that this natural remedy is safe for your specific health needs.

CHAPTER 4: CARDIOVASCULAR AND RESPIRATORY SYSTEMS.

HERBAL REMEDIES FOR CARDIOVASCULAR HEALTH.

HAWTHORN BERRY TONIC FOR HEART HEALTH.

The Hawthorn Berry Tonic is a traditional remedy known for its beneficial effects on cardiovascular health. Hawthorn berries contain a variety of bioactive compounds, including flavonoids and oligomeric proanthocyanidins, which are thought to enhance heart function, improve circulation, and support the overall health of the cardiovascular system.
Ingredients:

- 2 tablespoons dried hawthorn berries
- 2 cups water

Instructions:

- Add 2 tablespoons of dried hawthorn berries to a small saucepan.
- Pour 2 cups of water over the berries and bring the mixture to a simmer over medium heat.
- Reduce the heat and let the berries simmer gently for about 20 minutes. This allows the beneficial compounds in the berries to be extracted into the water.
- After simmering, strain the tonic to remove the berries, leaving a clear liquid.
- The tonic can be consumed warm or cooled down to room temperature.

What to Expect:
Drinking Hawthorn Berry Tonic can offer several benefits for heart health. It may help to regulate blood pressure, improve circulation, and strengthen the heart muscle. Some people also find that it helps to reduce symptoms of heart failure and angina. The tonic has a slightly sweet and tart flavor, making it a pleasant drink to enjoy daily. For best results, consider incorporating this tonic into your routine over a period of weeks or months, as the heart-supportive effects of hawthorn berries can take some time to manifest fully. As with any natural remedy, it's important to consult with a healthcare provider before starting, especially if you have a pre-existing heart condition or are taking medication for cardiovascular health, to ensure that it is appropriate for your specific health needs.

GARLIC INFUSION FOR BLOOD PRESSURE.

Garlic Infusion is a simple, natural remedy known for its potential to help regulate blood pressure. Garlic contains allicin, a compound that is believed to have a variety of health benefits, including the ability to improve heart health and lower blood pressure levels. This infusion uses fresh garlic to create a potent drink that can be included as part of a heart-healthy lifestyle.
Ingredients:

- 2-3 cloves of fresh garlic
- 1 cup boiling water

Instructions:

- Peel and finely mince 2-3 cloves of fresh garlic. The finer the mince, the more surface area is exposed, allowing more allicin to be released.
- Place the minced garlic in a heat-resistant cup or mug.
- Pour 1 cup of boiling water over the minced garlic, ensuring it's fully submerged.
- Cover and let the mixture steep for about 15 minutes. Covering the cup helps to trap the beneficial compounds released from the garlic.
- After steeping, strain the infusion to remove the garlic pieces, leaving a clear liquid.
- Optional: The taste of garlic infusion can be strong and pungent. To improve its palatability, you can add a teaspoon of honey or a few drops of lemon juice.

What to Expect:
Consuming Garlic Infusion can contribute to regulating blood pressure levels. The allicin and other beneficial compounds in garlic help to dilate blood vessels, improving circulation and potentially lowering high blood pressure. For those with hypertension, incorporating garlic into the diet or consuming this infusion regularly may aid in managing blood pressure levels. However, garlic is not a substitute for prescribed medication, and this infusion should be used as a complementary approach. It's important to monitor your blood pressure regularly and consult with a healthcare provider to ensure that any natural remedies you incorporate are safe and effective for your specific health needs. Garlic can also have a blood-thinning effect, so it's crucial to consult with a doctor if you're on blood-thinning medication.

GINKGO BILOBA TEA FOR CIRCULATION.

Ginkgo Biloba Tea is an herbal infusion made from the leaves of the Ginkgo Biloba tree, renowned for its ability to enhance blood circulation and cognitive function. The active compounds in Ginkgo Biloba, including flavonoids and terpenoids, are thought to increase blood flow by dilating blood vessels and reducing the stickiness of platelets. This makes Ginkgo

Biloba Tea an excellent choice for those looking to support their circulatory health and overall brain function.

Ingredients:

- 1-2 teaspoons dried Ginkgo Biloba leaves
- 1 cup boiling water

Instructions:

- Place 1-2 teaspoons of dried Ginkgo Biloba leaves in a tea infuser or directly in a cup.
- Pour 1 cup of boiling water over the leaves, ensuring they are fully submerged.
- Allow the tea to steep for about 10 minutes. This steeping time allows for the extraction of the beneficial compounds from the leaves.
- After steeping, remove the tea infuser or strain the tea to remove the loose leaves before drinking.
- Optional: Ginkgo Biloba Tea has a unique, slightly bitter taste. If desired, you can add honey or lemon to improve its flavor.

What to Expect:

Drinking Ginkgo Biloba Tea can provide several benefits for circulatory and cognitive health. You may notice an improvement in concentration and memory due to enhanced blood flow to the brain. Additionally, the increased circulation can benefit the entire body, potentially leading to improved energy levels and reduced symptoms of circulatory issues. Ginkgo Biloba Tea is a natural way to support vascular health and cognitive function, making it a valuable addition to a healthy lifestyle. However, Ginkgo Biloba can interact with certain medications, including blood thinners and anti-depressants, so it's important to consult with a healthcare provider before incorporating it into your routine, especially if you have existing health conditions or are taking medication.

Green Tea Infusion for Heart Health.

Green Tea Infusion is a simple yet powerful beverage, celebrated for its profound antioxidant benefits, especially for heart health. Rich in catechins, particularly epigallocatechin gallate (EGCG), green tea supports cardiovascular health by improving blood vessel function, reducing inflammation, and lowering the risk of heart disease. Regular consumption of green tea is associated with a lower risk of developing heart disease and stroke, making it a valuable addition to a heart-healthy lifestyle.

Ingredients:

- 1-2 teaspoons of green tea leaves
- 1 cup of hot water (about 160-180°F, not boiling to prevent bitterness)

Instructions:

- Place 1-2 teaspoons of green tea leaves in a tea infuser or directly in a heat-resistant cup.
- Pour 1 cup of hot water over the green tea leaves. The optimal temperature for green tea is between 160-180°F to extract the beneficial compounds without releasing excessive tannins, which can make the tea bitter.
- Allow the tea to steep for about 3 minutes. Adjust the steeping time according to your taste preference for a stronger or milder flavor.
- After steeping, remove the tea infuser or strain the tea to remove the loose leaves.
- Optional: Green tea has a naturally delicate and slightly grassy flavor. If desired, you can enhance its taste with a slice of lemon or a small amount of honey, although many prefer it plain to fully enjoy its health benefits.

What to Expect:

Drinking Green Tea Infusion regularly can offer significant antioxidant benefits for heart health. The catechins in green tea may help reduce oxidative stress and inflammation, lower blood pressure, and improve cholesterol levels, all of which contribute to cardiovascular health. Additionally, green tea's mild caffeine content can provide a gentle energy boost without the jittery effects associated with stronger caffeinated beverages. Enjoying 2-3 cups of green tea daily can be a part of a balanced diet to support heart health. However, it's important to consider individual caffeine sensitivity and limit intake if you are sensitive to caffeine or have been advised to avoid it. As always, incorporating a variety of healthy lifestyle choices, including a balanced diet and regular physical activity, enhances the benefits of green tea for heart health.

Garlic and Hawthorn Berry Capsules for Blood Pressure.

Garlic and Hawthorn Berry Capsules are a natural dietary supplement designed to support healthy blood pressure levels. Garlic is well-known for its cardiovascular benefits, including its ability to lower blood pressure and improve cholesterol levels. Hawthorn berries complement garlic by enhancing heart function and circulation, making this combination a potent aid for maintaining cardiovascular health.

Ingredients:

- Powdered garlic
- Powdered hawthorn berry
- Empty capsules

Instructions:

- Obtain high-quality powdered garlic and powdered hawthorn berry. You can find these powders at health food stores or online.
- In a bowl, mix equal parts of powdered garlic and powdered hawthorn berry. The exact amounts will depend on how many capsules you intend to make. A general guideline is to use 1 part garlic powder to 1 part hawthorn berry powder.
- Once the powders are thoroughly mixed, carefully fill empty capsules with the blend. A capsule machine can simplify this process and ensure consistent dosage.
- Store the filled capsules in a cool, dry place, ideally in a dark bottle to protect them from light.

Dosage:

- The typical dosage is one capsule taken 1-2 times daily, or as directed by a healthcare provider. It's important to start with a lower dose to assess your body's response.

What to Expect:

Taking Garlic and Hawthorn Berry Capsules daily can contribute to healthier blood pressure levels and overall cardiovascular health. Garlic's natural compounds, such as allicin, help to relax blood vessels and improve blood flow, while hawthorn berry strengthens heart muscle and enhances heart function. Over time, you may notice an improvement in your blood pressure readings and cardiovascular endurance. These capsules can be a convenient and effective way to incorporate these heart-healthy herbs into your daily routine. However, it's essential to consult with a healthcare provider before starting any new supplement, especially if you have existing health conditions or are taking medications, to ensure they are appropriate for your specific health needs and to avoid potential interactions.

BILBERRY TEA FOR CIRCULATION.

Bilberry Tea is a nourishing herbal infusion made from the dried fruits of the bilberry plant, closely related to blueberries. Rich in antioxidants, particularly anthocyanins, bilberry is revered for its ability to support blood circulation and eye health. Regular consumption of bilberry tea can help strengthen blood vessels, improve blood flow, and enhance night vision and overall eye health.

Ingredients:

- 1-2 teaspoons dried bilberry fruit
- 1 cup boiling water

Instructions:

- Place 1-2 teaspoons of dried bilberry fruit in a tea infuser or directly in a heat-resistant cup.

- Pour 1 cup of boiling water over the bilberries, ensuring they are fully submerged.
- Allow the bilberries to steep for about 10-15 minutes. The longer steeping time allows for a fuller extraction of the beneficial anthocyanins and other antioxidants.
- After steeping, remove the tea infuser or strain the tea to remove the bilberries.
- Optional: Bilberry tea has a naturally tart and slightly sweet flavor, reminiscent of blueberries. If desired, you can add honey or lemon to enhance its taste.

What to Expect:
Drinking Bilberry Tea regularly can provide significant benefits for circulation and eye health. The anthocyanins in bilberries help to improve the elasticity of blood vessels, enhancing blood flow and reducing the risk of circulatory problems. These antioxidants also support eye health by protecting against oxidative stress and improving visual acuity, especially in low-light conditions. Enjoy bilberry tea daily to harness its circulatory and vision-supporting benefits. However, it's important to note that while bilberry tea can complement a healthy lifestyle, it should not replace treatments or medications prescribed for circulatory or eye conditions. Always consult with a healthcare provider before incorporating new herbal teas into your routine, especially if you have existing health conditions or are taking medications.

Hibiscus Flower Infusion for Blood Pressure.

Hibiscus Flower Infusion is a vibrant and tangy beverage known for its potential benefits in managing blood pressure levels. Rich in antioxidants, bioflavonoids, and anthocyanins, hibiscus flowers can help promote heart health by lowering high blood pressure and reducing the risk of heart disease when consumed regularly.

Ingredients:
- 2 tablespoons dried hibiscus flowers
- 1 cup boiling water

Instructions:
- Place 2 tablespoons of dried hibiscus flowers in a tea infuser or directly in a heat-resistant cup.
- Pour 1 cup of boiling water over the hibiscus flowers, ensuring they are fully submerged.
- Allow the flowers to infuse for about 5-10 minutes. The infusion will turn a deep red color, indicating that the hibiscus has released its beneficial compounds.

- After infusing, remove the tea infuser or strain the tea to remove the flowers.
- Optional: Hibiscus tea has a naturally tart flavor that some may find similar to cranberries. You can sweeten it with honey or enhance it with a slice of lemon or lime for added flavor.

What to Expect:
Drinking Hibiscus Flower Infusion daily can contribute to managing blood pressure levels. Studies have shown that hibiscus can have a positive effect on lowering systolic and diastolic blood pressure, likely due to its bioactive compounds. Enjoying this tea regularly as part of a healthy diet and lifestyle may help in maintaining cardiovascular health. Additionally, its high antioxidant content can support overall well-being by combating oxidative stress. It's important to note that while hibiscus tea can be beneficial for blood pressure management, it should not replace any prescribed medications or treatments. Always consult with a healthcare provider before adding hibiscus tea to your regimen, especially if you have existing health conditions or are taking medication, as hibiscus can interact with certain drugs.

Cayenne Pepper Circulatory Boost Tonic.

Cayenne Pepper Circulatory Boost Tonic is a stimulating drink known for its ability to enhance blood circulation and support heart health. Cayenne pepper contains capsaicin, a compound that helps to improve blood flow throughout the body by expanding blood vessels and increasing the rate at which blood circulates. This simple tonic is easy to prepare and can be a powerful addition to a heart-healthy lifestyle.
Ingredients:

- A pinch of cayenne pepper (about 1/8 teaspoon)
- 1 cup warm water

Instructions:

- Add a pinch of cayenne pepper to 1 cup of warm water. The amount of cayenne can be adjusted according to your tolerance, but it's best to start with a small amount due to its potent heat.
- Stir the mixture thoroughly until the cayenne pepper is well dispersed in the water.
- Drink the tonic slowly. If you're new to consuming cayenne pepper, take small sips to gauge your body's reaction to the heat and potency of the pepper.

What to Expect:
Drinking the Cayenne Pepper Circulatory Boost Tonic can provide an immediate warming effect throughout the body, indicative of its circulatory

benefits. You may experience a slight increase in heart rate and warmth, signaling improved blood flow. Regular consumption can contribute to better circulation, enhanced metabolic rate, and overall cardiovascular health. Cayenne pepper is also known for its anti-inflammatory properties, which can further support heart health by reducing inflammation in the body.
It's important to use cayenne pepper cautiously, especially if you have a sensitive stomach, as it can cause gastrointestinal discomfort in some individuals. Always start with a small amount to assess your tolerance. Additionally, consult with a healthcare provider before incorporating cayenne pepper into your routine, especially if you have existing heart conditions or are taking medication, to ensure it is safe for your specific health situation.

CELERY SEED TEA FOR BLOOD PRESSURE.

Celery Seed Tea is a traditional herbal remedy often used to support healthy blood pressure levels. Celery seeds contain a variety of compounds, including phthalides, which are believed to help lower blood pressure by relaxing the blood vessel walls and improving blood flow. This tea is a simple and natural way to complement dietary and lifestyle approaches aimed at managing blood pressure.
Ingredients:

- 1 teaspoon celery seeds
- 1 cup boiling water

Instructions:

- Crush the celery seeds slightly to release their essential oils. This can be done using a mortar and pestle or the back of a spoon.
- Place the crushed celery seeds in a tea infuser or directly in a heat-resistant cup.
- Pour 1 cup of boiling water over the celery seeds, ensuring they are fully immersed.
- Allow the seeds to steep for about 10-15 minutes. The steeping time allows for the extraction of the beneficial compounds from the celery seeds into the water.
- After steeping, remove the tea infuser or strain the tea to remove the seeds.
- Optional: Celery seed tea has a distinct, somewhat bitter flavor. If desired, you can add honey or lemon to improve its taste.

What to Expect:
Regular consumption of Celery Seed Tea can be a beneficial addition to a heart-healthy lifestyle, particularly for those looking to support blood pressure management. The natural diuretic properties of celery seeds may also help in reducing fluid retention, further contributing to blood pressure

regulation. While celery seed tea can be a valuable part of a holistic approach to maintaining healthy blood pressure levels, it's important to use it as part of a comprehensive plan that includes a balanced diet, regular exercise, and any prescribed medications. As with any natural remedy, it's advisable to consult with a healthcare provider before incorporating celery seed tea into your routine, especially if you have existing health conditions or are taking medications, to ensure it is appropriate and safe for your specific health needs.

Cacao and Hawthorn Berry Heart Tonic.

Cacao and Hawthorn Berry Heart Tonic is a delicious and healthful drink designed to support heart health and improve circulation. Both ingredients are celebrated for their cardiovascular benefits: cacao is rich in flavonoids that can enhance heart function and lower blood pressure, while hawthorn berries have been used traditionally to strengthen the heart and vascular system. This tonic combines the best of both, offering a tasty way to support your heart health.

Ingredients:

- 1 teaspoon powdered cacao (ensure it's pure, unsweetened cacao for the full health benefits)
- 1 teaspoon dried hawthorn berries, crushed or whole
- 1 cup hot water

Instructions:

- If using whole dried hawthorn berries, lightly crush them to increase the surface area for infusion. This can be done with a mortar and pestle or the back of a spoon.
- Combine 1 teaspoon of powdered cacao with the crushed or whole dried hawthorn berries in a tea infuser or directly in a heat-resistant cup.
- Pour 1 cup of hot water over the cacao and hawthorn mixture, ensuring the ingredients are fully submerged.
- Allow the mixture to steep for about 10-15 minutes. Covering the cup during steeping can help retain the heat and ensure a stronger infusion.
- After steeping, remove the tea infuser or strain the tea to remove the hawthorn berries.
- Optional: Enhance the natural flavors by adding a touch of honey or a dash of cinnamon. Both add warmth and depth to the tonic, as well as additional health benefits.

What to Expect:

Drinking the Cacao and Hawthorn Berry Heart Tonic regularly can contribute to a healthier heart and improved circulation. The antioxidant properties of cacao can help reduce inflammation and improve cholesterol levels, while hawthorn berries work to enhance cardiac function and support blood vessel health. This tonic is a delightful way to enjoy the benefits of these powerful heart-healthy ingredients. The rich, slightly bitter taste of cacao beautifully complements the fruity, tangy flavor of hawthorn berries, making this tonic a pleasure to drink. As with any dietary supplement, it's wise to consult with a healthcare provider before adding this tonic to your routine, especially if you have existing health conditions or are taking medications, to ensure it complements your overall health plan.

FLAXSEED AND GARLIC CHOLESTEROL-LOWERING SPREAD.

The Flaxseed and Garlic Cholesterol-Lowering Spread is a nutritious and flavorful addition to any meal, designed specifically to aid in reducing cholesterol levels. Flaxseeds are rich in alpha-linolenic acid (ALA), a type of omega-3 fatty acid, and lignans, both of which have been shown to have a positive effect on heart health and cholesterol levels. Garlic, renowned for its health benefits, can also contribute to lowering cholesterol and improving cardiovascular health. Combined with olive oil, which is high in monounsaturated fats, this spread is not only heart-healthy but also delicious.
Ingredients:

- 2 tablespoons ground flaxseeds
- 2 cloves of garlic, crushed
- 2-3 tablespoons olive oil (adjust to desired consistency)

Instructions:

- Grind the flaxseeds using a coffee grinder or a food processor until they reach a fine consistency. Ground flaxseeds are more easily digested, allowing for better absorption of their nutrients.
- Crush 2 cloves of garlic using a garlic press or mince them finely with a knife.
- In a small bowl, mix the ground flaxseeds and crushed garlic together. Gradually add olive oil to the mixture, stirring until you achieve a spreadable consistency. The amount of olive oil can be adjusted based on your preference for a thinner or thicker spread.
- Optional: For added flavor, you can include a pinch of salt, some cracked black pepper, or a squeeze of lemon juice to the spread.
- Store the spread in an airtight container in the refrigerator. Use within a few days for best freshness and potency.

What to Expect:
Incorporating the Flaxseed and Garlic Cholesterol-Lowering Spread into your diet can help in managing cholesterol levels thanks to the beneficial

properties of its ingredients. Spread it on whole-grain bread, crackers, or use it as a flavorful addition to sandwiches and salads. Regular consumption of flaxseeds has been linked to lower levels of LDL (bad) cholesterol and an increase in HDL (good) cholesterol, while garlic can help reduce overall cholesterol levels and improve heart health. Olive oil's monounsaturated fats further contribute to cardiovascular wellness. This spread combines health benefits with great taste, making it an enjoyable way to support your heart health. As with any dietary change intended to address health issues, it's advisable to consult with a healthcare provider to ensure it aligns with your overall health plan and dietary needs.

HIBISCUS AND GREEN TEA BLEND FOR HEART HEALTH.

The Hibiscus and Green Tea Blend is a powerful combination that offers significant cardiovascular benefits. Both hibiscus flowers and green tea leaves are rich in antioxidants, particularly flavonoids that have been shown to support heart health by lowering blood pressure, reducing blood lipid levels, and improving overall vascular function. This refreshing and tangy tea blend is not only delicious but also a great way to support your heart health naturally.

Ingredients:

- 1 teaspoon dried hibiscus flowers
- 1 teaspoon green tea leaves
- 1 cup hot water (about 175°F for green tea to avoid bitterness)

Instructions:

- Combine 1 teaspoon of dried hibiscus flowers with 1 teaspoon of green tea leaves in a tea infuser or directly in a heat-resistant cup.
- Pour 1 cup of hot water over the hibiscus and green tea mixture. The optimal temperature for brewing green tea is about 175°F, which helps to extract the beneficial compounds without releasing excessive bitterness.
- Allow the tea to steep for about 3-5 minutes. Adjust the steeping time according to your preference for strength and flavor intensity.
- After steeping, remove the tea infuser or strain the tea to remove the hibiscus flowers and green tea leaves.
- Optional: You can add a natural sweetener like honey or a slice of lemon to enhance the flavor. However, many enjoy the natural tartness of hibiscus and the subtle astringency of green tea without any additions.

What to Expect:

Drinking the Hibiscus and Green Tea Blend regularly can offer a range of cardiovascular benefits. The antioxidants in both hibiscus and green tea help to protect the heart and blood vessels from oxidative stress and inflammation. Regular consumption may help lower high blood pressure, reduce cholesterol levels, and improve blood flow, contributing to overall cardiovascular health. This tea blend is a delightful, heart-healthy beverage choice that can be enjoyed hot or cold, making it a versatile addition to your daily routine. Remember, while this tea can complement a heart-healthy lifestyle, it's important to maintain a balanced diet, engage in regular physical activity, and follow any treatment plans prescribed by your healthcare provider for optimal cardiovascular health.

Rose Hip and Hibiscus Heart Health Tea.

Rose Hip and Hibiscus Heart Health Tea is a vibrant and tangy infusion known for its plethora of cardiovascular benefits. Both rose hips and hibiscus flowers are rich in vitamin C and antioxidants, making this tea an excellent choice for supporting heart health. The bioactive compounds in this blend can help lower blood pressure, reduce cholesterol levels, and strengthen the cardiovascular system.

Ingredients:

- 1 teaspoon dried rose hips
- 1 teaspoon dried hibiscus flowers
- 1 cup boiling water

Instructions:

- Combine 1 teaspoon of dried rose hips with 1 teaspoon of dried hibiscus flowers in a tea infuser or directly in a heat-resistant cup.
- Pour 1 cup of boiling water over the mixture, ensuring that the rose hips and hibiscus are fully submerged.
- Allow the blend to steep for about 5-10 minutes. The steeping time allows for the full extraction of the healthful antioxidants and vitamins.
- After steeping, remove the tea infuser or strain the tea to remove the solids.
- Optional: The natural tartness of the hibiscus and the fruity flavor of the rose hips create a delightful taste, but you can add honey or a slice of lemon for additional flavor if desired.

What to Expect:

Drinking Rose Hip and Hibiscus Heart Health Tea can provide significant cardiovascular benefits. The high vitamin C content and antioxidants present in both rose hips and hibiscus contribute to reducing oxidative stress and inflammation in the body, which are key factors in heart disease. Regular consumption of this tea may help manage blood pressure levels, support healthy cholesterol levels, and enhance overall cardiovascular health. This tea is not only beneficial for the heart but also supports immune function due to its high vitamin C content. Enjoy this heart-healthy tea as part of your daily routine to reap its full benefits. Remember, maintaining a balanced diet and engaging in regular physical activity are also crucial for cardiovascular health. As always, consult with a healthcare provider before introducing new herbal teas into your regimen, especially if you have existing health conditions or are taking medications.

OMEGA-3 RICH FLAXSEED DRINK.

The Omega-3 Rich Flaxseed Drink is a simple, yet incredibly nutritious beverage that provides a significant boost of omega-3 fatty acids, essential for heart health. Omega-3s are known for their role in reducing inflammation, lowering blood pressure, and decreasing triglyceride levels. Flaxseeds are one of the richest plant-based sources of alpha-linolenic acid (ALA), a type of omega-3 fatty acid, making this drink an excellent choice for supporting cardiovascular health.

Ingredients:

- 2 tablespoons flaxseeds
- 1 cup water or juice (choose juice with no added sugars for the healthiest option)

Instructions:

- Grind the flaxseeds using a coffee grinder or a high-speed blender until they reach a fine, powdery consistency. Freshly ground flaxseeds are recommended for optimal nutrient absorption.
- Mix the ground flaxseeds into 1 cup of water or your choice of juice. Stir well until the ground flaxseeds are fully dispersed.
- Let the mixture sit for a few minutes to allow the flaxseeds to swell and release their gel-like fiber, which is beneficial for digestive health.
- Stir again before drinking. The texture will be slightly thickened due to the soluble fiber in the flaxseeds.

What to Expect:

Incorporating the Omega-3 Rich Flaxseed Drink into your daily routine can offer multiple benefits for heart health. The ALA omega-3 fatty acids in flaxseeds can help reduce cardiovascular risk factors, including inflammation and high cholesterol. Additionally, the soluble fiber in flaxseeds supports healthy digestion and can help regulate blood sugar levels. This drink is a convenient way to increase your intake of essential nutrients that support overall health and well-being. For best results, consume this drink regularly as part of a balanced diet that includes a variety of nutrient-dense foods. Always ensure to maintain adequate hydration and consult with a healthcare provider before making significant changes to your diet, especially if you have existing health conditions or are taking medications.

NETTLE AND LEMON BALM TEA FOR CIRCULATION.

Nettle and Lemon Balm Tea is an herbal infusion that combines the nutritive benefits of nettle leaves with the calming and heart-supportive properties of lemon balm. Nettle is rich in vitamins and minerals that support blood health and circulation, while lemon balm can help reduce stress and anxiety, factors that can affect cardiovascular health. This tea is a gentle, natural way to support heart health and improve circulation.

Ingredients:

- 1 teaspoon dried nettle leaves
- 1 teaspoon dried lemon balm
- 1 cup boiling water

Instructions:

- Combine 1 teaspoon of dried nettle leaves with 1 teaspoon of dried lemon balm in a tea infuser or directly in a heat-resistant cup.
- Pour 1 cup of boiling water over the herbs, ensuring they are fully submerged.
- Allow the tea to steep for about 10 minutes. Covering the cup during steeping helps to retain the essential oils and beneficial compounds in the tea.
- After steeping, remove the tea infuser or strain the tea to remove the loose herbs.
- Optional: The tea has a naturally mild and pleasant flavor. However, if desired, you can add honey or a slice of lemon to enhance its taste.

What to Expect:

Regular consumption of Nettle and Lemon Balm Tea can offer several benefits for circulation and heart health. Nettle's high content of iron and vitamins supports healthy blood flow and oxygenation of the body, while lemon balm's calming effects can help to lower blood pressure and reduce stress, further benefiting heart health. This tea blend is a wonderful addition to a heart-healthy lifestyle, providing both nutritive support and stress relief. Enjoy this tea daily, especially in moments of relaxation or as part of your morning or evening routine, to harness its full benefits for circulation and overall well-being. Remember, maintaining a balanced diet, engaging in regular physical activity, and managing stress are also crucial for optimal heart health.

GARLIC AND HAWTHORN CARDIOVASCULAR TONIC.

The Garlic and Hawthorn Cardiovascular Tonic is a potent natural remedy designed to support cardiovascular function and promote heart health. Garlic is renowned for its ability to lower blood pressure, reduce cholesterol levels, and prevent arterial plaque formation. Hawthorn berries complement garlic by improving heart muscle function, increasing circulation, and stabilizing blood pressure. This tonic combines the cardiovascular benefits of both ingredients, offering a powerful aid to heart health.

Ingredients:

- 1-2 fresh garlic cloves
- 1 tablespoon dried hawthorn berries or 1 teaspoon hawthorn berry extract
- 1 cup water (if using dried berries)

Instructions:

- If using dried hawthorn berries: Boil 1 cup of water and add 1 tablespoon of dried hawthorn berries. Simmer for 10-15 minutes, then strain the berries from the water and let it cool to room temperature.
- For the garlic: Peel and finely mince 1-2 fresh garlic cloves.
- Combining ingredients:
  - If using dried berries: Mix the minced garlic into the cooled hawthorn berry infusion.
  - If using hawthorn berry extract: Mix the minced garlic with 1 teaspoon of hawthorn berry extract and add to a glass of water.
- Consume this mixture daily. If the taste is too strong, you can add a bit of honey to sweeten it naturally.

What to Expect:

Incorporating the Garlic and Hawthorn Cardiovascular Tonic into your daily routine can support heart health in several ways. You may notice improvements in blood pressure levels, a reduction in cholesterol, and overall enhanced cardiovascular function. Garlic's sulfur compounds, such as allicin, provide potent antioxidant and anti-inflammatory benefits, while hawthorn's bioflavonoids and oligomeric proanthocyanidins help to strengthen heart function and blood vessels.

It's important to introduce this tonic gradually into your diet and monitor your body's response, as both garlic and hawthorn can interact with certain medications, particularly blood thinners and heart medications. Always consult with a healthcare provider before starting any new health regimen, especially if you have pre-existing health conditions or are taking medication.

Respiratory Health Remedies.

Elderflower Tea for Respiratory Health.

Elderflower Tea is a gentle and aromatic beverage known for its beneficial effects on respiratory health. The delicate blossoms of the elder tree are rich in compounds that can help soothe irritation and inflammation in the respiratory tract, making it an excellent choice for relief during colds, coughs, and other respiratory ailments.

Ingredients:

- 1 tablespoon dried elderflowers
- 1 cup hot water

Instructions:

- Place 1 tablespoon of dried elderflowers in a tea infuser or directly in a cup.
- Pour 1 cup of boiling water over the elderflowers, ensuring they are fully submerged.
- Allow the elderflowers to infuse in the hot water for about 15 minutes. This steeping time allows the water to extract the elderflowers' beneficial properties effectively.
- If you used a tea infuser, remove it from the cup. If the elderflowers were added directly, strain the tea through a fine mesh sieve to remove the flowers before drinking.
- Optional: Enhance the flavor and therapeutic properties of the tea by adding a teaspoon of honey or a slice of lemon.

What to Expect:

Drinking Elderflower Tea can offer relief from symptoms associated with colds and respiratory infections, such as congestion, cough, and sore throat. The tea's natural anti-inflammatory and antiviral properties help support the body's immune response and promote healing. Elderflower Tea is also known for its diaphoretic effect, meaning it can help reduce fever by promoting sweating. Enjoying this tea during the cold and flu season can be a comforting and effective way to support respiratory health and overall wellness.

Thyme and Honey Cough Syrup.

Thyme and Honey Cough Syrup is a natural and effective remedy for soothing coughs and relieving throat irritation. Thyme is known for its antispasmodic and antibacterial properties, making it beneficial for treating respiratory issues, while honey is a natural cough suppressant and soothes sore throats. This homemade syrup combines the therapeutic benefits of both ingredients, offering a gentle yet potent solution for cough relief.

Ingredients:

- 1 tablespoon dried thyme
- 1 cup water
- Equal parts honey (approximately 1/2 cup, depending on the reduction of your infusion)

Instructions:

- In a small saucepan, bring 1 cup of water to a simmer.
- Add 1 tablespoon of dried thyme to the simmering water.
- Allow the mixture to simmer gently for about 15 minutes. This process extracts the medicinal properties of the thyme.
- After simmering, strain the mixture to remove the thyme, collecting the infused water in a clean container. Let it cool down to just above room temperature.
- Measure the thyme infusion and mix with an equal amount of honey. For example, if you have 1/2 cup of thyme infusion, mix it with 1/2 cup of honey.
- Stir the mixture thoroughly until the honey is completely dissolved.
- Transfer the syrup to a clean jar or bottle with a lid for storage.

Dosage:

- Take 1 teaspoon of the Thyme and Honey Cough Syrup as needed for cough relief. Do not exceed 4-5 teaspoons in a 24-hour period.

What to Expect:

The Thyme and Honey Cough Syrup can provide relief from coughing and soothe sore throats. You should notice a reduction in cough frequency and intensity, as well as alleviation of throat irritation shortly after taking the syrup. Thyme's antimicrobial properties can also help fight the underlying infection causing the cough. This natural remedy is suitable for adults and children over the age of one year. However, due to the risk of botulism, honey should not be given to infants under one year of age. Always consult with a healthcare provider if the cough persists or is accompanied by other symptoms like fever, as it may indicate a more serious condition. Store the cough syrup in a cool, dark place or in the refrigerator to maintain its potency and freshness for up to 2-3 weeks.

Lemon and Honey Sore Throat Soother.

Lemon and Honey Sore Throat Soother is a classic, natural remedy combining the antibacterial properties of honey with the vitamin C-rich, acidic nature of lemon to relieve sore throat symptoms.

Ingredients:

- Juice of 1 lemon
- 1 tablespoon honey

- 1 cup warm water

Instructions:

- Squeeze the juice of one lemon into a cup.
- Add 1 tablespoon of honey to the lemon juice.
- Pour 1 cup of warm water into the cup and stir well until the honey is fully dissolved.

What to Expect:

Drinking this mixture can provide immediate relief for a sore throat by coating the throat and easing irritation. The lemon helps to break up mucus, while the honey provides a soothing effect. This remedy is also hydrating and can boost your vitamin C intake, supporting overall immune function.

ELDERBERRY SYRUP FOR IMMUNE SUPPORT.

Elderberry Syrup is a time-honored natural remedy known for its immune-boosting properties. Elderberries are packed with vitamins and antioxidants that can help prevent and ease cold and flu symptoms. This homemade syrup combines the powerful benefits of elderberries with the soothing properties of honey, creating a potent immune support tonic.

Ingredients:

- 1/2 cup dried elderberries
- 2 cups water
- 1 cup honey

Instructions:

- Add 1/2 cup of dried elderberries to a saucepan with 2 cups of water.
- Bring the mixture to a boil, then reduce the heat and allow it to simmer gently for about 45 minutes. This slow simmering process helps to extract the beneficial compounds from the elderberries.
- After 45 minutes, remove the saucepan from the heat. Use a potato masher or the back of a spoon to mash the elderberries, releasing more of their juice.
- Strain the mixture through a fine mesh sieve or cheesecloth into a bowl, pressing the elderberries to extract as much liquid as possible. Discard the mashed elderberries.
- Allow the liquid to cool to lukewarm before adding 1 cup of honey. It's important that the liquid isn't too hot to preserve the natural enzymes and beneficial properties of the honey.
- Stir the honey into the elderberry liquid until it's fully dissolved.
- Transfer the elderberry syrup to a clean, airtight bottle or jar.

Dosage:

- For immune support, take 1 tablespoon of Elderberry Syrup daily. During times of illness or when you feel a cold coming on, the dosage can be increased to 1 tablespoon up to 4 times a day.

What to Expect:

Regular consumption of Elderberry Syrup can enhance your immune system's ability to fight off colds and flu. Many people report fewer and less severe symptoms when they start taking elderberry syrup at the first sign of illness. Additionally, the syrup's high antioxidant content supports overall health and well-being. Elderberry Syrup is generally safe for most people, but it's wise to consult with a healthcare provider before starting any new supplement, especially for children, pregnant or nursing women, or individuals with underlying health conditions. Store your elderberry syrup in the refrigerator, where it can be kept for up to two months.

Elderberry and Cinnamon Syrup for Immune Support.

Elderberry and Cinnamon Syrup is a potent homemade remedy that harnesses the immune-boosting properties of elderberries combined with the anti-inflammatory benefits of cinnamon, sweetened with honey for a pleasant taste and additional health benefits.

Ingredients:

- ½ cup dried elderberries
- 1 cinnamon stick
- 2 cups water
- ½ cup honey

Instructions:

- Combine ½ cup of dried elderberries and 1 cinnamon stick with 2 cups of water in a saucepan. Bring the mixture to a boil, then reduce the heat and let it simmer for about 20 minutes to reduce the liquid by half.
- Remove from heat and let the mixture cool slightly. Strain the liquid into a bowl, pressing the berries to extract all the juice.
- Discard the elderberries and cinnamon stick. While the liquid is still warm (but not hot), stir in ½ cup of honey until it dissolves completely.
- Transfer the syrup to a clean, airtight bottle or jar. Store in the refrigerator.

What to Expect:

Taking Elderberry and Cinnamon Syrup, especially during cold and flu season, can help enhance immune function and provide additional protection against common respiratory pathogens. The syrup can also soothe sore throats and coughs, making it a versatile remedy for seasonal ailments.

LEMON AND GINGER MORNING ELIXIR FOR IMMUNE BOOSTING.

The Lemon and Ginger Morning Elixir is a zesty and warming beverage that combines the immune-boosting power of lemon juice with the anti-inflammatory and antioxidant benefits of ginger, sweetened naturally with honey. It's the perfect way to start your day with a healthful kick.

Ingredients:

- Juice of 1 lemon
- 1 tablespoon grated ginger
- 1 tablespoon honey
- 1 cup warm water

Instructions:

- Squeeze the juice of one lemon into a cup.
- Add 1 tablespoon of freshly grated ginger.
- Stir in 1 tablespoon of honey until it dissolves in the mixture.
- Pour 1 cup of warm water into the cup and mix well to combine all the ingredients.

What to Expect:

Drinking this elixir in the morning can help boost your immune system, aiding in the fight against colds and flu. The combination of lemon and ginger also aids digestion and boosts your metabolism, while honey provides a soothing, antibacterial effect. It's a simple yet powerful drink to enhance overall well-being.

ROSEHIP TEA FOR VITAMIN C BOOST.

Rosehip Tea is a flavorful, nutrient-rich beverage made from the fruit of the rose plant, known for its exceptionally high vitamin C content, which supports immune system health and skin rejuvenation.

Ingredients:

- 1 tablespoon dried rosehips
- 1 cup hot water

Instructions:

- Place 1 tablespoon of dried rosehips in a cup.
- Pour 1 cup of hot water over the rosehips and let them infuse for 10 to 15 minutes.
- Strain the tea into another cup to remove the rosehips.

What to Expect:

Drinking Rosehip Tea provides a natural, potent source of vitamin C, essential for collagen production, immune health, and antioxidant protection. Its tangy flavor and health benefits make it a delightful beverage, suitable for daily consumption to boost your vitamin C intake naturally.

ROSEHIP AND HIBISCUS TEA FOR VITAMIN C.

Rosehip and Hibiscus Tea is an antioxidant-rich blend that combines the high k C content of rosehips with the refreshing and tangy taste of hibiscus flowers, offering a delightful way to boost your vitamin C intake naturally.
Ingredients:

- 1 tablespoon dried rosehips
- 1 tablespoon dried hibiscus flowers
- 1 cup hot water

Instructions:

- Mix 1 tablespoon each of dried rosehips and dried hibiscus flowers in a cup or tea infuser.
- Pour 1 cup of hot water over the blend and let it steep for 10 to 15 minutes.
- Strain the tea into another cup to remove the solids.

What to Expect:
This tea serves as a potent natural source of vitamin C, essential for immune support, collagen production, and antioxidant protection. Drinking Rosehip and Hibiscus Tea can also provide other health benefits, such as supporting heart health and promoting healthy skin. Its vibrant color and tart flavor make it a refreshing beverage for any time of day.

SEA BUCKTHORN BERRY AND ROSEHIP SYRUP FOR VITAMIN C.

The Sea Buckthorn Berry and Rosehip Syrup is a potent concoction designed to harness the incredible vitamin C content and antioxidant properties of sea buckthorn berries and rosehips. This homemade syrup is not only delicious but also a powerful immune booster, promoting skin health and overall vitality.
Ingredients:

- ½ cup dried sea buckthorn berries
- ½ cup dried rosehips
- 4 cups water
- 1 cup honey (or adjust to taste)

Instructions:

- Combine ½ cup of dried sea buckthorn berries and ½ cup of dried rosehips with 4 cups of water in a large saucepan. Bring the mixture to a boil.
- Reduce the heat and let the mixture simmer gently for about 30-45 minutes, or until the liquid has reduced by half, to concentrate the flavors and nutrients.

- Strain the mixture through a fine mesh strainer or cheesecloth into a large bowl, pressing on the solids to extract as much liquid as possible. Discard the solids.
- While the liquid is still warm (not hot), add 1 cup of honey to the strained liquid. Stir well until the honey is completely dissolved. Adjust the amount of honey based on your preferred sweetness.
- Pour the finished syrup into sterilized glass bottles or jars. Seal and store in the refrigerator.

How to Use:

- Consume 1-2 tablespoons of the Sea Buckthorn Berry and Rosehip Syrup daily, directly or diluted in water, tea, or added to smoothies.

What to Expect:

This syrup offers a high concentration of vitamin C, known for its immune-boosting and skin-enhancing benefits. Both sea buckthorn berries and rosehips are rich in antioxidants, which fight free radicals and support overall health. Regular consumption of this syrup can help improve immune function, contribute to healthier skin, and provide a general feeling of well-being. The addition of honey not only sweetens the syrup but also adds its own antibacterial and soothing properties, making this syrup a delightful way to support your health naturally.

Mullein Leaf Tea for Respiratory Congestion.

Mullein Leaf Tea is a traditional herbal remedy widely used for easing respiratory congestion and improving overall lung health. Mullein, with its natural anti-inflammatory and expectorant properties, helps in loosening phlegm and facilitating easier breathing. This gentle yet effective tea is suitable for addressing various respiratory issues, including coughs, colds, and bronchitis.

Ingredients:

- 1-2 teaspoons dried mullein leaves
- 1 cup boiling water

Instructions:

- Place 1-2 teaspoons of dried mullein leaves in a tea infuser or directly in a heat-resistant cup.
- Pour 1 cup of boiling water over the mullein leaves, making sure they are fully submerged.
- Cover and allow the tea to steep for about 15 minutes. Covering the cup helps to retain the volatile oils and medicinal properties of the herb.
- After steeping, remove the tea infuser or strain the tea to remove the loose leaves.

- Optional: Mullein tea has a mild, somewhat sweet flavor. If desired, you can add honey or lemon to enhance its taste and add further soothing properties for the throat.

What to Expect:
Drinking Mullein Leaf Tea can provide significant relief from respiratory congestion. You may notice a reduction in the thickness of phlegm and ease in breathing shortly after consuming the tea. Mullein's soothing effect on the respiratory tract can help alleviate coughing and irritation. For best results, drink 2-3 cups of mullein tea daily while experiencing respiratory symptoms. Mullein Leaf Tea is generally safe for most people. However, it's important to source the dried leaves from a reputable supplier to ensure they are clean and free of contaminants. As with any herbal remedy, it's advisable to consult with a healthcare provider before incorporating mullein tea into your routine, especially if you have existing health conditions, are pregnant or breastfeeding, or are taking medications. Remember, persistent or severe respiratory symptoms should be evaluated by a healthcare professional to rule out more serious conditions.

ELDERFLOWER AND YARROW IMMUNE BOOSTING TEA.

Elderflower and Yarrow Immune Boosting Tea is a traditional remedy known for its powerful immune-boosting properties. Combining elderflower, with its antiviral and anti-inflammatory benefits, with yarrow, known for its ability to induce sweating and reduce fever, this tea is particularly effective at the onset of cold or flu symptoms.

Ingredients:

- 1 tablespoon dried elderflowers
- 1 tablespoon dried yarrow
- 1 cup hot water

Instructions:

- Mix 1 tablespoon each of dried elderflowers and dried yarrow in a tea infuser or directly in a cup.
- Pour 1 cup of boiling water over the herbs and allow them to infuse for about 10 minutes. The steeping time allows for the active constituents to be released into the water.
- Remove the tea infuser or strain the tea to remove the herbs.

What to Expect:
Drinking Elderflower and Yarrow Immune Boosting Tea at the onset of cold or flu symptoms can help enhance the immune system's response, aiding in the faster recovery by alleviating symptoms such as fever, congestion, and sore throat. Elderflower acts as a natural diuretic and anti-inflammatory, while yarrow promotes sweating, which can be beneficial in reducing fevers.

Together, they create a synergistic effect that supports the body's natural defenses. It's recommended to consume this tea several times a day when feeling under the weather to maximize its therapeutic benefits.

Astragalus Root Decoction for Immune Boosting.

The Astragalus Root Decoction is a potent, health-enhancing beverage made from the slow simmering of dried astragalus root. Renowned in traditional Chinese medicine for its capability to bolster the immune system, astragalus offers a naturopathic means of enhancing bodily defenses and establishing a threshold of protective energy.

Ingredients:

- 1 tablespoon dried astragalus root
- 4 cups of water

Instructions:

- Combine 1 tablespoon of dried astragalus root with 4 cups of cold water in a saucepan.
- Bring the water to a gentle boil, then reduce the heat to a simmer.
- Cover and let the astragalus root simmer for about 40 minutes. This extensive time ensures a well-drawn decoction.
- After simmering, carefully strain the decoction into a cup or jar, removing any astragalus root.
- Drink and enjoy.

What to Expect:

Astragalus root decoction can help boost immune system health and vitality. Studies show the root may help increase white blood cell count, important fighters against infection in the body. The root's flavor may be strong in tea form, but helped along with the sweetening of honey to taste, if need be. Be sure to enjoy this decoction drink most often around cold and flu season, for bolstering the body's defenses. Though it can be recommended for any time of year for its nutritional benefits: vitamins, minerals, and antioxidants; plus, immune enhancing and overall increasing of well-being and vitality in the body, no matter the season.

Shiitake Mushroom Broth for Immune Boosting.

The Shiitake Mushroom Broth is a savory and healing concoction that leverages the immune-boosting properties of shiitake mushrooms, renowned for their ability to enhance immune function and support overall health. Infused with herbs, this broth is not only a delight to the senses but also a powerful ally in maintaining well-being.

Ingredients:

- 1 cup dried shiitake mushrooms

- 6 cups water
- 1 onion, quartered
- 2 cloves of garlic, crushed
- 1 piece of ginger (about 2 inches), sliced
- Optional herbs: 1 bay leaf, a sprig of thyme, or a piece of kombu seaweed
- Salt to taste

Instructions:

- Rinse the dried shiitake mushrooms under cold water to remove any debris.
- In a large pot, combine the rinsed mushrooms with 6 cups of water. Add the quartered onion, crushed garlic, sliced ginger, and any optional herbs you're using.
- Bring the mixture to a boil, then reduce the heat to a simmer. Cover and let it simmer for about 1 hour to allow the flavors to meld and the broth to become rich and aromatic.
- After simmering, strain the broth through a fine mesh sieve, discarding the solids. Season the clear broth with salt to taste.
- Serve the broth warm, or allow it to cool and store it in the refrigerator for up to a week.

What to Expect:

Drinking Shiitake Mushroom Broth can significantly support your immune system, thanks to the mushrooms' high content of beta-glucans, compounds known for their immune-modulating effects. This broth is also comforting and can be particularly beneficial during cold and flu season or whenever your immune system needs a boost. The addition of garlic and ginger not only enhances the flavor but also adds to the broth's immune-supporting properties with their natural antiviral and antibacterial characteristics. This broth can be enjoyed on its own or used as a base for soups and stews to incorporate these health benefits into various dishes.

ASTRAGALUS AND ELDERBERRY IMMUNE-BOOSTING SYRUP.

This immune-boosting syrup combines the adaptogenic benefits of astragalus root with the antiviral properties of elderberries, sweetened with honey to create a potent natural remedy for enhancing immune function.

Ingredients:

- ½ cup dried elderberries
- ¼ cup dried astragalus root
- 3 cups water
- 1 cup honey

Instructions:

- Combine ½ cup of dried elderberries and ¼ cup of dried astragalus root with 3 cups of water in a saucepan. Bring the mixture to a boil, then reduce the heat and simmer until the liquid is reduced by half, about 30 to 45 minutes.
- Remove from heat and let the mixture cool to room temperature. Strain the liquid, pressing the berries and astragalus to extract all the juice.
- Discard the solids. While the liquid is still lukewarm, add 1 cup of honey and stir until it is completely dissolved.
- Transfer the syrup to a clean, airtight bottle or jar. Store in the refrigerator.

How to Use:

- Take 1 tablespoon of the syrup daily to support immune function, especially during cold and flu season or whenever you feel the need for an immune boost.

What to Expect:

The Astragalus and Elderberry Immune-Boosting Syrup is a powerful tool for enhancing immune health. Astragalus root is known for its ability to support and strengthen the immune system, while elderberries provide critical antioxidants and vitamins that help fight off infections. Honey not only adds sweetness but also offers additional antibacterial and soothing properties. Together, these ingredients create a synergistic effect that can help ward off illnesses and maintain overall health.

ASTRAGALUS ROOT SOUP FOR IMMUNE STRENGTHENING.

Astragalus Root Soup integrates the immune-strengthening properties of astragalus root into a nourishing and warming meal. Astragalus is revered in traditional Chinese medicine for its ability to boost the body's defense mechanisms and enhance overall vitality. Adding astragalus root slices to soups not only imparts a subtle, sweet flavor but also infuses the dish with health-promoting benefits.

Ingredients:

- 2-3 slices of dried astragalus root (approximately 10-15 grams)
- Your choice of soup base (chicken, vegetable, or beef broth)
- Soup ingredients (vegetables, protein source like chicken, beef, or tofu, and any preferred grains or noodles)
- Seasonings to taste (garlic, ginger, onion, salt, pepper)

Instructions:

- Begin by preparing your chosen soup base. If using store-bought broth, pour it into a large pot. For homemade broth, prepare it according to your recipe.

- Add 2-3 slices of dried astragalus root to the pot. If the astragalus slices are large, you can break them into smaller pieces to distribute their flavor and benefits more evenly.
- Bring the soup to a boil, then reduce the heat to allow it to simmer. Add your chosen vegetables, protein source, and any grains or noodles at the appropriate times based on their cooking needs.
- Season the soup with garlic, ginger, onion, salt, and pepper according to your taste preferences. These additional ingredients can complement the health benefits of astragalus by providing extra nutrients and flavor.
- Let the soup simmer for at least 1 hour. This slow cooking process allows the astragalus root to release its beneficial compounds into the broth.
- Before serving, remove the astragalus root slices. They are not harmful to eat, but they can be fibrous and are generally used for their flavor and health properties rather than as a food source.

What to Expect:
Consuming Astragalus Root Soup can help strengthen the immune system, making it a great dietary addition, especially during cold and flu season or anytime you feel the need to boost your immune response. The soup's warmth and nutrients provide comfort and nourishment, while the astragalus root works to enhance your body's natural defenses. This soup is a delicious way to incorporate the benefits of astragalus into your diet, supporting overall health and well-being.

Olive Leaf Extract for Immune Boosting and Antiviral Support.

Olive Leaf Extract is derived from the leaves of the olive tree and is renowned for its immune-boosting and antiviral properties. This natural supplement contains oleuropein, a compound that has been shown to enhance the body's ability to fight infections and support overall health.
How to Use:
Select a high-quality olive leaf extract from a reputable source, ensuring it specifies the oleuropein content for effectiveness. Adhere to the dosing instructions provided on the product label, as concentrations and recommended doses can vary. Olive leaf extract is available in various forms, including capsules, liquid tinctures, and powders, allowing for flexibility in how it can be incorporated into your daily routine.
What to Expect:
Integrating olive leaf extract into your daily health regimen can bolster your immune system, offering protection against colds, flu, and other viral

infections. Its rich antioxidant content also provides cellular protection against oxidative stress, contributing to long-term health and prevention of chronic conditions. Additionally, olive leaf extract has been linked to cardiovascular benefits, such as improved blood pressure and cholesterol levels, due to its anti-inflammatory and antioxidative properties. The extract's broad-spectrum antimicrobial effects further make it an excellent supplement for enhancing your body's defenses. As with introducing any new supplement, consulting with a healthcare professional beforehand is recommended, especially for those with existing health conditions or those taking other medications, to ensure safety and appropriateness.

REISHI MUSHROOM IMMUNE ELIXIR.

The Reishi Mushroom Immune Elixir is a powerful tonic derived from simmering reishi mushroom slices, a medicinal mushroom revered for centuries in traditional medicine for its immune-boosting properties and potential to promote longevity. Known as the "mushroom of immortality," reishi is rich in compounds that support immune function, reduce stress, and enhance overall health.

Ingredients:

- A handful of dried reishi mushroom slices
- 4 cups of water

Instructions:

- Place a handful of dried reishi mushroom slices in a pot with 4 cups of water.
- Bring the water to a boil, then reduce the heat to a simmer.
- Let the reishi slices simmer for at least 2 hours. The longer you simmer the mushrooms, the more concentrated the decoction will become.
- After simmering, strain the liquid to remove the mushroom slices, resulting in a dark, richly flavored decoction.
- Serve the elixir warm, or allow it to cool and store it in the refrigerator for later use.

What to Expect:

Consuming the Reishi Mushroom Immune Elixir can significantly enhance immune system function, helping to protect against infections and diseases. Reishi mushrooms contain polysaccharides, triterpenes, and other compounds known for their health-promoting effects, including anti-inflammatory and antioxidant properties. Regular intake of this elixir may also help manage stress and promote a sense of calm, contributing to overall well-being and potentially increasing longevity. The taste of the decoction can be strong and woody, which some may find an acquired taste; however, its health benefits are well regarded. For those looking to support their immune health naturally, the Reishi Mushroom Immune Elixir offers a time-tested solution.

Eucalyptus Steam Inhalation for Sinus Relief.

Eucalyptus steam inhalation is a natural method to alleviate sinus congestion and discomfort. Eucalyptus essential oil contains compounds such as cineole (eucalyptol), which have decongestant properties and can help to clear the sinuses, reduce inflammation, and relieve nasal congestion. This method is simple, yet effective for providing quick relief from sinus pressure and congestion.

Instructions:

- Boil a pot of water and pour it into a heat-resistant bowl. Allow it to cool slightly just to ensure it's not too hot to cause steam burns.
- Add 2-3 drops of eucalyptus essential oil to the hot water. Ensure to use therapeutic-grade essential oil and avoid touching your face or eyes after handling the oil.
- Lean over the bowl and drape a towel over your head and the bowl to trap the steam.
- Close your eyes to avoid irritation and inhale the steam deeply through your nose for 5-10 minutes. Take breaks if needed, especially if the sensation is too intense.
- After inhaling the steam, gently blow your nose to clear out loosened mucus.

What to Expect:

Inhaling eucalyptus-infused steam can provide immediate relief by opening the nasal passages and clearing the sinuses. The warm steam helps to moisten the nasal passages, loosen mucus, and reduce the symptoms of congestion. Eucalyptus oil's anti-inflammatory properties can also help to soothe irritation in the nasal passages.

This method can be particularly beneficial during cold and flu season or for those with chronic sinus issues. For best results, you can perform eucalyptus steam inhalation once or twice a day as needed during periods of congestion. However, it's important to use caution with hot water to avoid burns and to test for any sensitivity to eucalyptus oil by inhaling a small amount before proceeding with a full session. If you have asthma or other respiratory conditions, consult with a healthcare provider before trying steam inhalation, as it may not be suitable for everyone.

Licorice Root Decoction for Sore Throat.

Licorice Root Decoction is a traditional remedy known for its soothing effect on sore throats. Licorice root contains glycyrrhizin, a compound that can

help reduce inflammation, soothe irritation, and alleviate pain, making it an excellent natural treatment for sore throats and other respiratory ailments.
Ingredients:

- 1 tablespoon dried licorice root
- 1 cup water

Instructions:

- Combine 1 tablespoon of dried licorice root with 1 cup of water in a small saucepan.
- Bring the mixture to a boil, then reduce the heat and allow it to simmer gently for about 30 minutes. This long simmering time helps to extract the beneficial compounds from the licorice root into the water.
- After simmering, strain the decoction to remove the licorice root pieces, leaving a clear liquid.
- Allow the decoction to cool to a comfortable drinking temperature.

What to Expect:
Drinking Licorice Root Decoction can provide quick relief for a sore throat. The soothing properties of licorice root can help to coat and calm the throat, reducing irritation and pain. Additionally, licorice root has mild antiviral and antimicrobial properties that can support the healing process of throat infections.
It's important to note that while licorice root is effective for sore throat relief, excessive consumption should be avoided, especially by those with high blood pressure, heart disease, or kidney disease, due to the potential for glycyrrhizin to cause water retention and increase blood pressure. Pregnant and nursing women should also avoid licorice root. As with any natural remedy, it's advisable to consult with a healthcare provider before incorporating licorice root decoction into your regimen, especially if you have existing health conditions or are taking medications. Drink this decoction as needed for sore throat relief, but limit your intake to avoid potential side effects.

CINNAMON AND HONEY IMMUNE BOOSTER.

The Cinnamon and Honey Immune Booster is a simple yet powerful concoction that harnesses the natural antibacterial and antioxidant properties of both ingredients. This mixture is known for its ability to support immune health, reduce inflammation, and provide a host of antioxidant benefits. Regular consumption can help fortify the body's defenses, especially during colder months or periods of increased stress.
Ingredients:

- 1 tablespoon cinnamon powder
- 2 tablespoons honey

Instructions:

- In a small bowl, mix 1 tablespoon of cinnamon powder with 2 tablespoons of honey until you achieve a smooth consistency.
- Store the mixture in an airtight container at room temperature.

How to Use:

- Consume 1 teaspoon of the Cinnamon and Honey Immune Booster mixture daily, either directly or mixed into a warm cup of water or tea.
- For an extra boost, you can take this mixture in the morning on an empty stomach or before bedtime.

What to Expect:

Incorporating the Cinnamon and Honey Immune Booster into your daily routine can offer several health benefits. Cinnamon is rich in anti-inflammatory compounds that can help reduce the risk of disease and infection, while honey is known for its antimicrobial properties that can enhance immune function. Together, they create a potent blend that not only boosts the immune system but also provides a sweet and spicy flavor that is both comforting and warming. This natural remedy is a delightful way to support your health and well-being throughout the year.

LICORICE AND MARSHMALLOW ROOT SYRUP FOR COUGH.

Licorice and Marshmallow Root Syrup is a natural remedy designed to soothe and alleviate cough symptoms. Licorice root has expectorant and anti-inflammatory properties, aiding in loosening mucus and soothing irritated throat tissues. Marshmallow root, rich in mucilage, forms a protective layer on the throat, further easing coughs and soreness. Combined with honey, known for its antibacterial and soothing effects, this syrup is a powerful remedy for coughs and throat irritation.

Ingredients:

- 1 tablespoon dried licorice root
- 1 tablespoon dried marshmallow root
- 2 cups water
- Honey (to taste, but typically about ½ cup)

Instructions:

- Combine 1 tablespoon of dried licorice root and 1 tablespoon of dried marshmallow root with 2 cups of water in a medium saucepan.
- Bring the mixture to a boil, then reduce the heat and simmer gently for about 30 minutes, allowing the water to reduce by half and the herbal properties to be fully extracted.
- After simmering, strain the liquid to remove the herb particles, transferring the clear liquid to a heat-resistant container.
- While the liquid is still warm (but not too hot), add honey to taste. A typical ratio is about ½ cup of honey for the reduced liquid, but you

can adjust this based on your preference for sweetness and consistency.

- Stir the mixture well until the honey is fully dissolved and incorporated into the herbal liquid.
- Allow the syrup to cool before transferring it to a clean, airtight bottle or jar for storage.

What to Expect:

Using Licorice and Marshmallow Root Syrup can provide significant relief from coughs and throat irritation. The syrup works by coating the throat, easing the cough reflex, and soothing inflammation. Additionally, the antimicrobial properties of honey complement the herbal benefits, offering a mild infection-fighting boost.

This syrup can be taken as needed, with a typical dosage being 1-2 teaspoons every few hours for cough relief. However, because licorice root can affect blood pressure and other conditions, it's important to use this remedy judiciously and consult a healthcare provider if you have hypertension, heart disease, or are pregnant, breastfeeding, or taking medications.

Store the syrup in the refrigerator, where it can be kept for up to a couple of weeks. Shake well before each use, as natural separation may occur.

MULLEIN AND PLANTAIN LEAF TEA FOR LUNG SUPPORT.

Mullein and Plantain Leaf Tea is a beneficial herbal infusion aimed at supporting lung health. Both mullein and plantain leaves are revered in herbal medicine for their respiratory benefits. Mullein is known for its soothing effect on the bronchial tubes and its ability to reduce inflammation, making it ideal for coughs and respiratory irritation. Plantain leaves, on the other hand, have expectorant properties that help in clearing mucus from the lungs, as well as antibacterial effects that can aid in combating infections.

Ingredients:

- 1 teaspoon dried mullein leaves
- 1 teaspoon dried plantain leaves
- 1 cup boiling water

Instructions:

- Combine 1 teaspoon of dried mullein leaves with 1 teaspoon of dried plantain leaves in a tea infuser or directly in a heat-resistant cup.
- Pour 1 cup of boiling water over the herbal mixture, making sure the leaves are fully submerged.
- Cover and allow the tea to steep for about 10-15 minutes. Covering the cup during steeping helps to preserve the volatile oils and beneficial compounds in the tea.
- After steeping, remove the tea infuser or strain the tea to remove the loose leaves.

- Optional: The tea has a natural, earthy flavor. If desired, you can add honey or lemon to enhance its taste, though many find it pleasant and soothing on its own.

What to Expect:
Drinking Mullein and Plantain Leaf Tea can offer relief for various respiratory issues, such as coughs, congestion, and irritation. The soothing properties of mullein combined with the mucus-clearing and antibacterial effects of plantain can significantly support lung health and ease breathing. Regular consumption of this tea, especially during times of respiratory distress or during cold and flu season, can help maintain healthy lung function and protect against irritation.
While this tea is generally safe for most individuals, it's always a good idea to consult with a healthcare provider before incorporating new herbal remedies into your routine, especially if you have existing health conditions or are taking medications. Enjoy this lung-supporting tea as part of a holistic approach to respiratory health.

PINE NEEDLE STEAM INHALATION FOR CONGESTION.

Pine Needle Steam Inhalation is an effective natural remedy used to relieve nasal and chest congestion. The essential oils in pine needles, including pinene, have decongestant properties that can help to open airways, loosen mucus, and ease breathing. This method harnesses the therapeutic benefits of pine to provide relief from colds, coughs, and sinus congestion.
Instructions:

- Bring a pot of water to a boil and then remove it from the heat. You'll need enough water to fill a large bowl, so approximately 2-4 cups should suffice.
- Add a handful of fresh pine needles to the hot water. If you have a specific type of pine in mind, make sure it's safe for inhalation, as some types can be toxic.
- Lean over the bowl and cover your head and the bowl with a large towel to trap the steam.
- Close your eyes to avoid irritation from the essential oils and inhale deeply through your nose for 5-10 minutes. Take breaks as needed if the heat or the scent becomes too intense.
- After inhaling the steam, gently blow your nose to clear out loosened mucus.

What to Expect:
The steam inhalation process helps to moisturize and open nasal passages, while the pine needle essential oils work to reduce inflammation and congestion in the respiratory tract. This can lead to immediate relief from

congestion, making it easier to breathe. The warmth from the steam also soothes irritation in the nasal passages and throat. It's important to use caution when handling boiling water to avoid burns, and to ensure that the pine needles you use are from non-toxic species. Additionally, people with asthma or other respiratory conditions should consult a healthcare provider before trying steam inhalation, as it may not be suitable for everyone. This natural remedy can be used once or twice daily as needed for congestion relief. Always stay hydrated and consider pairing steam inhalation with other remedies and treatments to fully address the underlying cause of your congestion.

HYSSOP DECOCTION FOR RESPIRATORY RELIEF.

Hyssop Decoction is a traditional herbal remedy used for centuries to alleviate respiratory conditions, including bronchitis, coughs, and congestion. Hyssop, a herb with potent expectorant, antiviral, and antibacterial properties, helps to clear mucus from the lungs, soothe irritated respiratory tracts, and combat infections. This decoction offers a natural way to support lung health and ease breathing difficulties.

Ingredients:

- 2 tablespoons dried hyssop
- 2 cups water

Instructions:

- Add 2 tablespoons of dried hyssop to 2 cups of water in a medium saucepan.
- Bring the mixture to a boil, then reduce the heat and allow it to simmer gently for about 20-30 minutes. This process extracts the active compounds from the hyssop, creating a potent medicinal liquid.
- After simmering, strain the liquid to remove the hyssop, leaving a clear decoction.
- Allow the decoction to cool to a comfortable drinking temperature.

What to Expect:

Drinking Hyssop Decoction can provide relief for various respiratory conditions. Its expectorant action helps to loosen and expel mucus, making it easier to breathe and reducing coughing spells. The antiviral and antibacterial properties of hyssop can also help in fighting off respiratory infections.

For respiratory relief, drink a warm cup of hyssop decoction 2-3 times daily. Since hyssop can stimulate the respiratory system, it's essential to use it cautiously, especially for those with epilepsy or pregnant women, as hyssop can have emmenagogue effects. As with any herbal remedy, it's wise to consult with a healthcare provider before incorporating hyssop into your health regimen, especially if you have existing health conditions or are taking other medications.

Anise Seed Tea for Coughs.

Anise Seed Tea is a traditional herbal remedy known for its expectorant properties, making it effective in soothing coughs and aiding in the clearance of mucus from the respiratory tract. Anise seeds contain anethole, a compound that helps loosen phlegm and ease coughing, while also providing a sweet, licorice-like flavor that makes this tea both medicinal and enjoyable.
Ingredients:

- 1 teaspoon anise seeds
- 1 cup boiling water

Instructions:

- Place 1 teaspoon of anise seeds in a tea infuser or directly in a heat-resistant cup.
- Pour 1 cup of boiling water over the anise seeds.
- Allow the seeds to steep for about 10-15 minutes. The steeping time allows for the extraction of the anethole and other beneficial compounds from the anise seeds.
- After steeping, remove the tea infuser or strain the tea to remove the seeds.
- Optional: If desired, you can add honey to sweeten the tea and enhance its cough-relieving properties. A slice of lemon can also be added for vitamin C and additional flavor.

What to Expect:
Drinking Anise Seed Tea can provide relief from coughing and help in expelling mucus from the respiratory system. Its natural expectorant properties make it an excellent choice for those suffering from coughs, whether due to a cold, flu, or bronchitis. The tea's warm and soothing nature can also provide comfort and relief from throat irritation. For best results, consider drinking Anise Seed Tea several times a day when experiencing cough symptoms. As with any herbal remedy, it's important to consult with a healthcare provider before incorporating it into your routine, especially if you are pregnant, nursing, or taking medication, as anise seeds can have estrogen-like effects and may interact with certain medications.

Coltsfoot Tea for Cough Relief.

Coltsfoot Tea, made from the leaves of the Coltsfoot plant (Tussilago farfara), has been traditionally used for centuries as a natural remedy for coughs and respiratory discomfort. Coltsfoot is known for its mucilage

content, which soothes the throat, and its expectorant properties, which help to loosen and expel phlegm from the respiratory tract.
Ingredients:

- 1-2 teaspoons dried coltsfoot leaves
- 1 cup boiling water

Instructions:

- Place 1-2 teaspoons of dried coltsfoot leaves in a tea infuser or directly in a heat-resistant cup.
- Pour 1 cup of boiling water over the coltsfoot leaves, ensuring they are fully submerged.
- Allow the leaves to infuse for about 10 minutes. The infusion time allows for the extraction of the beneficial compounds from the leaves.
- After infusing, remove the tea infuser or strain the tea to remove the leaves.
- Optional: Coltsfoot tea has a mild, somewhat earthy flavor. If desired, you can add honey or lemon to enhance its taste, though it's quite palatable on its own.

What to Expect:
Drinking Coltsfoot Tea can provide soothing relief for coughs and respiratory discomfort. The tea works by coating the throat, reducing irritation, and helping to loosen mucus, making it easier to clear the airways. This can be particularly beneficial during cold and flu season or for those with chronic respiratory conditions like bronchitis.
While coltsfoot tea can be effective for cough relief, it's important to use it cautiously and not for prolonged periods, as coltsfoot has been associated with liver toxicity and other adverse effects when used excessively. Pregnant or nursing women and individuals with liver conditions should avoid coltsfoot. As with any herbal remedy, it's advisable to consult with a healthcare provider before incorporating coltsfoot tea into your regimen, especially if you have existing health conditions or are taking medications.

LUNGWORT TEA FOR LUNG HEALTH.

Lungwort Tea, derived from the leaves of the Pulmonaria officinalis plant, is a traditional herbal remedy valued for its support of lung and respiratory health. The plant gets its name from its lung-shaped leaves, and historically, it was used in herbal medicine under the doctrine of signatures, which suggested that herbs resemble the body parts they are intended to treat. Lungwort contains compounds that are believed to have soothing, anti-inflammatory, and antioxidant properties, making it beneficial for conditions such as coughs, bronchitis, and other respiratory ailments.
Ingredients:

- 1-2 teaspoons dried lungwort leaves
- 1 cup boiling water

Instructions:

- Place 1-2 teaspoons of dried lungwort leaves in a tea infuser or directly in a heat-resistant cup.
- Pour 1 cup of boiling water over the lungwort leaves, ensuring they are fully submerged.
- Cover and allow the leaves to steep for about 10 minutes. Covering the cup during steeping helps to preserve the essential oils and beneficial compounds in the tea.
- After steeping, remove the tea infuser or strain the tea to remove the loose leaves.
- Optional: Lungwort tea has a mild, herbal flavor. If desired, you can add honey or lemon to enhance its taste, though many find it pleasant in its natural state.

What to Expect:

Drinking Lungwort Tea can provide support for lung and respiratory health. Its soothing properties may help to ease coughs and reduce irritation in the respiratory tract, offering relief for those with bronchitis or similar conditions. The antioxidant components of lungwort also contribute to its health benefits, potentially protecting lung tissue from damage and supporting overall respiratory function.

While lungwort tea can be a helpful addition to a respiratory health regimen, it's important to remember that it should not replace conventional treatments for serious conditions. Always consult with a healthcare provider before adding new herbal teas to your health routine, especially if you have existing health conditions or are taking medications. Enjoy lungwort tea as part of a balanced approach to respiratory health and well-being.

MULLEIN AND LICORICE ROOT SYRUP FOR BRONCHITIS.

Mullein and Licorice Root Syrup is a natural concoction designed to provide relief for respiratory conditions like bronchitis. Mullein is renowned for its expectorant properties, helping to loosen and expel mucus from the lungs, while licorice root acts as a soothing agent, reducing irritation and inflammation in the bronchial tubes. Combined with honey, this syrup serves as a powerful remedy for coughs, inflammation, and discomfort associated with bronchitis.

Ingredients:

- 2 tablespoons dried mullein leaves
- 1 tablespoon dried licorice root
- 2 cups water

- Honey (about 1 cup or to taste)

Instructions:

- Combine 2 tablespoons of dried mullein leaves and 1 tablespoon of dried licorice root with 2 cups of water in a saucepan.
- Bring the mixture to a boil, then reduce the heat and simmer gently for about 30 minutes. This process allows the water to reduce by half, intensifying the concentration of the herbal extracts.
- Strain the liquid through a fine mesh strainer or cheesecloth to remove all plant materials, ensuring you have a clear liquid left.
- While the liquid is still warm (but not too hot), mix in honey to taste. A good starting point is to add an equal amount of honey to the volume of liquid you have left, but you can adjust this according to your preference for sweetness and consistency.
- Stir the mixture well until the honey is completely dissolved. The syrup should have a thick consistency.
- Transfer the syrup to a clean, airtight bottle or jar for storage.

What to Expect:

Using Mullein and Licorice Root Syrup can offer soothing relief from the symptoms of bronchitis, including cough, inflammation, and irritation in the respiratory tract. The syrup works by coating the throat, reducing cough reflex, and helping to clear mucus from the lungs. Honey not only improves the taste but also brings additional antibacterial and soothing properties to the syrup. You can take 1-2 teaspoons of the syrup as needed, up to four times a day, for cough and throat irritation relief. However, it's important to note that while this natural remedy can be effective in alleviating symptoms, it should not replace medical treatment for severe or persistent conditions. Always consult with a healthcare provider if symptoms of bronchitis worsen or do not improve with home treatment. Store the syrup in the refrigerator, where it can be kept for up to a couple of weeks. Make sure to label the container with the date it was made. Shake well before each use, as natural separation may occur.

Pleurisy Root Tea for Chest Congestion.

Pleurisy Root Tea is crafted from the roots of the Pleurisy plant, also known as Butterfly Weed, which has been traditionally used to treat respiratory ailments, including chest congestion. Its name comes from its use in treating pleurisy, a condition that causes inflammation in the pleura surrounding the lungs. Pleurisy root acts as an expectorant, helping to loosen and expel phlegm, and possesses anti-inflammatory properties that can reduce discomfort and promote respiratory health.

Ingredients:

- 1 teaspoon dried pleurisy root

- 1 cup boiling water

Instructions:

- Place 1 teaspoon of dried pleurisy root in a tea infuser or directly in a heat-resistant cup.
- Pour 1 cup of boiling water over the pleurisy root, making sure it's fully submerged.
- Cover and allow the pleurisy root to steep for about 10-15 minutes. Covering the cup helps to retain the therapeutic volatile oils.
- After steeping, remove the tea infuser or strain the tea to remove the pleurisy root.
- Optional: Pleurisy root tea has a distinct, somewhat bitter flavor. If desired, you can add honey or lemon to improve its taste, though it is often consumed plain to maximize its medicinal benefits.

What to Expect:

Drinking Pleurisy Root Tea can offer relief from chest congestion by helping to break up phlegm and facilitating its expulsion from the respiratory system. The anti-inflammatory properties of pleurisy root may also help to reduce chest pain and discomfort associated with coughing. This tea is particularly beneficial during cold and flu season or for those suffering from respiratory conditions that lead to congestion.

While pleurisy root tea can be a helpful natural remedy, it's important to use it judiciously. Pleurisy root should be avoided by pregnant and nursing women and those with cardiac conditions, as it can stimulate the heart. Always consult with a healthcare provider before incorporating new herbal remedies into your regimen, especially if you have pre-existing health conditions or are taking medications. Enjoy pleurisy root tea as part of a comprehensive approach to respiratory health, and seek professional medical advice if symptoms persist or worsen.

LOBELIA INFLATA EXTRACT FOR ASTHMA RELIEF.

Lobelia Inflata, often referred to as Indian tobacco, is a traditional remedy used for its potential benefits in easing respiratory conditions, including asthma. The primary active component, lobeline, may act as an expectorant to clear mucus from the airways and has been suggested to have a bronchodilating effect, which can assist in alleviating symptoms of asthma attacks. However, the potency of Lobelia Inflata and the risk of toxicity at improper doses necessitate cautious use.

Instructions for Use:

Lobelia extract should be administered according to the product's instructions or under the guidance of a healthcare provider. Dosage and frequency depend on the extract's strength and individual health

considerations. Generally, a small amount of lobelia extract is diluted in water or another suitable liquid for oral consumption. It's crucial to start with the lowest possible dose to gauge individual tolerance.
What to Expect:
Appropriate use of Lobelia Inflata extract may offer symptomatic relief for asthma by relaxing respiratory muscles and facilitating mucus clearance from the lungs. Relief from asthma symptoms can vary; some individuals might experience immediate improvement, while others may notice benefits with consistent use over time.
Important Considerations:

- Lobelia Inflata can cause adverse effects, particularly at high doses, including but not limited to nausea, vomiting, diarrhea, and tremors. Adherence to recommended dosages is essential to minimize the risk of toxicity.
- This herbal remedy is contraindicated for pregnant and nursing women, individuals with heart disease, high blood pressure, or a sensitivity to tobacco.
- Lobelia should not be used as a substitute for prescribed asthma treatments. Consulting with a healthcare provider before using Lobelia Inflata extract is critical to ensure its safety and appropriateness for your health situation, particularly for those with asthma or other respiratory issues.
- Informing healthcare providers about all herbal supplements being taken is important to avoid potential drug interactions.

ANISE AND THYME COUGH SYRUP.

Anise and Thyme Cough Syrup combines the potent expectorant properties of anise seeds with the antibacterial and antispasmodic benefits of thyme. This natural syrup is designed to soothe coughs, loosen mucus, and support overall respiratory health. Honey adds a soothing texture and additional antimicrobial properties, making this syrup a comprehensive remedy for cough relief.
Ingredients:

- 1 tablespoon anise seeds
- 1 tablespoon dried thyme
- 1 cup water
- Honey (1/2 cup or to taste)

Instructions:

- Combine 1 tablespoon of anise seeds and 1 tablespoon of dried thyme with 1 cup of water in a saucepan.

- Bring the mixture to a boil, then reduce the heat and simmer gently for about 20 minutes. This process allows the water to absorb the medicinal properties of the herbs.
- Strain the mixture through a fine mesh sieve or cheesecloth to remove the herbs, collecting the infused liquid in a bowl.
- While the liquid is still warm, add 1/2 cup of honey, or adjust according to your preference for sweetness. Stir until the honey is completely dissolved into the herbal infusion.
- Transfer the syrup to a clean, airtight bottle or jar for storage.

What to Expect:
Anise and Thyme Cough Syrup can provide effective relief from coughs and respiratory discomfort. The anise seeds help to break up mucus, making it easier to expel, while thyme's antimicrobial properties can help fight the underlying infection causing the cough. Honey not only improves the flavor of the syrup but also offers additional cough-suppressing benefits. Take 1-2 teaspoons of the syrup as needed for cough relief. Because this is a natural remedy, it's suitable for frequent use, but always monitor your response to the syrup. This cough syrup can be stored in the refrigerator for up to two weeks.
It's important to note that while this homemade syrup can be a helpful remedy for mild coughs, it should not replace medical treatment for more serious respiratory conditions or persistent symptoms. As with any home remedy, individuals with allergies to the ingredients or those who are pregnant, nursing, or have pre-existing health conditions should consult a healthcare provider before use.

Elecampane Root Syrup for Lung Support.

Elecampane Root Syrup is a traditional herbal remedy renowned for its effectiveness in supporting respiratory health. Elecampane root contains inulin, a prebiotic fiber, along with several compounds such as alantolactone, which are thought to have expectorant, antimicrobial, and anti-inflammatory properties. This makes the syrup particularly beneficial for people with bronchitis, asthma, and other respiratory issues, as it helps to clear mucus from the lungs, soothe irritation, and combat infection.
Ingredients:

- 2 tablespoons chopped elecampane root
- 2 cups water
- Honey (about 1 cup, or to taste)

Instructions:

- Add 2 tablespoons of chopped elecampane root to 2 cups of water in a saucepan.

- Bring the mixture to a boil, then reduce the heat and simmer for about 30 minutes. The goal is to reduce the volume by half, concentrating the decoction and ensuring the active compounds are well extracted.
- Strain the decoction through a fine mesh strainer or cheesecloth to remove the elecampane root pieces, capturing the liquid in a clean bowl.
- While the liquid is still warm but not too hot, add honey to taste. A good starting point is to add an equal volume of honey to the liquid you have left, but you can adjust according to your preference for sweetness and consistency.
- Stir the mixture well until the honey is completely dissolved.
- Pour the finished syrup into a clean, airtight bottle or jar for storage.

What to Expect:
Taking Elecampane Root Syrup can significantly enhance respiratory health. Its expectorant properties help loosen and expel mucus, making breathing easier for individuals with congested lungs. The anti-inflammatory effects can soothe irritated respiratory tracts, while its antimicrobial action helps fight off infections.
For cough and respiratory support, take 1 teaspoon of the syrup up to three times a day. However, elecampane should be used with caution, especially by pregnant or nursing women, and individuals with pre-existing health conditions should consult a healthcare provider before using this remedy.
Store the syrup in the refrigerator, where it can keep for several weeks. Shake well before each use as natural separation may occur. This syrup offers a natural, holistic approach to improving lung health and alleviating respiratory discomfort.

Pine Needle and Eucalyptus Respiratory Steam.

Pine Needle and Eucalyptus Respiratory Steam combines the powerful decongestant properties of pine needles with the soothing, eucalyptol-rich vapors of eucalyptus leaves. This natural remedy is designed to clear respiratory passages, ease breathing, and provide relief from congestion, colds, and sinus infections. The steam inhalation method helps to deliver the therapeutic compounds directly to the respiratory system, offering immediate benefits.
Ingredients:
- A handful of fresh pine needles
- A handful of fresh eucalyptus leaves (or 2-3 drops of eucalyptus essential oil if fresh leaves are not available)
- A pot of boiling water

Instructions:

- Bring a pot of water to a boil and then remove it from the heat.
- Carefully add a handful of fresh pine needles and a handful of fresh eucalyptus leaves to the hot water. If using eucalyptus essential oil, add 2-3 drops to the water instead.
- Lean over the pot and drape a towel over your head and the pot to create a tent that traps the steam.
- Close your eyes to avoid irritation from the essential oils, and inhale the steam deeply through your nose for 5-10 minutes. Take breaks if needed, especially if the steam feels too intense.
- After the inhalation session, gently blow your nose to help clear loosened mucus and congestion.

What to Expect:
Inhaling the steam from pine needles and eucalyptus can significantly help to open up nasal passages, soothe irritated respiratory tracts, and promote easier breathing. The antimicrobial properties of both pine and eucalyptus also help to fight and prevent infection. This method can be particularly soothing during cold and flu season or for those with chronic respiratory conditions like asthma or bronchitis.
It's important to use caution with steam inhalation to avoid burns. Always keep a safe distance from the hot water, and adjust the heat as necessary to make the experience comfortable.
This natural remedy can be used once or twice daily as needed for respiratory relief. However, steam inhalation may not be suitable for everyone, including small children and those with certain health conditions, so consult a healthcare provider if you have concerns.

White Horehound Cough Syrup.

White Horehound Cough Syrup is a traditional herbal remedy used for centuries to soothe coughs and clear mucus from the respiratory tract. White horehound (Marrubium vulgare) has expectorant and anti-inflammatory properties, making it an effective natural treatment for coughs, colds, and bronchitis. When combined with honey, this syrup not only enhances the medicinal benefits but also improves the taste, making it easier to consume.
Ingredients:

- 2 tablespoons dried white horehound
- 2 cups water
- Honey (about 1 cup, or to taste)

Instructions:

- Add 2 tablespoons of dried white horehound to 2 cups of water in a saucepan.

- Bring the mixture to a boil, then reduce the heat and simmer for about 20 minutes. This process helps to extract the active compounds from the horehound.
- Strain the liquid through a fine mesh sieve or cheesecloth to remove the plant material, ensuring you collect the clear liquid in a bowl.
- While the liquid is still warm, add honey to taste. A ratio of equal parts liquid to honey is typical, but you can adjust this based on your preference for sweetness and syrup consistency.
- Stir until the honey is completely dissolved into the horehound infusion.
- Transfer the syrup to a clean, airtight bottle or jar for storage.

What to Expect:
Taking White Horehound Cough Syrup can provide relief from persistent coughs and help to expel mucus from the respiratory system. The syrup works by soothing the throat, reducing inflammation, and stimulating the removal of phlegm.
For cough relief, take 1 teaspoon of syrup up to three times a day. Because this is a natural remedy, it can be used as needed but should not be seen as a substitute for medical treatment if symptoms persist or in cases of severe respiratory conditions.
Store your White Horehound Cough Syrup in the refrigerator, where it can be kept for up to two weeks. Always consult with a healthcare provider before starting any new herbal remedy, especially if you have existing health conditions, are pregnant, nursing, or taking medication.

MINT AND EUCALYPTUS CHEST RUB.

Mint and Eucalyptus Chest Rub is a natural remedy designed to provide respiratory relief and soothe symptoms of congestion, coughs, and colds. The menthol from mint leaves offers cooling and soothing properties, while eucalyptus leaves contain eucalyptol, known for its decongestant and antimicrobial effects. When combined with a carrier oil and beeswax, these herbs create a chest rub that can help open airways and ease breathing.
Ingredients:

- ¼ cup fresh mint leaves or 2 tablespoons dried mint
- ¼ cup fresh eucalyptus leaves or 2 tablespoons dried eucalyptus
- ½ cup carrier oil (such as coconut oil, olive oil, or almond oil)
- 2 tablespoons beeswax pellets

Instructions:

- Infuse the Carrier Oil:
    - Combine the mint and eucalyptus leaves with the carrier oil in a double boiler or a heat-safe bowl over a pot of simmering water.

    - Gently heat the mixture for 2-3 hours to allow the oil to infuse with the properties of the herbs. Avoid boiling. If using a slow cooker, you can set it to low for the same duration.
    - After infusion, strain the oil through a fine mesh sieve or cheesecloth to remove the herb particles, collecting the infused oil in a clean container.
- Make the Chest Rub:
    - Return the infused oil to the double boiler and add the beeswax pellets.
    - Heat the mixture gently until the beeswax is completely melted, stirring well to ensure it is thoroughly combined with the oil.
    - Once melted and mixed, carefully pour the mixture into small tins or jars.
    - Allow the mixture to cool and solidify at room temperature.

What to Expect:
Using the Mint and Eucalyptus Chest Rub can offer soothing relief for respiratory discomfort. Apply a small amount of the rub to the chest, neck, or back and gently massage it into the skin. The menthol from the mint and the eucalyptol from the eucalyptus will help to open the airways, making breathing easier, while the warmth from the rub can soothe muscle tension and discomfort.
This chest rub is a great natural alternative to over-the-counter vapor rubs, free from synthetic ingredients. However, it's important to patch test a small amount on the skin first to check for any allergic reactions, especially if you have sensitive skin or are prone to allergies. Keep the rub away from the eyes, inside of the nose, and other sensitive areas.
Store the chest rub in a cool, dry place. If properly stored, it should last for up to a year. Always consult with a healthcare provider before using herbal remedies, especially for children, pregnant or nursing women, or individuals with pre-existing health conditions.

Ivy Leaf Extract for Bronchial Support.

Ivy Leaf Extract is widely recognized for its efficacy in supporting bronchial health and providing relief from coughs. Extracted from the leaves of the ivy plant (Hedera helix), this natural remedy contains saponins, which have expectorant, anti-inflammatory, and spasmolytic properties. These qualities make ivy leaf extract particularly beneficial for treating conditions such as bronchitis and chronic obstructive pulmonary disease (COPD), as it helps to loosen mucus, reduce cough severity, and soothe the bronchial passages.

Instructions:

- Ivy leaf extract is typically available in several forms, including syrups, lozenges, and capsules. Follow the dosage instructions provided on the product packaging or as directed by a healthcare provider.
- For syrups, a common dosage is 1-2 teaspoons (5-10 ml) taken 2-3 times a day.
- If using lozenges, one may be taken several times a day as needed for cough relief.
- Capsule dosages can vary, so it's important to adhere to the recommended amount on the label.

What to Expect:

Taking Ivy Leaf Extract can offer significant relief for those suffering from bronchial and respiratory conditions. Its mucolytic action helps break down mucus, making it easier to clear the airways, while its soothing properties can help alleviate coughing fits and irritation in the throat and bronchial tubes. Users often report a reduction in the frequency and intensity of coughs, as well as improved breathing, within a few days of consistent use.

Ivy leaf extract is generally considered safe for most people, including children, when used according to the recommended dosages. However, it's always wise to consult with a healthcare provider before starting any new supplement, especially for individuals with pre-existing health conditions, pregnant or nursing women, and young children, to ensure its safety and appropriateness for their specific health needs.

COLTSFOOT AND HONEY SYRUP FOR PERSISTENT COUGHS.

Coltsfoot and Honey Syrup is a traditional remedy favored for its effectiveness in soothing persistent coughs and clearing mucus from the respiratory tract. Coltsfoot, known for its expectorant properties, helps to loosen mucus, making it easier to expel, while honey acts as a natural demulcent, soothing the throat and reducing coughing. This combination makes the syrup a potent remedy for cough relief.

Ingredients:

- 2 tablespoons dried coltsfoot leaves
- 1 cup water
- Honey (1/2 cup or to taste)

Instructions:

- Add 2 tablespoons of dried coltsfoot leaves to 1 cup of water in a saucepan.
- Bring the mixture to a boil, then reduce the heat and simmer for about 15-20 minutes, allowing the water to extract the beneficial compounds from the coltsfoot leaves.

- Strain the mixture through a fine mesh sieve or cheesecloth to remove the coltsfoot leaves, collecting the liquid in a clean container.
- While the liquid is still warm, add 1/2 cup of honey, or adjust according to your preference for sweetness. Stir until the honey is completely dissolved.

What to Expect:
Taking Coltsfoot and Honey Syrup can offer immediate and effective relief from persistent coughs and assist in clearing mucus from the respiratory tract. The combination of coltsfoot's expectorant properties and honey's natural soothing effects makes this syrup a potent remedy for alleviating cough symptoms and enhancing respiratory comfort. The syrup works by loosening mucus, facilitating easier expulsion, and soothing the throat to reduce the urge to cough. Suitable for taking up to three times daily, the dosage can be adjusted based on the severity of symptoms and individual response to the treatment. However, it's crucial to approach the use of coltsfoot with caution due to its pyrrolizidine alkaloids content, which can be harmful in large quantities or with prolonged use, making it unsuitable for pregnant or nursing women and individuals with liver disease. Always consult a healthcare provider before incorporating new herbal remedies into your regimen, especially for persistent or severe health issues. The syrup should be stored in the refrigerator and can last up to two weeks; remember to shake well before each use due to natural separation.

OREGANO AND THYME ANTIMICROBIAL STEAM.

Oregano and Thyme Antimicrobial Steam therapy combines the powerful antimicrobial properties of oregano and thyme, making it an effective natural remedy for clearing respiratory passages and combating infections. Both herbs are rich in essential oils such as thymol and carvacrol, which have been shown to have significant antibacterial and antiviral effects. This steam therapy can help alleviate symptoms of congestion, sinusitis, and other respiratory conditions by opening up nasal passages and lungs, providing relief and promoting healing.
Instructions:

- Bring a pot of water to a boil and then remove it from the heat.
- Add a handful of fresh oregano and thyme leaves to the hot water. If fresh herbs are not available, dried herbs can also be used, but fresh is preferred for their higher essential oil content.
- Lean over the pot and cover your head and the pot with a towel to create a tent that traps the steam.

- Close your eyes to avoid irritation and inhale the steam deeply through your nose for 5-10 minutes. Take breaks if necessary, especially if the steam feels too intense.
- After completing the steam inhalation, gently blow your nose to clear out loosened mucus and debris.

What to Expect:

Inhaling the steam infused with oregano and thyme can provide an immediate sensation of relief in the respiratory passages, making breathing easier. The warm, moist air helps to loosen mucus, while the antimicrobial properties of the herbs work to reduce inflammation and fight off pathogens causing infections. Regular use, especially during the onset of respiratory symptoms, can aid in quicker recovery and alleviate discomfort associated with congestion and infections. It's a natural, soothing way to enhance respiratory health without the use of pharmaceuticals. However, steam inhalation should be approached with caution to avoid burns or irritation, and it's important to consult with a healthcare provider if symptoms persist or if you have a pre-existing respiratory condition. This natural remedy is supportive of overall respiratory health and can be a pleasant addition to your wellness routine during cold and flu season or whenever respiratory support is needed.

CHAPTER 5: MUSCULOSKELETAL AND NERVOUS SYSTEMS.

HERBAL REMEDIES FOR PAIN AND INFLAMMATION.

TURMERIC AND BLACK PEPPER JOINT HEALTH MIX.

The Turmeric and Black Pepper Joint Health Mix is a simple yet potent combination designed to support joint health and reduce inflammation. Turmeric contains curcumin, a powerful anti-inflammatory and antioxidant compound, while black pepper contains piperine, which enhances the absorption of curcumin, making this blend especially effective for managing joint pain and inflammation.

Ingredients:

- 1 teaspoon turmeric powder
- A pinch of black pepper

Instructions:

- Mix 1 teaspoon of turmeric powder with a pinch of black pepper in a small bowl or container. Ensure the two are well combined.
- This mixture can be added to various meals or drinks. Incorporate it into smoothies, teas, soups, or any dish where turmeric's warm, earthy flavor would complement the other ingredients.
- For a direct approach, you can also mix this blend into a glass of warm water or milk (dairy or plant-based) and drink it, especially before bedtime or in the morning.

What to Expect:

Regularly incorporating the Turmeric and Black Pepper Joint Health Mix into your diet can help reduce inflammation associated with joint pain and improve overall joint health. The anti-inflammatory benefits of this blend may also support other aspects of health, including heart health, brain function, and digestive health. It's a natural, holistic approach to managing inflammation and supporting body wellness. Remember, consistency is key to seeing the benefits, and it's always wise to consult with a healthcare provider, especially if you have existing health conditions or take medications, to ensure this blend is right for you.

CINNAMON AND HONEY ANTI-INFLAMMATORY PASTE.

Cinnamon and Honey Anti-Inflammatory Paste is a potent blend that leverages the anti-inflammatory and antioxidant properties of both ingredients to combat inflammation and enhance overall health.

Ingredients:

- 1 tablespoon cinnamon powder
- 2 tablespoons honey

Instructions:

- In a small bowl, mix 1 tablespoon of cinnamon powder with 2 tablespoons of honey until a smooth paste is formed.
- Consume a small amount of this paste daily, approximately ½ to 1 teaspoon.

What to Expect:

Regular consumption of this paste can help reduce inflammation in the body, potentially providing relief from conditions like arthritis, heart disease, and more. Cinnamon's antimicrobial properties, combined with honey's healing abilities, also support immune health. This natural remedy is not only beneficial for its anti-inflammatory effects but also promotes general wellness.

TURMERIC AND BLACK PEPPER CAPSULES FOR ANTI-INFLAMMATORY BENEFITS.

Turmeric and Black Pepper Capsules are a powerful combination that harnesses turmeric's anti-inflammatory properties enhanced by black pepper, which increases the absorption of curcumin, the active ingredient in turmeric.

Ingredients:

- Turmeric powder
- Black pepper (ground)
- Empty capsules

Instructions:

- Mix turmeric powder with a pinch of ground black pepper. The recommended ratio is approximately ¼ teaspoon of black pepper for every tablespoon of turmeric powder.
- Carefully open the empty capsules and fill them with the turmeric and black pepper mixture. A capsule machine can simplify this process and ensure consistent dosages.
- Close the capsules.

What to Expect:

Taking these capsules regularly can significantly reduce inflammation and pain associated with conditions like arthritis, digestive issues, and general inflammation. The black pepper enhances the bioavailability of curcumin, making the capsules more effective than turmeric alone.

TURMERIC, BLACK PEPPER, AND COCONUT OIL PASTE FOR INFLAMMATION.

This paste combines the anti-inflammatory powers of turmeric with the bioavailability-enhancing effects of black pepper and the healthy fats of coconut oil, creating a synergistic blend that maximizes the body's absorption of turmeric's active compound, curcumin.

Ingredients:

- 2 tablespoons turmeric powder
- 1 teaspoon black pepper, ground
- 3 tablespoons coconut oil, melted

Instructions:

- In a small bowl, mix 2 tablespoons of turmeric powder with 1 teaspoon of ground black pepper.
- Add 3 tablespoons of melted coconut oil to the turmeric and black pepper mixture. Stir well until a smooth paste is formed.
- Store the paste in a clean, airtight jar in the refrigerator.

How to Use:

- Consume a small amount of this paste, about ¼ to ½ teaspoon, daily. It can be added to warm beverages, smoothies, or used as a condiment in meals.

What to Expect:

Using this paste daily can help reduce inflammation, relieve pain, and support overall health. The combination of turmeric and black pepper has been shown to enhance curcumin absorption significantly, while coconut oil provides a healthy fat source that further assists in the absorption of turmeric's soluble compounds. This paste is beneficial for those dealing with chronic inflammation, joint pain, or anyone looking to support their general well-being.

GINGER AND TURMERIC ANTI-INFLAMMATORY JUICE.

This potent juice combines the powerful anti-inflammatory effects of fresh ginger and turmeric roots, both of which are known for their medicinal benefits, including reducing inflammation and enhancing overall health.

Ingredients:

- 4 inches of fresh ginger root
- 4 inches of fresh turmeric root
- 2 cups of water or coconut water (optional, for dilution)
- Juice of 1 lemon (optional, for flavor)

- 1 tablespoon honey (optional, for sweetness)

Instructions:

- Peel the ginger and turmeric roots to remove the outer skin.
- Roughly chop the roots into smaller pieces to fit your juicer.
- Juice the ginger and turmeric roots. If you don't have a juicer, you can blend the pieces with a small amount of water and then strain the mixture through a fine-mesh sieve or cheesecloth to extract the juice.
- (Optional) Mix the juice with 2 cups of water or coconut water to dilute the strong flavors.
- (Optional) Add the juice of 1 lemon and 1 tablespoon of honey to enhance the flavor and support immune function.
- Stir the mixture thoroughly until the honey dissolves and all the flavors are well combined.

Serving Suggestion:

- Drink a small glass (about 2-4 ounces) of this ginger and turmeric juice daily, especially in the morning on an empty stomach, to maximize its absorption and healing benefits.

What to Expect:

Drinking this ginger and turmeric anti-inflammatory juice can support reducing bodily inflammation, leading to relief from aches, pains, and some chronic inflammation-related conditions. Ginger and turmeric contain powerful antioxidants and health-promoting properties that can also improve digestion, boost immune support, and contribute to overall health and vitality. The blend may have a back warming and somewhat pungent spice, which can be softened by the lemon's acidity and the honey's sweetness. Drink it consistently to enjoy its unique and specific medicinal positive aspects.

TURMERIC AND GINGER ANTI-INFLAMMATORY DRINK.

The Turmeric and Ginger Anti-Inflammatory Drink is a warming and healing beverage that combines the potent anti-inflammatory properties of turmeric with the digestive and immune-boosting benefits of ginger. This drink is perfect for reducing inflammation, soothing digestive discomfort, and enhancing overall immunity.

Ingredients:

- 1 teaspoon turmeric powder
- 1 teaspoon grated ginger
- 1 cup warm water or milk (almond milk, coconut milk, or dairy milk work well)
- Optional: Honey or maple syrup to taste
- Optional: A pinch of black pepper to enhance turmeric absorption

Instructions:

- Combine 1 teaspoon of turmeric powder and 1 teaspoon of freshly grated ginger in a cup.
- Pour 1 cup of warm water or your choice of milk over the turmeric and ginger. Stir well to combine.
- If desired, add a pinch of black pepper to the mixture. Black pepper contains piperine, which significantly enhances the absorption of curcumin, the active compound in turmeric.
- Sweeten with honey or maple syrup to taste, if desired.
- Stir the drink well before drinking. Enjoy it warm.

What to Expect:
Drinking the Turmeric and Ginger Anti-Inflammatory Drink can help reduce bodily inflammation, which is beneficial for those suffering from conditions like arthritis, muscle soreness, or chronic pain. Ginger adds to the anti-inflammatory effects and aids in digestion and nausea relief. This drink is also known for its immune-boosting properties, making it a great beverage to incorporate into your routine, especially during cold and flu season. The warm, spicy flavor is not only comforting but also offers therapeutic benefits.

TURMERIC, GINGER, AND BLACK PEPPER ANTI-INFLAMMATORY PASTE.

The Turmeric, Ginger, and Black Pepper Anti-inflammatory Paste is a potent combination designed to harness the powerful anti-inflammatory and antioxidant effects of its ingredients. Turmeric contains curcumin, a compound known for its anti-inflammatory properties, while ginger adds additional anti-inflammatory and digestive benefits. Black pepper contains piperine, which significantly enhances the absorption of curcumin, making this blend highly effective for reducing inflammation and supporting overall health.

Ingredients:

- 2 tablespoons turmeric powder
- 1 tablespoon freshly grated ginger
- 1 teaspoon black pepper, ground
- Water (enough to form a paste)

Instructions:

- In a small bowl, mix together 2 tablespoons of turmeric powder, 1 tablespoon of freshly grated ginger, and 1 teaspoon of ground black pepper.
- Gradually add water to the mixture, stirring continuously, until you achieve a paste-like consistency. Aim for a mixture that is thick enough to be spreadable but not too runny.
- Store the paste in an airtight container in the refrigerator.

How to Use:

- Consume about ½ to 1 teaspoon of the paste daily. You can add it directly to warm water or milk to make a drink, incorporate it into your cooking, or even blend it into smoothies.
- For an enhanced anti-inflammatory effect, you can also add a teaspoon of this paste to warm teas or dishes that complement its flavors, such as curries, soups, or stews.

What to Expect:

Regular consumption of the Turmeric, Ginger, and Black Pepper Anti-inflammatory Paste can provide significant relief from inflammation and pain, particularly for conditions like arthritis, digestive issues, and muscle soreness. The paste may also support immune function and promote overall well-being. Its natural ingredients work synergistically to offer a holistic approach to managing inflammation and improving health. Remember to start with a small amount to ensure your body's tolerance and gradually increase as needed.

TURMERIC GOLDEN MILK FOR INFLAMMATION.

Turmeric Golden Milk is a traditional Ayurvedic drink known for its anti-inflammatory and antioxidant properties. The main ingredient, turmeric, contains curcumin, a compound that has been extensively studied for its health benefits, particularly in reducing inflammation. The addition of black pepper enhances the absorption of curcumin, making this beverage not only delicious but also a powerful remedy for combating inflammation throughout the body.

Ingredients:

- 1 cup of milk (dairy or plant-based)
- 1 teaspoon turmeric powder
- A pinch of black pepper

Instructions:

- Warm a cup of your chosen milk in a small saucepan over medium heat. Avoid boiling to preserve the nutrients.
- Stir in 1 teaspoon of turmeric powder and a pinch of black pepper. The black pepper is crucial as it contains piperine, which significantly enhances the absorption of curcumin by the body.
- Heat the mixture for a few minutes, stirring occasionally, until it is warm and thoroughly mixed. Be careful not to let it boil.
- Once warm, pour the golden milk into a cup.

What to Expect:

Drinking Turmeric Golden Milk can provide soothing relief and contribute to reducing inflammation in the body. This drink is especially beneficial for individuals experiencing joint pain, stiffness, or inflammatory conditions. The warmth of the milk combined with the therapeutic properties of turmeric creates a comforting beverage that can be enjoyed any time of day, particularly in the evening as it can promote relaxation and support a good night's sleep. Regular consumption of golden milk can be a part of a healthy lifestyle aimed at managing inflammation and enhancing overall wellness. While turmeric golden milk is generally safe for most people, those with specific health conditions or on certain medications should consult with a healthcare provider before incorporating it regularly into their diet, due to turmeric's potent biological effects.

GINGER COMPRESS FOR MUSCLE PAIN.

A Ginger Compress is a traditional remedy used to alleviate muscle pain and soreness. Ginger, known for its potent anti-inflammatory and analgesic properties, can help to reduce pain and improve circulation to the affected area. The warmth of the compress also aids in relaxing tight muscles and enhancing the therapeutic effects of ginger.

Instructions:

- Grate fresh ginger until you have approximately 2 tablespoons.
- Wrap the grated ginger in a thin cloth or cheesecloth, making a secure pouch to prevent the ginger from falling out.
- Heat water in a pot until it's hot but not boiling. Remove from heat.
- Place the ginger pouch in the hot water for about 1 minute to allow the ginger's properties to infuse into the water and the pouch to warm up.
- Carefully remove the ginger pouch from the water, squeezing out excess water. Ensure the pouch is not too hot to avoid burns.
- Apply the warm ginger compress directly to the sore muscles. You can leave it on for 15-30 minutes, re-warming the pouch as necessary by dipping it back into the hot water for a few seconds.

What to Expect:

Applying a Ginger Compress to sore muscles can provide immediate relief by warming the area, which helps to reduce pain and stiffness. The ginger's anti-inflammatory properties aid in reducing swelling and discomfort, while its natural heat improves blood circulation to the affected area, promoting faster healing. This treatment is especially beneficial for muscle soreness after exercise, strains, or chronic muscle pain. It's a natural and effective way to address muscle pain without the use of pharmaceutical pain relievers.

Always test the temperature of the compress on the inside of your wrist before applying it to the affected area to ensure it's comfortably warm and not too hot. While ginger compresses are generally safe, individuals with sensitive skin should proceed with caution, as the ginger can cause irritation to some. If any discomfort or irritation occurs, remove the compress immediately. For persistent or severe muscle pain, consult with a healthcare provider to rule out any underlying conditions.

White Willow Bark Decoction for Pain Relief.

White Willow Bark Decoction is a time-honored natural remedy for pain relief, leveraging the analgesic and anti-inflammatory properties of white willow bark. Rich in salicin, a compound that the body converts into salicylic acid (similar to the active ingredient in aspirin), this decoction can effectively alleviate headaches, reduce inflammation, and soothe general aches and pains without the synthetic additives found in over-the-counter pain relievers.
Ingredients:

- 1 tablespoon dried white willow bark
- 2 cups water

Instructions:

- Combine 1 tablespoon of dried white willow bark with 2 cups of water in a saucepan.
- Bring the mixture to a boil, then reduce the heat and simmer for about 20-30 minutes. This allows the salicin in the bark to be fully extracted into the water.
- After simmering, strain the liquid to remove all solid pieces of bark, resulting in a clear decoction.
- Let the decoction cool to a comfortable drinking temperature before consuming.

What to Expect:
Drinking White Willow Bark Decoction can offer significant relief from headaches, muscle aches, and inflammation-related discomfort. Its natural salicin content acts as a pain reliever and anti-inflammatory agent, providing a gentle yet effective alternative to conventional medications. The effects may take a bit longer to manifest compared to standard painkillers, with relief typically felt within an hour or so after consumption.
While white willow bark is a natural and effective pain relief option, it's important to approach its use with caution. Individuals with allergies to aspirin or other salicylates should avoid white willow bark. Similarly, due to its blood-thinning properties, it should not be used in conjunction with blood thinners or by individuals with certain health conditions without consulting a healthcare provider. Pregnant or nursing women and children should also avoid white willow bark.
As with any herbal remedy, moderation is key, and it's advisable to consult with a healthcare provider before incorporating white willow bark decoction into your health regimen, especially if you have existing health conditions or

are taking medication. This natural decoction offers a holistic approach to managing pain and inflammation, supporting overall well-being.

BOSWELLIA RESIN EXTRACT FOR JOINT PAIN.

Boswellia Resin Extract, derived from the sap of the Boswellia tree, is a natural supplement celebrated for its powerful anti-inflammatory properties. It's particularly valued for its efficacy in treating joint pain and inflammation associated with conditions like osteoarthritis and rheumatoid arthritis. The active components in Boswellia, known as boswellic acids, are thought to inhibit inflammatory pathways in the body, thereby reducing pain and improving mobility in affected joints.

Usage:

- Follow the dosage instructions on the label of the commercially prepared Boswellia extract. The recommended dose can vary depending on the concentration of the extract.

What to Expect:

Taking Boswellia Resin Extract can lead to noticeable improvements in joint pain and inflammation. Many users report reduced stiffness and increased joint mobility with regular use. Boswellia's anti-inflammatory effects can be particularly beneficial for those suffering from chronic joint conditions, providing a natural alternative or complement to traditional pain management therapies.

While Boswellia is generally well-tolerated, it's important to consider potential interactions with other medications and the possibility of allergic reactions in susceptible individuals. It's advisable to consult with a healthcare provider before beginning any new supplement, especially for individuals with existing health conditions or those taking other medications. Unlike immediate relief painkillers, the benefits of Boswellia may accumulate over time, with optimal effects typically observed after a few weeks of consistent use.

Boswellia Resin Extract offers a promising natural solution for managing joint pain and inflammation, supporting individuals in maintaining an active and comfortable lifestyle. Its use as part of a comprehensive approach to joint health, including physical therapy, exercise, and a balanced diet, can enhance overall well-being and quality of life for those affected by joint pain.

ARNICA SALVE FOR BRUISES AND SPRAINS.

Arnica Salve is a natural remedy widely used for its remarkable healing properties, especially in treating bruises, sprains, and muscle soreness. Arnica, derived from the flowers of the Arnica montana plant, contains anti-inflammatory and pain-relieving compounds that help to reduce swelling and speed up the healing process of soft tissue injuries. When infused in a carrier oil and blended with beeswax, it creates a potent salve that can be applied directly to the skin for localized relief.

Ingredients:

- ¼ cup dried arnica flowers
- 1 cup carrier oil (e.g., olive oil, coconut oil, or almond oil)
- ¼ cup beeswax pellets

Instructions:

- Infuse the dried arnica flowers in the carrier oil. Combine the arnica flowers and carrier oil in a double boiler and gently heat for 2-3 hours to allow the arnica's properties to infuse into the oil. Do not let the oil boil.
- Strain the oil through a fine mesh strainer or cheesecloth to remove the arnica flowers, capturing the infused oil in a clean container.
- Add the beeswax pellets to the infused oil. Return the mixture to the double boiler and gently heat, stirring occasionally, until the beeswax is completely melted and combined with the oil.
- Once fully blended, carefully pour the mixture into small tins or jars. Allow it to cool and solidify before securing the lids.
- Label the containers with the contents and date.

What to Expect:

Applying Arnica Salve to bruises, sprains, and sore muscles can provide significant relief. The salve works by reducing inflammation and pain in the affected area, promoting faster healing. You may notice a reduction in bruising and swelling within a few days of consistent application.

It's crucial to note that Arnica Salve should not be applied to broken skin or open wounds due to the risk of irritation. Some individuals may be sensitive to arnica; it's advisable to do a patch test on a small area of skin before widespread use. If any adverse reaction occurs, discontinue use immediately.

Arnica Salve is a valuable addition to any home remedy kit for natural and effective treatment of minor injuries. However, for severe injuries or persistent pain, consulting a healthcare provider is recommended.

COMFREY POULTICE FOR JOINT PAIN.

Comfrey Poultice is a traditional remedy renowned for its healing properties, particularly in relieving joint pain. Comfrey, a plant with a long history of medicinal use, contains allantoin, a compound that promotes cell regeneration and reduces inflammation. This makes it an excellent choice for treating sore joints, sprains, and bruises. Applying a poultice made from fresh comfrey leaves directly to the affected area can provide targeted pain relief and support the healing process.

Instructions:

- Gather a handful of fresh comfrey leaves. Ensure the leaves are clean and free from pesticides.
- Using a mortar and pestle or a food processor, crush the comfrey leaves into a fine paste. If needed, add a small amount of water to help form the paste.
- Spread the comfrey paste on a piece of clean cloth or gauze large enough to cover the affected joint.
- Apply the poultice to the sore joint, securing it with a wrap or bandage. Be sure not to wrap it too tightly, allowing the skin to breathe.
- Leave the poultice on for up to an hour, monitoring for any adverse reactions. If irritation occurs, remove the poultice immediately.

What to Expect:

Applying a Comfrey Poultice can provide soothing relief from joint pain and inflammation. The allantoin in comfrey facilitates the healing process by stimulating cell growth and repair, which can be particularly beneficial for joint and muscle injuries. Many users report a significant reduction in pain and improved mobility after poultice application.

While comfrey is effective in treating external aches and pains, it should not be applied to broken skin or open wounds. Additionally, due to the presence of pyrrolizidine alkaloids (PAs) in comfrey, which can be harmful if absorbed in large amounts over time, it's recommended to use this remedy for short-term relief and not on a continuous basis. Pregnant or nursing women should avoid using comfrey.

As with any herbal remedy, it's wise to consult with a healthcare provider before using comfrey, especially if you have pre-existing conditions or are taking medications. Comfrey Poultice offers a natural and gentle option for joint pain relief, complementing a holistic approach to health and wellness.

EPSOM SALT AND LAVENDER BATH FOR MUSCLE RELAXATION.

An Epsom Salt and Lavender Bath is a therapeutic bathing experience that combines the muscle-relaxing properties of Epsom salts with the calming effects of lavender essential oil. Epsom salts, rich in magnesium sulfate, help to soothe sore muscles, reduce inflammation, and draw out toxins from the body. Lavender essential oil adds a layer of relaxation and stress relief, enhancing the overall bathing experience to calm the mind while easing muscle tension.

Instructions:

- Fill your bathtub with warm water, adjusting the temperature to your preference. Ensure it's warm enough to dissolve the Epsom salts but not too hot to prevent skin irritation.
- Add 1-2 cups of Epsom salts directly to the bathwater. Stir the water with your hand or a spoon to help dissolve the salts thoroughly.
- Add 5-10 drops of lavender essential oil to the bath. To promote even distribution of the oil, you can first mix the lavender oil with a carrier oil (like coconut or jojoba oil) or with a small amount of liquid soap before adding it to the bath.
- Once the Epsom salts have dissolved and the lavender oil is added, step into the bath and soak for 20-30 minutes. Use this time to relax fully, breathing in the soothing aroma of lavender.

What to Expect:

Soaking in an Epsom Salt and Lavender Bath can provide immediate relief from muscle soreness and tension. The magnesium in Epsom salts helps to relax muscles and improve circulation, while lavender oil's calming properties can reduce stress and promote a sense of well-being. After the bath, you should feel physically relaxed and mentally calm, with a noticeable reduction in muscle soreness. This bath is especially beneficial after a long day or a strenuous workout to aid recovery and promote restful sleep.

While Epsom salt baths are generally safe for most people, those with sensitive skin should start with a lower concentration of salts and essential oils to gauge their skin's reaction. Pregnant women and individuals with health conditions should consult with a healthcare provider before incorporating Epsom salt baths into their routine. Enjoy this soothing and restorative bath as a natural way to unwind and care for your body.

Herbal Remedies for Nervous System Health.

Bacopa Monnieri (Brahmi) Tea for Cognitive Function.

Bacopa Monnieri, also known as Brahmi, is a revered herb in Ayurvedic medicine, celebrated for its remarkable benefits in enhancing memory and cognitive function. Rich in bacosides, compounds that are believed to improve neuron communication, Bacopa Monnieri is thought to boost brain function, enhance learning and memory, and reduce anxiety, making it an excellent natural nootropic.

Ingredients:

- 1-2 teaspoons dried Bacopa Monnieri (Brahmi) leaves
- 1 cup boiling water

Instructions:

- Place 1-2 teaspoons of dried Bacopa Monnieri leaves in a tea infuser or directly in a heat-resistant cup.
- Pour 1 cup of boiling water over the Brahmi leaves, ensuring they are fully submerged.
- Allow the tea to steep for about 10-15 minutes. The longer steeping time allows for the full extraction of the bacosides and other beneficial compounds.
- After steeping, remove the tea infuser or strain the tea to remove the loose leaves.
- Optional: Brahmi tea has a distinct, somewhat earthy flavor. If desired, you can add honey or lemon to enhance its taste, though many prefer it plain to fully enjoy its cognitive benefits.

What to Expect:

Drinking Bacopa Monnieri (Brahmi) Tea can lead to improvements in cognitive function over time. Users may notice enhanced memory, increased focus and concentration, and reduced stress and anxiety levels. Brahmi works gradually, and consistent use over several weeks to months is typically required to experience its full cognitive enhancing effects.

While Bacopa Monnieri is generally considered safe for most individuals, it's important to consult with a healthcare provider before starting any new supplement regimen, especially for those with pre-existing health conditions or those taking medications, as Brahmi can interact with certain drugs. Brahmi tea offers a natural, gentle way to support brain health and cognitive function, making it a valuable addition to a healthy lifestyle focused on mental well-being.

Ginkgo Biloba Leaf Tea for Brain Health.

Ginkgo Biloba Leaf Tea is derived from the leaves of the Ginkgo Biloba tree, one of the oldest living tree species known for its therapeutic properties, especially in enhancing brain health and improving circulation. Rich in flavonoids and terpenoids, Ginkgo Biloba has been shown to increase blood flow to the brain, which can help improve cognitive functions such as memory, focus, and processing speed. It's also believed to have antioxidant properties that protect the brain from oxidative stress.

Ingredients:

- 1-2 teaspoons dried Ginkgo Biloba leaves
- 1 cup boiling water

Instructions:

- Place 1-2 teaspoons of dried Ginkgo Biloba leaves in a tea infuser or directly in a heat-resistant cup.
- Pour 1 cup of boiling water over the Ginkgo Biloba leaves, making sure they are fully submerged.
- Allow the leaves to infuse for about 10 minutes. This steeping time allows the beneficial compounds to be extracted into the water.
- After steeping, remove the tea infuser or strain the tea to remove the leaves.
- Optional: Ginkgo Biloba tea has a unique, somewhat bitter taste. If desired, you can add a natural sweetener like honey or a slice of lemon to enhance its flavor.

What to Expect:

Drinking Ginkgo Biloba Leaf Tea regularly can offer several benefits for brain health and circulation. Users may notice improved memory, enhanced cognitive functions, and increased mental clarity. Additionally, the improved blood circulation can contribute to overall vitality and wellness.

While Ginkgo Biloba is beneficial for many, it's important to approach its use with caution, especially for individuals on blood thinners or those with clotting disorders, due to its blood-thinning properties. Pregnant or nursing women should also avoid Ginkgo Biloba. As with any herbal supplement, it's advisable to consult with a healthcare provider before incorporating Ginkgo Biloba tea into your routine, particularly if you have existing health conditions or are taking medication.

Ginkgo Biloba Leaf Tea offers a natural and gentle way to support brain health and enhance cognitive functions, making it a valuable addition to a health-conscious lifestyle.

GOTU KOLA TEA FOR COGNITIVE ENHANCEMENT.

Gotu Kola Tea is made from the leaves of the Gotu Kola plant (Centella asiatica), a revered herb in Ayurvedic and traditional Chinese medicine known for its potent cognitive-enhancing properties. Gotu Kola is believed to improve memory, boost brain function, and reduce anxiety, making it an excellent choice for those looking to naturally support their cognitive health.

Ingredients:

- 1-2 teaspoons dried Gotu Kola leaves
- 1 cup boiling water

Instructions:

- Place 1-2 teaspoons of dried Gotu Kola leaves in a tea infuser or directly in a heat-resistant cup.

- Pour 1 cup of boiling water over the Gotu Kola leaves, ensuring they are fully submerged.
- Allow the tea to steep for about 10 minutes. This allows enough time for the active compounds in Gotu Kola to infuse into the water.
- After steeping, remove the tea infuser or strain the tea to remove the loose leaves.
- Optional: Gotu Kola tea has a mild, slightly earthy flavor. You can add honey or a slice of lemon to enhance its taste if desired, though many enjoy it in its pure form to fully appreciate its benefits.

What to Expect:
Regular consumption of Gotu Kola Tea can lead to noticeable improvements in cognitive function. Users often report enhanced memory, increased focus, and a reduction in anxiety levels. Gotu Kola's adaptogenic properties also help the body manage stress more effectively, further supporting mental clarity and well-being.
While Gotu Kola is generally safe for most people, it's important to consult with a healthcare provider before starting any new herbal supplement, especially for individuals with pre-existing health conditions, pregnant or nursing women, or those taking medications, as Gotu Kola can interact with certain drugs.
Incorporating Gotu Kola Tea into your daily routine can be a simple and effective way to naturally support your cognitive health and enhance brain function, contributing to overall mental agility and performance.

LEMON VERBENA TEA FOR NERVOUS SYSTEM SUPPORT.

Lemon Verbena Tea, made from the fragrant leaves of the Lemon Verbena plant (Aloysia citrodora), is cherished for its delightful citrus scent and its calming effects on the nervous system. This herbal tea is known to soothe anxiety, reduce stress, and promote relaxation without inducing drowsiness, making it an excellent choice for those seeking natural ways to support mental well-being and nervous system health.
Ingredients:

- 1-2 teaspoons dried Lemon Verbena leaves
- 1 cup boiling water

Instructions:

- Place 1-2 teaspoons of dried Lemon Verbena leaves in a tea infuser or directly in a heat-resistant cup.
- Pour 1 cup of boiling water over the leaves, ensuring they are fully immersed in the water.

- Cover and allow the tea to steep for about 5-10 minutes. Covering the cup helps to retain the essential oils and aroma of the tea, enhancing its flavor and therapeutic properties.
- After steeping, remove the tea infuser or strain the tea to remove the loose leaves.
- Optional: Lemon Verbena tea has a naturally sweet and lemony flavor that many enjoy on its own. However, you can add a teaspoon of honey or a slice of lemon if you prefer a slightly sweeter or more tangy taste.

What to Expect:

Drinking Lemon Verbena Tea can provide a sense of calm and relaxation, making it a perfect beverage to unwind after a stressful day or to enjoy any time you need a mental reset. Its gentle soothing properties can help ease nervous tension, reduce anxiety, and improve sleep quality when consumed before bedtime.

Lemon Verbena is generally considered safe for most people, but as with any herbal tea, it's wise to start with a small amount to ensure you do not have an adverse reaction. If you are pregnant, nursing, or have a serious medical condition, consult with a healthcare provider before incorporating Lemon Verbena Tea into your routine.

Incorporating Lemon Verbena Tea into your daily regimen can be a delightful and effective way to support nervous system health, promote relaxation, and enhance overall well-being with the added benefit of its refreshing citrus flavor.

CHAPTER 6: SPECIFIC HEALTH CONCERNS FOR MEN AND WOMEN.

HERBAL REMEDIES FOR WOMEN'S HEALTH.

RED CLOVER AND SAGE MENOPAUSAL SUPPORT TEA.

Red Clover and Sage Menopausal Support Tea is a herbal infusion specifically formulated to alleviate symptoms associated with menopause. Red clover is rich in isoflavones, plant-based compounds that mimic the effects of estrogen in the body, helping to balance hormone levels and relieve hot flashes, night sweats, and other menopausal symptoms. Sage, on the other hand, has been traditionally used for its cooling properties and ability to reduce excessive sweating and hot flashes.

Ingredients:

- 1 teaspoon dried red clover blossoms
- 1 teaspoon dried sage leaves
- 1 cup boiling water

Instructions:

- Combine 1 teaspoon of dried red clover blossoms with 1 teaspoon of dried sage leaves in a tea infuser or directly in a heat-resistant cup.
- Pour 1 cup of boiling water over the herbal mixture, ensuring the herbs are fully submerged.
- Cover and allow the tea to steep for about 10-15 minutes. Covering the cup during steeping helps to preserve the volatile oils and beneficial compounds in the tea.
- After steeping, remove the tea infuser or strain the tea to remove the loose herbs.
- Optional: The tea has a mild, pleasant flavor, but you can add honey or lemon to enhance its taste if desired.

What to Expect:

Drinking Red Clover and Sage Menopausal Support Tea can offer significant relief from menopausal symptoms. The isoflavones in red clover help to balance hormone levels, potentially reducing the frequency and intensity of hot flashes and night sweats. Sage contributes to this effect by providing a cooling sensation and further helping to manage excessive sweating. Many women report feeling a sense of overall well-being and reduced discomfort after incorporating this tea into their daily routine.

While this herbal tea can be beneficial for menopausal support, it's important to note that individual responses to herbs can vary. Starting with a small amount and monitoring your body's reaction is advisable. Additionally,

consult with a healthcare provider before adding new herbal remedies to your regimen, especially if you have existing health conditions, are taking medications, or if you have hormone-sensitive conditions, as the phytoestrogens in red clover may not be appropriate for everyone.
Incorporating Red Clover and Sage Menopausal Support Tea into your daily routine can be a natural and gentle way to navigate the challenges of menopause and enhance your overall quality of life during this transitional period.

Chasteberry (Vitex) and Black Cohosh Hormone Balancing Tonic.

Chasteberry (Vitex) and Black Cohosh Hormone Balancing Tonic is a potent herbal remedy designed to help balance female hormones naturally. Chasteberry, derived from the Vitex agnus-castus plant, has been traditionally used to alleviate symptoms associated with menstrual disorders and menopausal changes by regulating the pituitary gland's function. Black Cohosh, from the Actaea racemosa plant, is known for its ability to ease menopausal symptoms like hot flashes, mood swings, and sleep disturbances. Together, these tinctures create a synergistic blend that supports hormonal balance and overall female reproductive health.
Ingredients:

- Chasteberry (Vitex) tincture
- Black Cohosh tincture
- Water or juice for dilution (optional)

Instructions:

- Mix equal parts of Chasteberry (Vitex) tincture and Black Cohosh tincture. A typical starting dosage might be 20 drops of each tincture, but you should refer to the specific dosing recommendations on the tincture bottles as concentrations can vary.
- The mixed tinctures can be taken directly under the tongue for rapid absorption, or they can be diluted in a small amount of water or juice if preferred.
- Take this tonic once or twice daily, or as directed by a healthcare provider. Consistency is key for observing the best results.

What to Expect:
Regular use of the Chasteberry and Black Cohosh Hormone Balancing Tonic can lead to an improvement in hormonal balance over time. Women may notice a reduction in premenstrual syndrome (PMS) symptoms, decreased frequency and severity of menopausal hot flashes, improved mood stability, and overall better menstrual health.
It's important to note that while this tonic can offer significant benefits, the effects may take several weeks to become noticeable. Additionally, because

these herbs influence hormonal levels, they may not be suitable for everyone, especially those with hormone-sensitive conditions, those who are pregnant or breastfeeding, or those currently taking hormonal medications, including birth control or hormone replacement therapy. Always consult with a healthcare professional before starting any new supplement, particularly when addressing hormonal concerns, to ensure it's appropriate for your specific health situation.

Incorporating the Chasteberry (Vitex) and Black Cohosh Hormone Balancing Tonic into your wellness routine can provide a natural and supportive approach to managing hormonal imbalances and enhancing reproductive health.

BLACK COHOSH AND SAGE MENOPAUSE SYMPTOM RELIEF TEA.

Black Cohosh and Sage Menopause Symptom Relief Tea is an herbal blend designed specifically for women going through menopause. This tea combines the hormone-balancing effects of black cohosh with the sweat-reducing and calming properties of sage, offering a natural remedy to alleviate common menopausal symptoms such as hot flashes, night sweats, and mood swings.

Ingredients:

- 1 teaspoon dried black cohosh root
- 1 teaspoon dried sage leaves
- 1 cup boiling water

Instructions:

- Combine 1 teaspoon of dried black cohosh root and 1 teaspoon of dried sage leaves in a tea infuser or directly in a heat-resistant cup.
- Pour 1 cup of boiling water over the herbal mixture, ensuring the herbs are fully submerged.
- Allow the tea to steep for about 10-15 minutes. Covering the cup during steeping helps to preserve the essential oils and beneficial compounds in the tea.
- After steeping, remove the tea infuser or strain the tea to remove the loose herbs.
- Optional: The tea has a robust, somewhat bitter flavor. You can add a natural sweetener like honey or a slice of lemon to enhance its taste if desired.

What to Expect:

Drinking Black Cohosh and Sage Menopause Symptom Relief Tea can offer significant relief from menopausal symptoms. The black cohosh works by mimicking the effects of estrogen in the body, which can help balance hormone levels and reduce symptoms like hot flashes and mood swings. Sage

is known for its ability to decrease excessive sweating and hot flashes, making it particularly beneficial for night sweats.
While this herbal tea can be beneficial for menopausal support, it's important to note that individual responses to herbs can vary. It's also crucial to use black cohosh with caution, as it may interact with certain medications and is not recommended for women with a history of hormone-sensitive conditions. Always consult with a healthcare provider before adding new herbal remedies to your regimen, especially if you have existing health conditions or are taking medications.
Incorporating Black Cohosh and Sage Menopause Symptom Relief Tea into your daily routine can be a natural and effective way to navigate the challenges of menopause and improve your overall quality of life during this transitional period.

Dong Quai and Red Raspberry Leaf Tonic for Menstrual Health.

Dong Quai and Red Raspberry Leaf Tonic is a synergistic herbal blend designed to support menstrual health and alleviate discomfort associated with menstrual cycles. Dong Quai, often referred to as "female ginseng," is renowned for its ability to balance estrogen levels and improve blood circulation. Red Raspberry Leaf is celebrated for its uterine toning properties, making it an excellent herb for reducing menstrual cramps and regulating menstrual cycles. Together, these herbs create a tonic that not only supports the reproductive system but also promotes overall female hormonal balance.
Ingredients:

- 1 teaspoon dong quai root (dried and chopped)
- 1 teaspoon red raspberry leaves (dried)
- 1 cup boiling water

Instructions:

- Combine 1 teaspoon of chopped dong quai root and 1 teaspoon of dried red raspberry leaves in a tea infuser or directly in a heat-resistant cup.
- Pour 1 cup of boiling water over the herbs, ensuring they are fully submerged.
- Allow the mixture to steep for about 10-15 minutes. Covering the cup during steeping helps to preserve the essential oils and beneficial compounds in the tea.
- After steeping, remove the tea infuser or strain the tea to remove the loose herbs.
- Optional: The tea has a distinct, somewhat earthy flavor. You can add a natural sweetener like honey or a slice of lemon to enhance its taste if desired.

What to Expect:
Drinking Dong Quai and Red Raspberry Leaf Tonic can offer significant relief from menstrual discomfort and contribute to a healthier menstrual cycle. Women may notice reduced severity of menstrual cramps, more regulated cycles, and an overall sense of hormonal balance. Dong Quai's circulatory benefits also help in alleviating symptoms of menstrual stagnation, such as bloating and mood swings.
While this herbal tonic can be beneficial for many women, it's important to use caution, as dong quai can increase photosensitivity and should not be used by those with hormone-sensitive conditions without consulting a healthcare provider. Similarly, pregnant women should avoid dong quai due to its potential to stimulate the uterus. Always consult with a healthcare provider before incorporating new herbal remedies into your regimen, especially if you have existing health conditions or are taking medications.
Incorporating Dong Quai and Red Raspberry Leaf Tonic into your wellness routine can be a powerful natural approach to enhancing menstrual health and navigating the challenges of the menstrual cycle with greater ease and comfort.

Chaste Tree (Vitex) Berry Extract for Hormonal Balance.

Chaste Tree Berry Extract, derived from the Vitex agnus-castus plant, is a natural supplement widely recognized for its ability to promote hormonal balance in women. By influencing the pituitary gland, it helps regulate the production of hormones such as progesterone and estrogen, making it particularly beneficial for addressing issues related to menstrual cycles, premenstrual syndrome (PMS), and fertility.
Usage Instructions:

- Follow the specific dosage instructions provided on the chaste tree berry extract product you purchase, as concentrations and formulations can vary widely between brands.
- The extract is typically taken once daily, either in the morning or evening, depending on the product's recommendation.

What to Expect:
Regular intake of Chaste Tree Berry Extract can lead to an improvement in hormonal balance, which may manifest as more regular menstrual cycles, reduced symptoms of PMS (such as mood swings, breast tenderness, and cramping), and an overall sense of well-being related to hormonal health. Some women also find it supportive for fertility challenges linked to hormonal imbalances.

While the benefits of Chaste Tree Berry Extract can be significant, it's important to remember that results may take several months to become fully apparent. Consistency is key in achieving the desired hormonal balance.
Chaste Tree Berry Extract is generally well-tolerated, but it's advisable to consult with a healthcare provider before starting any new supplement, especially for individuals with pre-existing health conditions, those taking hormonal medications, or those who are pregnant or breastfeeding. This is particularly important as Chaste Tree can interact with hormonal treatments and contraceptives.
Incorporating Chaste Tree Berry Extract into your routine can provide a natural approach to managing hormonal imbalances, supporting reproductive health, and enhancing overall well-being. However, monitoring your body's response and consulting with healthcare professionals ensures that this supplement is a suitable and effective choice for your individual health needs.

MOTHERWORT TEA FOR MENOPAUSAL SYMPTOMS.

Motherwort Tea, made from the leaves of the Leonurus cardiaca plant, is a traditional herbal remedy valued for its efficacy in easing menopausal symptoms. Motherwort is known for its calming properties, ability to improve heart function, and effectiveness in reducing symptoms such as hot flashes, anxiety, and heart palpitations. Its name, derived from its use in childbirth and women's health, reflects its affinity for supporting female reproductive health, especially during the menopause transition.
Ingredients:

- 1-2 teaspoons dried motherwort
- 1 cup boiling water

Instructions:

- Place 1-2 teaspoons of dried motherwort in a tea infuser or directly in a heat-resistant cup.
- Pour 1 cup of boiling water over the dried motherwort, ensuring it's fully submerged.
- Cover and allow the tea to steep for about 15 minutes. Covering the cup helps to retain the therapeutic volatile oils.
- After steeping, remove the tea infuser or strain the tea to remove the loose herbs.
- Optional: Motherwort tea has a bitter taste, which might be off-putting to some. You can add honey or a slice of lemon to mitigate the bitterness and enhance the flavor.

What to Expect:
Drinking Motherwort Tea can provide relief from menopausal symptoms by promoting relaxation, reducing heart palpitations, and easing hot flashes. The

herb's calming effect can also help mitigate anxiety and improve sleep quality, making it particularly beneficial for women experiencing stress or sleep disturbances associated with menopause.
While Motherwort Tea is beneficial for easing menopausal symptoms, it's important to use caution, as it may interact with certain medications, especially those related to heart conditions and blood pressure. Pregnant women should avoid motherwort due to its uterine stimulating properties. Always consult with a healthcare provider before incorporating new herbal teas into your regimen, particularly if you have existing health conditions or are taking medications.
Incorporating Motherwort Tea into your daily routine can be a natural and gentle way to manage menopausal symptoms and support overall well-being during this transitional period. However, individual experiences with herbal remedies can vary, so monitoring your body's response and consulting with healthcare professionals is advisable to ensure the best approach for your health needs.

CRANBERRY JUICE FOR URINARY TRACT HEALTH.

Cranberry Juice, particularly when unsweetened, is a well-known natural remedy for maintaining urinary tract health. Cranberries contain compounds called proanthocyanidins, which have been shown to prevent bacteria, especially E. coli, from adhering to the walls of the urinary tract. This mechanism is beneficial in preventing the onset of urinary tract infections (UTIs) and supporting overall urinary health.
Instructions:

- Opt for unsweetened cranberry juice to avoid the high sugar content found in many commercial cranberry juice drinks. The added sugars can negate the health benefits and potentially contribute to other health issues.
- Drinking about 8 to 16 ounces of unsweetened cranberry juice daily is recommended for urinary tract health maintenance. You can adjust the amount based on your personal health goals and response to the juice.

What to Expect:
Regular consumption of unsweetened cranberry juice can contribute to a healthy urinary tract by reducing the risk of UTIs. Many individuals find that incorporating cranberry juice into their daily routine helps minimize the frequency of UTIs and enhances overall urinary comfort.
While cranberry juice is effective for urinary tract health maintenance, it's not a substitute for medical treatment in the case of an existing UTI. If you

suspect you have a UTI, it's important to consult with a healthcare provider for appropriate treatment.
Additionally, cranberry juice may interact with certain medications, such as blood thinners. If you are taking medication, particularly warfarin or similar blood thinners, consult with a healthcare provider before adding cranberry juice to your routine.
Incorporating unsweetened cranberry juice into your daily regimen can be a simple and natural way to support urinary tract health. It's a proactive measure that complements a healthy lifestyle and hydration practices.

Evening Primrose Oil Capsules for PMS.

Evening Primrose Oil Capsules are a popular natural remedy derived from the seeds of the Evening Primrose plant (Oenothera biennis), celebrated for their ability to alleviate symptoms associated with premenstrual syndrome (PMS). Rich in gamma-linolenic acid (GLA), a type of omega-6 fatty acid, Evening Primrose Oil is thought to play a role in reducing inflammation and balancing hormones, which can significantly ease PMS symptoms such as mood swings, breast tenderness, bloating, and irritability.
Usage Instructions:

- Follow the dosage instructions provided on the packaging of the Evening Primrose Oil capsules you purchase, as the concentration of GLA can vary between brands.
- Capsules are typically taken once or twice daily, with or without food, but following specific product recommendations is best for optimal results.

What to Expect:
Regular intake of Evening Primrose Oil Capsules can lead to a reduction in the severity and duration of PMS symptoms. Many women report feeling less discomfort and experiencing fewer mood fluctuations during their menstrual cycle after incorporating Evening Primrose Oil into their routine. The benefits of Evening Primrose Oil may take several menstrual cycles to become fully apparent, so consistency is crucial.
While Evening Primrose Oil is well-tolerated by many, it's essential to be aware of potential interactions with medications, especially blood thinners and drugs affecting seizure threshold. Pregnant women or those planning to become pregnant should consult with a healthcare provider before taking Evening Primrose Oil, as there is insufficient evidence regarding its safety during pregnancy.
As with any supplement, consulting with a healthcare provider before starting Evening Primrose Oil is advisable, especially for individuals with pre-existing health conditions or those taking other medications. Evening Primrose Oil Capsules offer a natural approach to managing PMS symptoms,

contributing to improved well-being and quality of life during the menstrual cycle.

Raspberry Leaf Tea for Menstrual Cramps.

Raspberry Leaf Tea, made from the leaves of the red raspberry plant (Rubus idaeus), is a time-honored herbal remedy renowned for its benefits in female reproductive health. Particularly noted for its ability to ease menstrual cramps, raspberry leaf tea contains fragarine and tannins, which are thought to strengthen and tone the uterine muscles, helping to alleviate the pain associated with menstrual cramps.

Ingredients:

- 1-2 teaspoons dried raspberry leaves
- 1 cup boiling water

Instructions:

- Place 1-2 teaspoons of dried raspberry leaves in a tea infuser or directly in a heat-resistant cup.
- Pour 1 cup of boiling water over the raspberry leaves, ensuring they are fully submerged.
- Allow the tea to steep for about 10-15 minutes. The longer steeping time allows the beneficial compounds to be fully extracted into the water.
- After steeping, remove the tea infuser or strain the tea to remove the loose leaves.
- Optional: Raspberry leaf tea has a somewhat earthy, mildly sweet flavor. If desired, you can enhance its taste with honey or a slice of lemon.

What to Expect:

Drinking Raspberry Leaf Tea can offer significant relief from menstrual cramps due to its muscle-relaxing and uterine-toning properties. Many women report a decrease in the severity and duration of cramps when consuming the tea regularly, especially when started a few days before the onset of menstruation.

While Raspberry Leaf Tea is generally safe and beneficial for most women, it's always wise to consult with a healthcare provider before starting any new herbal remedy, particularly for those with existing health conditions, pregnant women, or those currently taking medications.

Incorporating Raspberry Leaf Tea into your wellness routine can be a natural and effective way to manage menstrual cramps and support overall reproductive health. Its gentle action and nutritional benefits make it a supportive herbal ally for women at various stages of life.

Red Clover Infusion for Menopausal Support.

Red Clover Infusion is a natural remedy rich in isoflavones, plant-based compounds that mimic the effects of estrogen in the body. This makes it particularly beneficial for women going through menopause, as it can help alleviate symptoms such as hot flashes, night sweats, and hormonal imbalances. Red clover is also known for its potential to improve bone density and promote heart health, making it a supportive herb during the menopausal transition.

Ingredients:

- 1-2 teaspoons dried red clover flowers
- 1 cup boiling water

Instructions:

- Place 1-2 teaspoons of dried red clover flowers in a tea infuser or directly in a heat-resistant cup.
- Pour 1 cup of boiling water over the red clover flowers, ensuring they are fully submerged.
- Cover and allow the infusion to steep for about 15-20 minutes. Covering the cup during steeping helps to preserve the beneficial compounds.
- After steeping, remove the tea infuser or strain the tea to remove the loose flowers.
- Optional: Red clover infusion has a mild, sweet taste. If desired, you can add honey or a slice of lemon to enhance its flavor.

What to Expect:

Regular consumption of Red Clover Infusion can provide relief from common menopausal symptoms. The isoflavones in red clover help to balance hormone levels, potentially reducing the frequency and severity of hot flashes and night sweats. Additionally, its natural phytoestrogens can support bone health, reducing the risk of osteoporosis associated with menopause.

While Red Clover Infusion offers many benefits for menopausal support, it's important to note that women with hormone-sensitive conditions, such as certain types of breast cancer, should use caution and consult with a healthcare provider before incorporating it into their regimen. Similarly, because red clover can act like estrogen in the body, it may interact with hormone medications and other treatments.

Incorporating Red Clover Infusion into your daily routine can be a gentle and natural way to navigate the challenges of menopause and support overall well-being during this significant life transition. However, individual responses to herbal remedies can vary, so monitoring your body's reaction and consulting with healthcare professionals is advisable to ensure the best approach for your health needs.

RASPBERRY LEAF AND NETTLE TEA FOR PREGNANCY.

Raspberry Leaf and Nettle Tea is a nourishing herbal blend known for its beneficial effects during pregnancy. Raspberry leaf is celebrated for its ability to tone and strengthen the uterine muscles, potentially aiding in a smoother labor and delivery. Nettle leaves, rich in vitamins and minerals such as iron, calcium, and magnesium, support overall pregnancy health, enhancing energy levels and ensuring a rich blood supply. Together, these herbs create a supportive tonic for expectant mothers.

Ingredients:

- 1 teaspoon dried raspberry leaves
- 1 teaspoon dried nettle leaves
- 1 cup boiling water

Instructions:

- Combine 1 teaspoon of dried raspberry leaves and 1 teaspoon of dried nettle leaves in a tea infuser or directly in a heat-resistant cup.
- Pour 1 cup of boiling water over the herbal mixture, ensuring the leaves are fully submerged.
- Cover and allow the tea to steep for about 10-15 minutes. Covering the cup helps to preserve the essential nutrients and flavors of the tea.
- After steeping, remove the tea infuser or strain the tea to remove the loose leaves.
- Optional: The tea has a mild, earthy flavor. If desired, you can add honey or a slice of lemon to enhance its taste, though many prefer it plain to fully enjoy its health benefits.

What to Expect:

Drinking Raspberry Leaf and Nettle Tea during pregnancy can offer several benefits, including enhanced uterine health, improved circulation, and increased nutrient intake. Raspberry leaf's uterine-toning properties may contribute to a more efficient labor, while nettle's nutritional profile supports overall health and vitality during pregnancy.

It's generally recommended to begin drinking this tea in the second trimester of pregnancy, as raspberry leaf is best avoided in the first trimester due to its uterine-stimulating properties. As with any herbal remedy during pregnancy, it's crucial to consult with a healthcare provider or a midwife before incorporating Raspberry Leaf and Nettle Tea into your routine, to ensure it's appropriate for your individual health circumstances and pregnancy journey. While many women report positive effects on their pregnancy and labor experience from drinking this tea, it's important to listen to your body and adjust your consumption based on personal tolerance and healthcare advice. This herbal tea can be a valuable part of a holistic approach to pregnancy care, offering a natural way to support your body as it prepares for childbirth and motherhood.

Angelica Root Tea for Menstrual Support.

Angelica Root Tea, made from the root of the Angelica sinensis plant, often referred to as Dong Quai or "female ginseng," is a traditional herbal remedy prized for its ability to support menstrual health. Angelica root is known for its warming properties, ability to improve blood circulation, and balance female hormones, making it particularly effective in alleviating menstrual discomfort such as cramps, irregular cycles, and premenstrual syndrome (PMS).

Ingredients:

- 1 teaspoon dried angelica root
- 1 cup boiling water

Instructions:

- Place 1 teaspoon of dried angelica root in a tea infuser or directly in a heat-resistant cup.
- Pour 1 cup of boiling water over the angelica root, ensuring it is fully submerged.
- Cover and allow the tea to steep for about 10-15 minutes. The cover helps to retain the essential oils and active compounds in the tea.
- After steeping, remove the tea infuser or strain the tea to remove the loose root pieces.
- Optional: Angelica root tea has a distinct, somewhat bitter taste. You can add honey or a slice of lemon to improve its flavor, although some people appreciate the tea's natural taste for its warming and invigorating properties.

What to Expect:

Drinking Angelica Root Tea can provide significant relief from menstrual discomfort. The herb's natural compounds work to relax muscle tissues, reducing cramps, and its hormone-balancing effects can help regulate menstrual cycles and alleviate PMS symptoms. Additionally, its circulatory benefits may reduce the heaviness of menstrual flow and improve overall wellbeing during your period.

While Angelica Root Tea is beneficial for menstrual support, it's important to use it with caution. Angelica root can increase photosensitivity and should not be used in conjunction with blood thinners or by individuals with bleeding disorders. It is also not recommended for pregnant women due to its potential to stimulate the uterus. Always consult with a healthcare provider before starting any new herbal remedy, especially if you have existing health conditions or are taking medication.

Incorporating Angelica Root Tea into your routine can be a natural and effective way to manage menstrual discomfort and support reproductive health. However, individual responses to herbal remedies can vary, so monitoring your body's reaction and consulting with healthcare professionals is advisable to ensure the best approach for your health needs.

FENUGREEK SEED INFUSION FOR LACTATION SUPPORT.

Fenugreek Seed Infusion is a widely recommended herbal remedy for breastfeeding mothers seeking to enhance milk production. Fenugreek seeds are high in phytoestrogens and diosgenin, which are thought to mimic the effects of estrogen in the body, stimulating milk ducts and enhancing lactation. This natural approach has been used for centuries across various cultures due to its effectiveness and general safety.

Ingredients:

- 1-2 tablespoons fenugreek seeds
- 1 cup boiling water

Instructions:

- Place 1-2 tablespoons of fenugreek seeds in a tea infuser or directly in a heat-resistant cup.
- Pour 1 cup of boiling water over the fenugreek seeds, ensuring they are fully submerged.
- Cover and allow the seeds to steep for about 10-15 minutes. Covering the cup helps to retain the heat and ensures a strong infusion.
- After steeping, remove the tea infuser or strain the infusion to remove the seeds.
- Optional: Fenugreek seed infusion has a distinctive, somewhat bitter taste. You can add honey or lemon to improve its flavor, though many find the natural sweetness of the seeds to be pleasant enough on its own.

What to Expect:

Regular consumption of Fenugreek Seed Infusion can lead to an increase in milk production within a few days to a week. Many breastfeeding mothers report significant improvements in their milk supply, which can help support the nutritional needs of their infants.

While fenugreek is generally safe for most individuals, it's important to start with a small amount to monitor your body's response. Some may experience mild gastrointestinal symptoms, and fenugreek can also affect the smell of urine, giving it a maple syrup-like odor. Pregnant women should avoid fenugreek due to its potential uterine stimulating effects. Additionally,

individuals with diabetes should be cautious, as fenugreek can lower blood sugar levels.
As with any supplement intended to affect milk supply, consulting with a lactation consultant or healthcare provider is advisable before starting fenugreek, especially if you have pre-existing conditions or are taking medications. Fenugreek Seed Infusion offers a natural, effective way to support lactation and enhance the breastfeeding experience.

Dong Quai and Red Clover Tea for Hormonal Balance.

Dong Quai and Red Clover Tea is a herbal blend specifically designed to support hormonal balance and overall women's health. Dong Quai, often called "female ginseng," is revered in traditional Chinese medicine for its ability to nourish the blood and balance female hormones, making it beneficial for menstrual irregularities and menopausal symptoms. Red Clover is rich in isoflavones, plant-based compounds that mimic estrogen, helping to alleviate menopausal symptoms such as hot flashes and osteoporosis risk.
Ingredients:

- 1 teaspoon dried Dong Quai root
- 1 teaspoon dried Red Clover flowers
- 1 cup boiling water

Instructions:

- Combine 1 teaspoon of dried Dong Quai root and 1 teaspoon of dried Red Clover flowers in a tea infuser or directly in a heat-resistant cup.
- Pour 1 cup of boiling water over the herbs, ensuring they are fully submerged.
- Cover and allow the tea to steep for about 15-20 minutes. The longer steeping time allows for the full extraction of beneficial compounds.
- After steeping, remove the tea infuser or strain the tea to remove the loose herbs.
- Optional: The tea has a distinct, herbal flavor. If desired, you can add honey or a slice of lemon to enhance its taste.

What to Expect:
Drinking Dong Quai and Red Clover Tea can offer significant support for hormonal balance, especially for women experiencing menstrual discomfort or undergoing menopausal transition. Users may notice a reduction in symptoms such as cramps, hot flashes, and mood swings, along with improved overall well-being.
While this tea is beneficial for many, it's important to approach its use with caution, particularly for those with hormone-sensitive conditions or individuals taking blood thinners, as Dong Quai can potentially increase the

risk of bleeding. Pregnant or nursing women should avoid this tea due to the potent effects of Dong Quai and Red Clover on hormones.
Always consult with a healthcare provider before incorporating new herbal remedies into your regimen, especially for those with existing health conditions or concerns. Dong Quai and Red Clover Tea can be a natural and gentle way to support women's health and hormonal balance, but individual responses can vary, making professional guidance crucial.

VITEX (CHASTE TREE) BERRY TEA FOR PMS.

Vitex (Chaste Tree) Berry Tea is a natural remedy recognized for its effectiveness in alleviating symptoms of Premenstrual Syndrome (PMS). The berries of the Vitex agnus-castus plant contain active compounds that regulate the pituitary gland, which in turn, helps balance hormone levels in the body. This hormonal regulation can lead to a reduction in PMS symptoms such as mood swings, breast tenderness, bloating, and cramps.
Ingredients:

- 1 teaspoon dried vitex (chaste tree) berries
- 1 cup boiling water

Instructions:

- Place 1 teaspoon of dried vitex berries in a tea infuser or directly in a heat-resistant cup.
- Pour 1 cup of boiling water over the berries, making sure they are fully submerged.
- Allow the tea to steep for about 10-15 minutes. The steeping time allows for the extraction of the beneficial compounds from the berries.
- After steeping, remove the tea infuser or strain the tea to remove the berries.
- Optional: Vitex berry tea has a slightly bitter, earthy flavor. If desired, you can add honey or lemon to enhance its taste.

What to Expect:
Drinking Vitex Berry Tea can provide relief from PMS symptoms over time. It's important to note that the effects of vitex are usually observed after consistent use for a few months. Many women report a significant reduction in the severity of their PMS symptoms, including fewer mood swings, lessened cramps, and reduced breast tenderness.
While Vitex Berry Tea is beneficial for many women, it's important to consult with a healthcare provider before incorporating it into your regimen, especially for those with hormone-sensitive conditions, those who are pregnant or nursing, or individuals on hormonal medications. Vitex may

interact with certain medications, including birth control pills and hormone therapies.
Incorporating Vitex (Chaste Tree) Berry Tea into your daily routine can be a gentle, natural way to manage PMS symptoms and support overall hormonal balance, contributing to improved menstrual health and well-being.

CRAMP BARK AND GINGER TEA FOR MENSTRUAL CRAMPS.

Cramp Bark and Ginger Tea is a powerful herbal remedy designed to alleviate menstrual cramps and discomfort. Cramp bark, as its name suggests, is highly valued for its antispasmodic properties, making it effective in relieving uterine muscle spasms. Ginger, known for its anti-inflammatory and analgesic qualities, complements cramp bark by reducing inflammation and pain associated with menstrual cramps. Together, these herbs create a soothing tea that can provide significant relief during menstruation.
Ingredients:

- 1 teaspoon cramp bark
- 1 inch fresh ginger, thinly sliced
- 1 cup boiling water

Instructions:

- Combine 1 teaspoon of cramp bark and the thinly sliced fresh ginger in a tea infuser or directly in a heat-resistant cup.
- Pour 1 cup of boiling water over the mixture, ensuring the herbs are fully submerged.
- Cover and allow the tea to steep for about 15-20 minutes. The extended steeping time is necessary for extracting the full benefits from the cramp bark and ginger.
- After steeping, remove the tea infuser or strain the tea to remove the herbs and ginger slices.
- Optional: The tea has a robust, somewhat spicy flavor from the ginger, which can be softened with a teaspoon of honey or a dash of lemon juice to enhance its taste.

What to Expect:
Drinking Cramp Bark and Ginger Tea during menstruation can offer quick relief from cramps and discomfort. The antispasmodic effect of cramp bark directly targets the uterus, easing muscle contractions, while ginger's anti-inflammatory properties help to reduce overall pain and discomfort. Many women find that sipping on this tea before or during the onset of cramps provides substantial relief, allowing for more comfortable and manageable menstrual periods.
While this tea is generally safe for most individuals, it's always prudent to consult with a healthcare provider before adding new herbal remedies to your health regimen, especially if you have existing medical conditions, are

pregnant or nursing, or are taking medications. As with any natural remedy, individual results may vary, and it may take a couple of cycles to fully gauge the tea's effectiveness for your specific needs.
Incorporating Cramp Bark and Ginger Tea into your routine can be a natural, effective way to manage menstrual cramps, offering a comforting and therapeutic option for those seeking relief from menstrual discomfort.

SHATAVARI AND ASHWAGANDHA WOMEN'S WELLNESS TONIC.

Shatavari and Ashwagandha Women's Wellness Tonic is a nourishing blend that combines two of Ayurveda's most revered herbs for supporting women's health. Shatavari, often called the "Queen of Herbs," is celebrated for its ability to balance female hormones and support reproductive health. Ashwagandha, known as the "Indian Ginseng," provides strength, energy, and stress relief. Together, these herbs create a tonic that promotes hormonal balance, enhances vitality, and supports overall wellness in women.
Ingredients:

- 1 teaspoon shatavari powder
- 1 teaspoon ashwagandha powder
- 1 cup warm milk (dairy or plant-based) or water

Instructions:

- Mix 1 teaspoon of shatavari powder and 1 teaspoon of ashwagandha powder in a cup.
- Add the mixture to 1 cup of warm milk or water. Stir well to ensure the powders are completely dissolved.
- Optional: Enhance the flavor and nutritional value by adding a natural sweetener like honey or maple syrup, and a pinch of cinnamon or cardamom.

What to Expect:
Drinking the Shatavari and Ashwagandha Women's Wellness Tonic can lead to various health benefits, including improved hormonal balance, reduced symptoms of PMS and menopause, enhanced energy levels, and a strengthened stress response. Shatavari's nourishing properties specifically support the female reproductive system, while ashwagandha's adaptogenic qualities help the body manage stress and promote overall vitality.
This tonic is ideally consumed daily, either in the morning to start your day with a boost of energy or in the evening to unwind and prepare for a restful night's sleep. Consistent use over time is key to experiencing the full benefits of these powerful herbs.
While this tonic is beneficial for many, it's important to consult with a healthcare provider before incorporating new herbal supplements into your routine, especially for those with existing health conditions, those who are

pregnant or breastfeeding, or individuals on medication. Both shatavari and ashwagandha are generally well-tolerated, but like any supplement, they may not be suitable for everyone.

Incorporating the Shatavari and Ashwagandha Women's Wellness Tonic into your daily routine can be a simple and effective way to support your health and well-being, leveraging the ancient wisdom of Ayurveda to enhance modern living.

YARROW AND GINGER TEA FOR MENSTRUAL CRAMPS.

Yarrow and Ginger Tea is a potent herbal remedy that combines the powerful anti-inflammatory and antispasmodic properties of yarrow with the warming, pain-relieving effects of ginger. This blend is particularly effective in alleviating menstrual cramps, reducing inflammation, and promoting relaxation during menstruation. Yarrow, with its ability to regulate blood flow and relieve spasms, and ginger, known for its gastrointestinal and pain-relieving benefits, make this tea an excellent choice for women seeking natural relief from menstrual discomfort.

Ingredients:

- 1 teaspoon dried yarrow flowers
- 1 inch fresh ginger, thinly sliced or 1 teaspoon ginger powder
- 1 cup boiling water

Instructions:

- Combine 1 teaspoon of dried yarrow flowers and the thinly sliced fresh ginger (or ginger powder) in a tea infuser or directly in a heat-resistant cup.
- Pour 1 cup of boiling water over the yarrow and ginger, ensuring the ingredients are fully submerged.
- Cover and allow the tea to steep for about 10-15 minutes. Covering the cup helps to retain the essential oils and active compounds in the tea.
- After steeping, remove the tea infuser or strain the tea to remove the loose herbs and ginger slices.
- Optional: The tea has a strong, somewhat bitter flavor, which can be softened with a teaspoon of honey or a dash of lemon juice to enhance its taste.

What to Expect:

Drinking Yarrow and Ginger Tea during menstruation can provide significant relief from cramps and discomfort. The antispasmodic action of yarrow helps to ease uterine contractions, while ginger's anti-inflammatory properties reduce pain and bloating. Many women find that sipping on this tea before or during the onset of menstrual cramps provides substantial relief, allowing for more comfortable and manageable periods.

While this tea is generally safe for most individuals, it's always prudent to consult with a healthcare provider before adding new herbal remedies to your health regimen, especially if you have existing medical conditions, are pregnant or nursing, or are taking medications. Yarrow, in particular, should be used with caution by those with allergies to plants in the Asteraceae family and may interact with blood-thinning medications due to its potential to affect blood clotting.

Incorporating Yarrow and Ginger Tea into your routine can be a natural, effective way to manage menstrual cramps, offering a comforting and therapeutic option for those seeking relief from menstrual discomfort.

MOTHERWORT AND DONG QUAI MENSTRUAL RELIEF TONIC.

The Motherwort and Dong Quai Menstrual Relief Tonic is a synergistic blend designed to alleviate menstrual discomfort and promote hormonal balance. Motherwort (Leonurus cardiaca) is renowned for its ability to ease menstrual cramps and heart palpitations, while Dong Quai (Angelica sinensis), often referred to as "female ginseng," is used for its hormone-regulating and blood-circulating properties. Together, these tinctures create a potent remedy for supporting menstrual health and well-being.

Ingredients:

- Motherwort tincture
- Dong Quai tincture

Instructions:

- Mix equal parts of motherwort and dong quai tinctures. A typical dosage might start with 10-20 drops of each tincture, but it's essential to refer to the dosing recommendations provided on the tincture bottles, as potency can vary.
- The mixed tinctures can be taken directly under the tongue for rapid absorption or diluted in a small amount of water or tea if preferred.
- Take the tonic 1-3 times daily, especially during the week before and during menstruation, or as directed by a healthcare provider.

What to Expect:

The Motherwort and Dong Quai Menstrual Relief Tonic can offer significant relief from menstrual discomfort, including cramps, bloating, and mood swings. By promoting hormonal balance and improving blood flow, this tonic may also help to regulate menstrual cycles and reduce the severity of PMS symptoms.

While this tonic is beneficial for many women, it's important to exercise caution and consult with a healthcare provider before starting any new herbal supplement, especially for those with existing health conditions, those who are pregnant or breastfeeding, or individuals taking medications, as herbs can interact with certain drugs.

Regular use of the Motherwort and Dong Quai Tonic can provide a natural and supportive approach to managing menstrual health, contributing to improved comfort and well-being during menstruation. However, individual responses to herbal remedies can vary, so monitoring your body's reaction and consulting with healthcare professionals is advisable to ensure the best approach for your health needs.

YARROW AND RED CLOVER MENSTRUAL RELIEF TEA.

Yarrow and Red Clover Menstrual Relief Tea is a herbal blend crafted to offer natural relief from menstrual discomfort and help regulate menstrual cycles. Yarrow, with its antispasmodic properties, effectively reduces cramping and discomfort, while red clover, rich in isoflavones, works to balance hormone levels, addressing symptoms of hormonal imbalance such as irregular cycles and PMS.

Ingredients:

- 1 teaspoon dried yarrow flowers
- 1 teaspoon dried red clover blossoms
- 1 cup boiling water

Instructions:

- Mix 1 teaspoon of dried yarrow flowers and 1 teaspoon of dried red clover blossoms in a tea infuser or directly in a heat-resistant cup.
- Pour 1 cup of boiling water over the herbs, ensuring they are fully submerged.
- Cover and allow the tea to steep for about 10-15 minutes. Covering during steeping helps to retain the essential oils and medicinal properties of the herbs.
- After steeping, remove the tea infuser or strain the tea to remove the loose herbs.
- Optional: The tea has a mild, pleasant flavor, but you can add honey or lemon to enhance its taste if desired.

What to Expect:

Drinking Yarrow and Red Clover Menstrual Relief Tea can offer significant relief from menstrual cramps and discomfort. The tea's natural compounds can help to relax the uterus, reduce inflammation, and alleviate pain. Additionally, the hormonal balancing effects of red clover may lead to more regular and less painful menstrual cycles over time.

While this tea is beneficial for menstrual support, it's important to note that individuals with hormone-sensitive conditions should use caution and

consult with a healthcare provider before incorporating red clover into their regimen. Similarly, yarrow should be avoided by pregnant women due to its potential to stimulate the uterus.
Incorporating Yarrow and Red Clover Menstrual Relief Tea into your routine during menstruation can provide a comforting and effective way to manage discomfort and support overall menstrual health, making it a valuable addition to your wellness toolkit.

SHATAVARI ROOT MILK FOR REPRODUCTIVE HEALTH.

Shatavari Root Milk is a traditional Ayurvedic tonic revered for its ability to support female reproductive health and vitality. Shatavari, also known as Asparagus racemosus, is considered a powerful rejuvenative herb for women, known for its phytoestrogenic properties that help balance hormone levels, nourish the reproductive tissues, and enhance fertility. When simmered in milk with a touch of honey, it creates a nurturing and soothing beverage that supports overall well-being.
Ingredients:

- 1 teaspoon powdered shatavari root
- 1 cup milk (dairy or plant-based)
- 1 teaspoon honey (or to taste)

Instructions:

- Add 1 teaspoon of powdered shatavari root to 1 cup of milk in a small saucepan. You can use dairy milk or any plant-based milk of your choice.
- Gently heat the mixture on a low flame, bringing it to a simmer. Avoid boiling to preserve the delicate nutrients in the shatavari and milk.
- Simmer for about 5-10 minutes, allowing the shatavari powder to infuse into the milk.
- Remove from heat and strain the mixture to remove any large particles of shatavari root, if necessary.
- Stir in 1 teaspoon of honey to sweeten the milk. Adjust the amount of honey according to your taste preference.
- Enjoy the shatavari root milk warm.

What to Expect:
Consuming Shatavari Root Milk can offer numerous benefits for female reproductive health, including hormonal balance, enhanced fertility, and improved vitality. It's particularly beneficial during various phases of a woman's life, including menstruation, pregnancy, lactation, and menopause. The tonic's nourishing properties also make it an excellent choice for overall immune support and stress reduction.

While Shatavari Root Milk is safe for most individuals, it's important to consult with a healthcare provider before incorporating it into your routine, especially if you are pregnant, nursing, or have any health conditions. Shatavari can affect hormone levels, so it's crucial to ensure it's appropriate for your individual health situation.
Incorporating Shatavari Root Milk into your daily or weekly routine can be a simple yet effective way to support and enhance female reproductive health and overall vitality, leveraging the ancient wisdom of Ayurveda for modern wellness.

HERBAL REMEDIES FOR MEN'S HEALTH.

SAW PALMETTO EXTRACT FOR PROSTATE HEALTH.

Saw Palmetto Extract, derived from the berries of the Serenoa repens tree, is widely recognized for its beneficial effects on prostate health. It's particularly noted for its ability to support urinary function and reduce the symptoms of benign prostatic hyperplasia (BPH), commonly known as an enlarged prostate. The active compounds in saw palmetto, including fatty acids and phytosterols, are believed to help reduce inflammation and inhibit the conversion of testosterone to dihydrotestosterone (DHT), a hormone linked to prostate enlargement.
Usage:

- Follow the dosage instructions provided on the packaging of the commercially prepared saw palmetto extract. A common dosage is between 160 mg to 320 mg per day, taken in divided doses, but it's important to adhere to the manufacturer's or your healthcare provider's recommendations.

What to Expect:
Regular intake of saw palmetto extract can lead to an improvement in urinary symptoms associated with BPH, such as decreased urinary frequency, improved urinary flow, and reduced nighttime urination. Many users report noticeable benefits within a few weeks to months of consistent use.
Saw palmetto extract is generally well-tolerated, with minimal side effects reported. However, some individuals may experience mild gastrointestinal upset. It's also important to note that while saw palmetto is beneficial for supporting prostate health, it should not replace medical treatment for those with diagnosed prostate conditions. Always consult with a healthcare provider before starting any new supplement, especially if you have pre-existing health conditions or are taking medications.
Given that saw palmetto can interact with hormone-related medications and therapies, including those for prostate cancer, it's crucial to discuss its use

with a healthcare professional to ensure it's appropriate for your specific health situation.
Incorporating saw palmetto extract into your daily routine can be a proactive approach to maintaining prostate health and managing symptoms of BPH, contributing to overall quality of life and well-being.

Nettle Leaf Tea for Urinary Health.

Nettle Leaf Tea, made from the leaves of the Urtica dioica plant, is a well-regarded herbal remedy for supporting urinary tract health. Rich in vitamins, minerals, and phytonutrients, nettle leaves have diuretic properties that help to flush out the urinary tract, reducing the risk of urinary infections and supporting overall kidney and bladder function. This tea is particularly beneficial for those looking to naturally support their urinary system.
Ingredients:

- 1-2 teaspoons dried nettle leaves
- 1 cup boiling water

Instructions:

- Place 1-2 teaspoons of dried nettle leaves in a tea infuser or directly in a heat-resistant cup.
- Pour 1 cup of boiling water over the nettle leaves, ensuring they are fully submerged.
- Cover and allow the tea to steep for about 10 minutes. Covering the cup during steeping helps to preserve the beneficial compounds in the tea.
- After steeping, remove the tea infuser or strain the tea to remove the loose leaves.
- Optional: Nettle leaf tea has a rich, earthy flavor. If desired, you can add honey or lemon to enhance its taste.

What to Expect:
Drinking Nettle Leaf Tea can offer several benefits for urinary tract health. The diuretic action of nettle helps to cleanse the urinary system, promoting healthy kidney function and reducing the risk of urinary tract infections. Additionally, the anti-inflammatory properties of nettle can help to alleviate symptoms associated with conditions like benign prostatic hyperplasia (BPH) and lower urinary tract symptoms (LUTS).
Nettle leaf is generally safe for most individuals, but it's always wise to consult with a healthcare provider before incorporating new herbal remedies into your health regimen, especially if you have existing medical conditions or are taking medications.

Incorporating Nettle Leaf Tea into your daily routine can be an effective and natural way to support urinary tract health, enhance kidney function, and maintain overall well-being.

PYGEUM BARK EXTRACT FOR PROSTATE SUPPORT.

Pygeum Bark Extract, derived from the bark of the African cherry tree (Prunus africana), is a natural supplement widely recognized for its benefits in supporting prostate health. This herbal extract has been used traditionally and in modern herbal practices to alleviate symptoms associated with benign prostatic hyperplasia (BPH) such as frequent urination, night-time urination, and difficulty starting and maintaining urination. Pygeum contains active compounds that help reduce prostate enlargement and inflammation, improving urinary function.

Usage:

- Follow the dosage instructions provided on the packaging of the commercially prepared pygeum extract. The standard dosage often ranges from 100 mg to 200 mg daily, divided into two doses, but it's essential to adhere to the manufacturer's or your healthcare provider's recommendations.

What to Expect:

Incorporating pygeum extract into your routine can lead to improvements in prostate health and urinary function. Many men report a decrease in symptoms associated with BPH, such as reduced urgency and frequency of urination, especially during the night. Additionally, pygeum may contribute to overall urinary tract health and function.

Benefits from pygeum extract are typically observed after consistent use for a period of several weeks to months. It's important to maintain regular intake as directed to achieve the best outcomes.

While pygeum bark extract is generally well-tolerated, some individuals may experience mild gastrointestinal discomfort. As with any supplement, it's advisable to consult with a healthcare provider before starting pygeum, especially for individuals with pre-existing health conditions, those taking medications, or if you have concerns about potential interactions.

Consulting with a healthcare provider is also crucial to ensure that symptoms are not related to a more serious condition. Pygeum bark extract offers a natural option for men seeking to support their prostate health and manage symptoms associated with benign prostatic hyperplasia, contributing to improved quality of life and well-being.

PUMPKIN SEED OIL FOR URINARY HEALTH.

Pumpkin Seed Oil, extracted from the seeds of the pumpkin (Cucurbita pepo), is a nutrient-rich supplement known for its benefits in supporting urinary health. Rich in antioxidants, zinc, and phytoestrogens, pumpkin seed oil has been shown to improve bladder function and reduce symptoms of urinary disorders. Its use is particularly beneficial for those experiencing overactive bladder, benign prostatic hyperplasia (BPH), and urinary incontinence, offering a natural approach to enhancing urinary tract function.
Usage:

- Consume cold-pressed pumpkin seed oil as directed, typically 1 to 2 tablespoons daily. It can be taken directly or added to salads, smoothies, or other cold dishes to avoid degrading its nutritional value with heat.

What to Expect:
Regular consumption of cold-pressed pumpkin seed oil can lead to improvements in urinary health, including enhanced bladder control, reduced frequency of urination, and alleviation of symptoms associated with BPH. The oil's anti-inflammatory properties and nutritional content support overall bladder and prostate health.
Benefits are usually observed after consistent use over a period of several weeks. It's important to maintain a regular intake as part of your daily routine to achieve the best results.
While pumpkin seed oil is generally safe and well-tolerated, individuals with allergies to pumpkin seeds should avoid it. As with any dietary supplement, it's wise to consult with a healthcare provider before incorporating pumpkin seed oil into your regimen, especially for those with underlying health conditions or those taking medications.
Pumpkin seed oil offers a convenient and natural option for supporting urinary health and enhancing the quality of life for individuals experiencing urinary tract issues.

UVA URSI LEAF TEA FOR URINARY TRACT INFECTIONS.

Uva Ursi Leaf Tea, derived from the leaves of the Arctostaphylos uva-ursi plant, is a traditional herbal remedy known for its effectiveness in supporting urinary tract health. Uva ursi leaves contain arbutin, a compound that converts into hydroquinone in the body, exerting antiseptic and antibacterial effects on the urinary tract. This makes uva ursi tea particularly beneficial for the treatment and prevention of urinary tract infections (UTIs). However, due to its potent properties, uva ursi is recommended for short-term use only.
Ingredients:

- 1-2 teaspoons dried uva ursi leaves
- 1 cup boiling water

Instructions:

- Place 1-2 teaspoons of dried uva ursi leaves in a tea infuser or directly in a heat-resistant cup.
- Pour 1 cup of boiling water over the leaves, ensuring they are fully submerged.
- Cover and allow the tea to steep for about 10-15 minutes. The cover helps to maintain the temperature and ensures a potent infusion.
- After steeping, remove the tea infuser or strain the tea to remove the leaves.
- Optional: Uva ursi tea has a strong, slightly bitter taste. While it's best consumed plain to maximize its benefits, a small amount of honey can be added to improve its palatability if necessary.

What to Expect:

Drinking Uva Ursi Leaf Tea can provide relief from the symptoms associated with urinary tract infections, such as burning sensation during urination and urgency. Its antibacterial action helps to cleanse the urinary tract, promoting healing and preventing further infections.

It's important to note that uva ursi should not be used for prolonged periods (no longer than one week) due to potential liver toxicity and other side effects from its active compounds. Also, uva ursi is not recommended during pregnancy, breastfeeding, or for individuals with kidney disorders.

While Uva Ursi Leaf Tea can be an effective remedy for UTIs, it's crucial to consult with a healthcare provider before use, especially if symptoms persist, as medical treatment may be necessary. Additionally, drinking plenty of water and maintaining good urinary hygiene can complement the benefits of uva ursi in supporting urinary tract health.

Incorporating Uva Ursi Leaf Tea into your health regimen can offer a natural and targeted approach to managing urinary tract infections, but due diligence and healthcare guidance are essential to ensure safety and effectiveness.

TRIBULUS TERRESTRIS TEA FOR LIBIDO.

Tribulus Terrestris Tea, made from the dried fruits or leaves of the Tribulus terrestris plant, is commonly used as a natural remedy to support male libido and vitality. The herb is reputed for its ability to enhance sexual function and increase testosterone levels naturally, making it a popular choice among men looking to improve their sexual health and overall energy levels.

Ingredients:

- 1-2 teaspoons dried Tribulus terrestris (fruits or leaves)
- 1 cup boiling water

Instructions:

- Place 1-2 teaspoons of dried Tribulus terrestris in a tea infuser or directly in a heat-resistant cup.
- Pour 1 cup of boiling water over the Tribulus terrestris, ensuring the herb is fully submerged.
- Cover and allow the tea to steep for about 10-15 minutes. Covering the cup helps to retain the essential oils and active compounds in the tea.
- After steeping, remove the tea infuser or strain the tea to remove the loose herb.
- Optional: Tribulus terrestris tea has a somewhat earthy, slightly bitter taste. You can add honey or lemon to improve its flavor, although many prefer to drink it plain to fully appreciate its effects.

What to Expect:
Drinking Tribulus Terrestris Tea may lead to an improvement in libido and sexual vitality over time. The herb is believed to work by increasing the levels of luteinizing hormone, which signals the body to produce more testosterone. Increased testosterone levels are associated with enhanced libido, improved sexual performance, and increased energy levels.
While Tribulus Terrestris is generally considered safe for most individuals, it's important to note that results can vary, and the effectiveness of the herb for boosting testosterone levels and improving sexual function has been met with mixed scientific reviews. Additionally, individuals with hormone-sensitive conditions should use caution, and consulting with a healthcare provider before starting any new herbal supplement is advisable, especially for those with underlying health conditions or those taking medications.
Incorporating Tribulus Terrestris Tea into your routine can be a natural way to support libido and vitality, but it should be part of a holistic approach to health that includes a balanced diet, regular exercise, and good lifestyle choices for optimal sexual health and overall well-being.

Saw Palmetto Berry Tea for Prostate Health.

Saw Palmetto Berry Tea is derived from the berries of the Serenoa repens plant and is widely recognized for its benefits in supporting prostate health. Saw palmetto is particularly noted for its use in reducing symptoms of benign prostatic hyperplasia (BPH), such as urinary frequency and urgency. The active compounds in saw palmetto berries help to inhibit the conversion of testosterone into dihydrotestosterone (DHT), a hormone associated with prostate enlargement.
Ingredients:

- 1-2 teaspoons dried saw palmetto berries
- 1 cup boiling water

Instructions:

- Place 1-2 teaspoons of dried saw palmetto berries in a tea infuser or directly in a heat-resistant cup.
- Pour 1 cup of boiling water over the berries, ensuring they are fully submerged.
- Cover and allow the tea to steep for about 10-15 minutes. Covering the cup during steeping helps to preserve the volatile oils and medicinal properties of the berries.
- After steeping, remove the tea infuser or strain the tea to remove the berries.
- Optional: Saw palmetto berry tea has a distinct, slightly bitter taste. If desired, you can add honey or a slice of lemon to improve its flavor.

What to Expect:

Drinking Saw Palmetto Berry Tea may contribute to improved prostate health and relief from symptoms associated with BPH. Regular consumption can help reduce urinary problems and support overall urinary function. However, it's important to note that benefits from saw palmetto might take several weeks to become noticeable.

While Saw Palmetto Berry Tea is beneficial for prostate health, it's crucial to consult with a healthcare provider before incorporating it into your routine, especially for individuals with existing medical conditions, those undergoing surgery, or those taking medications, as saw palmetto can interact with certain drugs.

Incorporating Saw Palmetto Berry Tea into your daily regimen can be a natural approach to supporting prostate health. However, it should not replace medical treatment for prostate issues but rather complement traditional therapies under the guidance of a healthcare professional.

Lycopene-rich Tomato Juice for Prostate Health.

Lycopene-rich Tomato Juice is a nutritious and natural way to support prostate health. Lycopene, a powerful antioxidant found in tomatoes, has been extensively studied for its potential to reduce the risk of prostate cancer and alleviate symptoms of prostate conditions such as benign prostatic hyperplasia (BPH). Consuming tomato juice, especially when made fresh, ensures a high intake of lycopene along with other beneficial nutrients.

Ingredients:

- 4-6 ripe tomatoes (depending on size)
- A pinch of salt (optional)
- Fresh herbs (such as basil or parsley, optional for flavor)

Instructions:

- Wash the tomatoes thoroughly under running water.

- Cut the tomatoes into quarters and remove the stems.
- Place the tomato quarters into a blender. For added flavor, you can also include fresh herbs like basil or parsley.
- Blend the tomatoes (and herbs, if using) until smooth.
- Strain the tomato mixture using a fine mesh sieve or cheesecloth to remove the seeds and skin, resulting in a smooth juice. This step is optional if you prefer a more fibrous juice.
- Add a pinch of salt to enhance the flavor, if desired.
- Serve the tomato juice immediately, or chill it in the refrigerator for a refreshing drink.

What to Expect:

Regular consumption of Lycopene-rich Tomato Juice can contribute to improved prostate health. The antioxidant properties of lycopene help protect cells from damage and may lower the risk of prostate cancer. Additionally, lycopene's anti-inflammatory effects can support the overall health of the prostate gland.

While drinking tomato juice is a beneficial and delicious way to increase your lycopene intake, it's important to incorporate it as part of a balanced diet rich in fruits, vegetables, and other nutrient-dense foods for overall health and well-being.

It's also worth noting that the body absorbs lycopene more effectively from cooked or processed tomatoes, such as tomato paste, sauce, or juice, especially when consumed with a small amount of healthy fats (like olive oil), enhancing lycopene's bioavailability.

Incorporating Lycopene-rich Tomato Juice into your daily routine can be an enjoyable and natural way to support prostate health. However, for individuals with specific health conditions or dietary restrictions, consulting with a healthcare provider before making significant dietary changes is advisable.

Zinc-rich Pumpkin Seed Snack for Male Fertility.

Pumpkin seeds are a nutritional powerhouse, especially rich in zinc, an essential mineral crucial for male fertility and prostate health. Zinc plays a vital role in testosterone production, sperm formation, and sperm motility, making pumpkin seeds an excellent dietary addition for men looking to improve their reproductive health. Additionally, pumpkin seeds contain other beneficial nutrients like magnesium, antioxidants, and fatty acids.

Ingredients:

- Raw or roasted pumpkin seeds

Instructions:

- For Raw Pumpkin Seeds: Simply measure out a portion (about a handful or 1/4 cup) of raw pumpkin seeds to eat as a snack. They can be consumed as is or added to salads, yogurts, or smoothies for a nutritional boost.
- For Roasted Pumpkin Seeds: If you prefer roasted pumpkin seeds, you can easily make them at home. Preheat your oven to 300°F (150°C). Spread the pumpkin seeds on a baking sheet in a single layer. For added flavor, you can lightly toss them with olive oil and sprinkle with salt or your favorite spices before roasting. Bake for about 20-30 minutes or until golden and crunchy, stirring occasionally to ensure even roasting.

What to Expect:

Incorporating pumpkin seeds into your diet can provide a significant boost in zinc intake, supporting male fertility by enhancing testosterone levels and improving sperm quality. Regular consumption of pumpkin seeds may also contribute to better prostate health due to their zinc content and anti-inflammatory properties.

Pumpkin seeds are not only beneficial for fertility and prostate health but also offer general health benefits, including improved heart health, better sleep quality (due to their magnesium content), and enhanced immune function.

It's easy to integrate pumpkin seeds into your daily diet as a snack or as an addition to meals. Their rich, nutty flavor and crunchy texture make them a satisfying and healthful snack choice.

While pumpkin seeds are a healthy food option, it's always a good idea to maintain a balanced diet and consult with a healthcare provider if you have specific health concerns or dietary requirements. Eating a variety of nutrient-dense foods is key to overall health and well-being

PUMPKIN SEED AND SAW PALMETTO BLEND FOR PROSTATE HEALTH.

The combination of pumpkin seeds and saw palmetto extract is a potent natural remedy for supporting prostate health. Pumpkin seeds are rich in zinc, a mineral essential for prostate function and health, while saw palmetto extract is widely recognized for its ability to improve symptoms of benign prostatic hyperplasia (BPH) and support overall urinary tract function. Together, they offer a synergistic approach to maintaining prostate health and preventing common prostate issues.

Ingredients:

- 1 tablespoon ground pumpkin seeds
- 1 teaspoon saw palmetto extract

Instructions:

- Grind the pumpkin seeds into a fine powder using a coffee grinder or a mortar and pestle.
- In a small bowl, mix 1 tablespoon of the ground pumpkin seeds with 1 teaspoon of saw palmetto extract. The extract is typically available in liquid form, which can easily be mixed with the ground seeds.
- Consume the mixture directly, or if preferred, you can add it to a smoothie, yogurt, or juice to make it more palatable.
- This blend should be consumed once daily, preferably with a meal to enhance absorption of the nutrients and compounds.

What to Expect:
Regular consumption of the pumpkin seed and saw palmetto blend may lead to an improvement in prostate health and urinary function. The nutrients and bioactive compounds in both ingredients work together to reduce inflammation, inhibit the conversion of testosterone to dihydrotestosterone (DHT), a contributing factor in prostate enlargement and support the overall health of the urinary tract.
While many men report positive effects on their prostate health after incorporating this blend into their daily regimen, it's important to remember that individual results can vary. It's also crucial to consult with a healthcare provider before starting any new supplement regimen, especially if you have existing health conditions or are taking medications, to ensure that this natural remedy is appropriate and safe for your specific health needs.
The pumpkin seed and saw palmetto blend is a natural, non-invasive option for supporting prostate health, but it should complement a comprehensive approach to health that includes regular medical check-ups, a balanced diet, and physical activity.

Nettle Root Extract for Male Vitality.

Nettle Root Extract, derived from the root of the Urtica dioica (stinging nettle) plant, is a natural supplement esteemed for its ability to support overall male vitality and health. Rich in bioactive compounds, nettle root is particularly noted for its benefits in promoting prostate health, enhancing urinary function, and potentially supporting testosterone levels. Its mechanism involves inhibiting the enzyme that converts testosterone into dihydrotestosterone (DHT), a hormone associated with prostate enlargement and hair loss.
Usage:

- Follow the dosage instructions provided on the nettle root extract product you purchase. Dosages can vary depending on the concentration of the extract, but a common recommendation is between 250 mg to 500 mg taken twice daily.

- Nettle root extract can be found in various forms, including capsules, tinctures, and powders. Choose the form that best fits your preference and lifestyle.

What to Expect:

Incorporating nettle root extract into your daily regimen can lead to several benefits for male vitality and health:

- Prostate Support: Regular use may help manage symptoms associated with benign prostatic hyperplasia (BPH), such as urinary frequency and urgency.
- Testosterone Balance: By inhibiting the conversion of testosterone to DHT, nettle root may help maintain healthier testosterone levels, which is crucial for energy, libido, and muscle mass.
- Anti-inflammatory Benefits: Nettle root has anti-inflammatory properties that can contribute to overall well-being and reduce discomfort from conditions such as joint pain.

While nettle root extract is generally considered safe for most individuals, it's important to start with a lower dose to assess tolerance. As with any supplement, there can be potential interactions with medications or conditions, so consulting with a healthcare provider before starting nettle root extract, especially for those with existing health conditions or those taking medications, is advisable.

Regular consumption of nettle root extract as part of a balanced lifestyle that includes a nutritious diet and regular exercise can support male vitality and contribute to a sense of overall well-being.

MACA ROOT POWDER FOR MALE ENERGY AND LIBIDO.

Maca Root Powder, derived from the root of the Lepidium meyenii plant native to the high Andes of Peru, is a traditional remedy known for its ability to enhance energy, stamina, and libido. Rich in nutrients including vitamins, minerals, amino acids, and phytonutrients, maca is considered an adaptogen, helping the body to adapt to and mitigate stressors, thereby supporting overall vitality and well-being.

Usage:

- Incorporate 1-2 teaspoons of maca root powder into your daily diet by mixing it into smoothies, water, juices, or even yogurt. You can also add it to oatmeal or homemade energy bars for an extra boost.
- Start with a smaller dose to assess your body's response, then gradually increase as needed. Since maca is a food product, it's generally safe for most people in moderate amounts.

What to Expect:

Consuming maca root powder regularly can lead to several benefits, particularly for men looking to enhance their energy levels and libido:

- Increased Energy: Many users report a significant boost in energy and endurance, making maca an excellent supplement for athletes or anyone seeking to improve their physical performance.
- Enhanced Libido: Maca has been traditionally used to increase sexual desire and improve libido in both men and women. It's considered a natural aphrodisiac.
- Mood Improvement: The adaptogenic qualities of maca may help improve mood and reduce anxiety, contributing to a better sense of overall well-being.

While maca is widely regarded as safe and beneficial, it's important to note that individual results can vary. As with any supplement, those with pre-existing health conditions or who are taking medications should consult with a healthcare provider before adding maca root powder to their regimen, especially if they have hormone-sensitive conditions.

Maca root powder offers a natural, nourishing way to support male energy, stamina, and libido. Its versatility makes it easy to incorporate into your daily diet, providing a simple yet effective approach to enhancing your overall vitality.

Saw Palmetto and Pygeum Africanum Extract for Prostate Health.

Combining Saw Palmetto and Pygeum Africanum extracts is a strategic approach to supporting prostate health and improving urinary function. Saw Palmetto, derived from the berry of the Serenoa repens tree, and Pygeum Africanum, extracted from the bark of the African cherry tree, are both recognized for their beneficial effects on the prostate gland and the urinary tract. These extracts work synergistically to reduce symptoms associated with benign prostatic hyperplasia (BPH) such as frequent urination, nighttime urination, and difficulty starting and maintaining urination.

Usage:

- Follow the dosage instructions on the labels of the commercially prepared Saw Palmetto and Pygeum Africanum extracts. A common dosage for Saw Palmetto is 160 mg twice daily, and for Pygeum Africanum, 100 mg daily, but these can vary based on the product's concentration and formulation.
- These extracts are typically available in capsule or liquid form, making them easy to incorporate into your daily routine.

What to Expect:

Regular intake of Saw Palmetto and Pygeum Africanum extracts can lead to noticeable improvements in prostate health and urinary function:

- Prostate Health: Both extracts are known to help reduce the size of the prostate gland or prevent further enlargement, addressing the root cause of BPH symptoms.
- Urinary Function: Many men experience relief from symptoms of BPH, such as reduced urinary frequency, increased urinary flow, and decreased nighttime urination.
- Overall Well-being: Improving prostate health and urinary function can significantly enhance quality of life and overall well-being.

While these herbal supplements are generally considered safe, it's important to consult with a healthcare provider before starting any new supplement regimen, especially if you have existing health conditions or are taking medications. This is crucial to ensure that the supplements will not interact adversely with medications or conditions.
Incorporating Saw Palmetto and Pygeum Africanum extracts into your health regimen can offer a natural, effective way to support prostate health and improve urinary function. However, maintaining a healthy lifestyle, including a balanced diet and regular exercise, is also important for optimal prostate health and general well-being.

FLAXSEED AND PUMPKIN SEED PROSTATE HEALTH SMOOTHIE.

This Flaxseed and Pumpkin Seed Prostate Health Smoothie is a nutritious and delicious way to support prostate health. Both flaxseeds and pumpkin seeds are rich in essential nutrients that benefit the prostate. Flaxseeds contain lignans and omega-3 fatty acids, which have been shown to have anti-inflammatory and anti-cancer properties. Pumpkin seeds are a good source of zinc, a mineral crucial for prostate health and hormonal balance.
Ingredients:

- 2 tablespoons ground flaxseeds
- 2 tablespoons raw pumpkin seeds
- 1 cup unsweetened almond milk (or any milk of your choice)
- 1 banana
- ½ cup mixed berries (such as blueberries, strawberries, or raspberries)
- A handful of spinach or kale (optional, for added nutrients)
- Ice cubes (optional, for a colder smoothie)

Instructions:

- Prep the Seeds: For easier blending and better nutrient absorption, grind the flaxseeds using a coffee grinder or spice mill. You can add the pumpkin seeds whole or grind them slightly.
- Combine Ingredients: In a blender, add the ground flaxseeds, pumpkin seeds, almond milk, banana, mixed berries, and leafy greens (if using). If you prefer a colder smoothie, add a few ice cubes.

- Blend: Blend on high until the smoothie reaches your desired consistency. If the smoothie is too thick, you can add more almond milk to thin it out.
- Serve: Pour the smoothie into a glass and enjoy immediately to take advantage of the full nutritional benefits.

What to Expect:

Consuming this Flaxseed and Pumpkin Seed Prostate Health Smoothie regularly can provide nutritional support for the prostate, thanks to the anti-inflammatory properties and essential nutrients from its ingredients. The lignans in flaxseeds and the zinc in pumpkin seeds are particularly beneficial for maintaining a healthy prostate and supporting overall male health.

This smoothie is not only packed with ingredients beneficial for prostate health but also contributes to your daily intake of fruits and vegetables, promoting overall well-being. It's a tasty, healthful way to start your day or as a nourishing snack.

Remember, while dietary strategies can support prostate health, they should complement regular medical check-ups and consultations with healthcare professionals, especially for those with existing prostate conditions or concerns.

Ginseng and Ginkgo Biloba Tonic for Male Vitality.

The Ginseng and Ginkgo Biloba Tonic is a potent natural remedy designed to enhance male vitality, energy levels, and cognitive function. Ginseng, known for its adaptogenic properties, helps to increase energy and reduce stress, while Ginkgo Biloba is celebrated for its ability to improve circulation and cognitive abilities. Together, these extracts offer a synergistic effect that can bolster physical health and mental sharpness.

Ingredients:

- Ginseng extract
- Ginkgo Biloba extract

Instructions:

- Preparation: Mix equal parts of Ginseng and Ginkgo Biloba extracts. The exact dosage can vary depending on the concentration of the extracts used, so it's important to refer to the manufacturer's instructions for each. A general guideline might be to mix 1 ml (about 20 drops) of each extract in a small glass of water or juice.
- Consumption: Take the mixed tonic once or twice daily, as directed. It's often recommended to take herbal tonics like this in the morning or early afternoon to benefit from their energizing effects without interfering with sleep.

- Duration: To observe the tonic's full benefits, consistent use over several weeks to months is suggested.

What to Expect:

- Enhanced Vitality: Regular intake of the Ginseng and Ginkgo Biloba Tonic may lead to increased energy levels and a reduction in fatigue, making daily activities and physical exercise feel more manageable.
- Improved Cognitive Function: Ginkgo Biloba's positive effects on circulation and neural health can result in better memory, focus, and overall cognitive performance.
- Stress Reduction: Ginseng's adaptogenic qualities help the body better manage stress, potentially leading to improved mood and well-being.

While the Ginseng and Ginkgo Biloba Tonic is generally safe for most adults, individuals taking blood thinners or those with a history of hormone-sensitive conditions should consult with a healthcare provider before use, due to potential interactions and contraindications.

Incorporating this tonic into your wellness routine can offer a natural boost to vitality and cognitive function, supporting a more energetic and focused lifestyle. Remember, the best results come from a holistic approach to health that includes a balanced diet, regular physical activity, and adequate rest.

EPIMEDIUM (HORNY GOAT WEED) AND MACA LIBIDO BOOSTER.

The combination of Epimedium (commonly known as Horny Goat Weed) and Maca root powder creates a powerful libido booster that also enhances energy levels. Both herbs have a long history of use in traditional medicine for increasing sexual desire and improving overall vitality. Epimedium is believed to support erectile function and sexual health through its active compounds that affect hormone levels and blood flow. Maca root, often referred to as Peruvian Ginseng, is known for its ability to increase stamina, energy, and sexual desire without impacting hormone levels directly.

Ingredients:

- 1 teaspoon powdered Epimedium (Horny Goat Weed)
- 1 teaspoon Maca root powder
- Smoothie or drink of your choice

Instructions:

- Measure out 1 teaspoon of powdered Epimedium and 1 teaspoon of Maca root powder.
- Add both powders to your preferred smoothie or drink. These powders blend well with various ingredients, so feel free to experiment with different recipes according to your taste preferences.
- Blend thoroughly to ensure the powders are well incorporated into the drink.

- Consume this libido-boosting blend once daily, or as desired, to support sexual health and energy.

What to Expect:
Incorporating the Epimedium and Maca Libido Booster into your daily routine can lead to an increase in libido and energy over time. Many individuals report enhanced sexual desire, improved stamina, and a greater sense of overall well-being after regular consumption of this blend.
While both Epimedium and Maca are generally considered safe for most individuals, it's important to be mindful of potential side effects. Epimedium may interact with certain medications and conditions, particularly those related to blood pressure and cardiovascular health. Maca is well-tolerated, but it's advisable to start with a lower dose to assess tolerance.
Before adding any new supplements to your regimen, especially those aimed at enhancing sexual health, it's crucial to consult with a healthcare provider to ensure they are appropriate for your health status and needs.
The Epimedium and Maca Libido Booster offers a natural approach to enhancing libido and vitality, making it a popular choice for individuals seeking to improve their sexual health and energy levels naturally.

GREEN TEA AND PUMPKIN SEED PROSTATE HEALTH BLEND.

The Green Tea and Pumpkin Seed Prostate Health Blend is an innovative and healthful concoction designed to support prostate health. Green tea is celebrated for its high antioxidant content, particularly epigallocatechin gallate (EGCG), which has been studied for its potential to reduce the risk of prostate cancer and support overall prostate health. Pumpkin seeds are rich in zinc, a mineral essential for prostate function and health. Together, these ingredients create a tea blend that not only supports prostate health but also provides a boost in antioxidants and essential nutrients.
Ingredients:

- 1-2 teaspoons green tea leaves
- 1 tablespoon ground pumpkin seeds
- 1 cup boiling water

Instructions:

- Grind pumpkin seeds to a fine powder using a coffee grinder or mortar and pestle.
- Combine 1-2 teaspoons of green tea leaves with 1 tablespoon of ground pumpkin seeds in a tea infuser or directly in a heat-resistant cup.
- Pour 1 cup of boiling water over the mixture, ensuring the ingredients are fully submerged.

- Allow the blend to steep for about 3-5 minutes for green tea and up to 10 minutes for the pumpkin seeds to ensure optimal extraction of their beneficial compounds.
- After steeping, remove the tea infuser or strain the tea to remove the loose leaves and pumpkin seed particles.
- Optional: You can add honey or lemon to enhance the flavor of the tea.

What to Expect:
Incorporating the Green Tea and Pumpkin Seed Prostate Health Blend into your daily routine can contribute to improved prostate health. The antioxidant properties of green tea may help protect prostate cells from oxidative stress, while the zinc from pumpkin seeds supports prostate function and reduces the risk of prostate enlargement.
It's important to consume this blend regularly to observe its benefits. Additionally, maintaining a balanced diet and a healthy lifestyle further supports prostate health and overall well-being.
While this blend is beneficial for prostate health, it's always advisable to consult with a healthcare provider before introducing any new supplements or herbs into your regimen, especially for individuals with existing health conditions or those taking medications.
The Green Tea and Pumpkin Seed Prostate Health Blend offers a natural and enjoyable way to support prostate health, combining the therapeutic properties of both ingredients into a soothing and nutritious beverage.

EPIMEDIUM (HORNY GOAT WEED) TEA FOR LIBIDO ENHANCEMENT.

Epimedium Tea, made from the leaves of the Epimedium plant, commonly known as Horny Goat Weed, is a traditional herbal remedy celebrated for its libido-enhancing properties. Rich in icariin, a compound that supports blood flow and improves sexual function, Epimedium Tea is a natural choice for those looking to boost their libido and enhance sexual health without relying on synthetic supplements.
Ingredients:

- 1-2 teaspoons dried Epimedium (Horny Goat Weed) leaves
- 1 cup boiling water

Instructions:

- Place 1-2 teaspoons of dried Epimedium leaves in a tea infuser or directly in a heat-resistant cup.
- Pour 1 cup of boiling water over the leaves, ensuring they are fully submerged.
- Cover and allow the tea to steep for about 10-15 minutes. Covering the cup helps to preserve the active compounds in the tea.

- After steeping, remove the tea infuser or strain the tea to remove the loose leaves.
- Optional: Epimedium tea has a slightly bitter taste. You can add honey or lemon to improve its flavor, though many prefer to drink it plain to experience its full effects.

What to Expect:
Consuming Epimedium Tea can lead to an increase in libido and overall sexual well-being. The active components in the herb work to enhance blood flow, which is essential for sexual arousal and performance. Additionally, its use may support endurance and energy levels, contributing to a more satisfying sexual experience.
While Epimedium Tea is beneficial for libido enhancement, it's important to note that individual responses to herbs can vary. It's also crucial to use Epimedium responsibly, as excessive consumption may lead to side effects. Individuals with heart conditions, low blood pressure, or those taking medications should consult with a healthcare provider before adding Epimedium Tea to their regimen, to ensure its safe use.
Incorporating Epimedium (Horny Goat Weed) Tea into your routine can offer a natural and holistic approach to boosting libido and enhancing sexual health, aligning with traditional herbal practices for wellness and vitality.

SAW PALMETTO AND NETTLE ROOT EXTRACT FOR PROSTATE HEALTH.

The combination of Saw Palmetto and Nettle Root Extract is widely recognized for its benefits in supporting prostate health and improving urinary function. Saw Palmetto is known for its ability to inhibit the conversion of testosterone to dihydrotestosterone (DHT), a hormone associated with prostate enlargement. Nettle Root, on the other hand, offers anti-inflammatory properties and can help alleviate symptoms of benign prostatic hyperplasia (BPH), such as urinary frequency and urgency.
Usage:

- Follow the dosage instructions provided on the packaging of the saw palmetto and nettle root extract products. A common approach is to take the recommended dose of each extract once or twice daily, but this can vary based on the concentration of the products.
- These extracts are often available in capsule or liquid form, making them convenient to incorporate into your daily routine.

What to Expect:
Regular intake of Saw Palmetto and Nettle Root Extract can lead to an improvement in prostate health and urinary function. Many men report reduced symptoms of BPH, such as less frequent urination at night, improved urinary flow, and overall enhanced comfort.

It's important to note that while these supplements can provide relief and support for prostate health, they may not replace medical treatments for more severe prostate conditions. Additionally, results can vary from person to person and may take several weeks to become noticeable.
Before starting any new supplement regimen, especially for specific health conditions like prostate health, consulting with a healthcare provider is advisable. This is particularly important for individuals with pre-existing medical conditions, those taking medications, or anyone undergoing treatment for prostate issues.
Incorporating Saw Palmetto and Nettle Root Extract into your health regimen can be an effective, natural approach to maintaining prostate health and supporting urinary function, contributing to overall well-being and quality of life.

POMEGRANATE JUICE FOR ANTIOXIDANT SUPPORT.

Pomegranate Juice is a nutrient-dense beverage, renowned for its high content of antioxidants, particularly punicalagins and anthocyanins. These powerful compounds help neutralize harmful free radicals in the body, reducing oxidative stress and supporting overall health. Regular consumption of pomegranate juice is especially beneficial for men's health, offering cardiovascular benefits, supporting prostate health, and potentially improving erectile function due to enhanced blood flow.
Instructions:

- For the freshest and most beneficial juice, choose ripe pomegranates. You'll need about 2-3 large pomegranates for one cup of juice.
- Cut the pomegranates in half and scoop out the arils (seeds) into a bowl. Be careful as the juice can stain.
- Use a manual juicer or press the arils in a sieve over a bowl to extract the juice. For a less labor-intensive method, you can also blend the arils briefly and then strain the mixture to remove the pulp.
- Drink the juice freshly made, or store it in an airtight container in the refrigerator for 2-3 days to maintain its antioxidant properties.

What to Expect:
Drinking pomegranate juice regularly can contribute to a significant increase in your antioxidant intake, supporting cellular health and reducing the risk of chronic diseases. Men may find specific health benefits in terms of improved cardiovascular health, thanks to the juice's ability to improve cholesterol profiles and lower blood pressure. Additionally, the antioxidants in pomegranate juice have been linked to prostate health, with studies suggesting a role in reducing the risk of prostate cancer and supporting the treatment of BPH symptoms.

While pomegranate juice is a healthful addition to most diets, it's rich in natural sugars and calories, so moderation is key, especially for those monitoring their sugar intake or managing conditions like diabetes. Furthermore, pomegranate juice can interact with certain medications, similar to grapefruit juice, by affecting their metabolism in the body. If you're taking medication, especially for hypertension or cholesterol, consult with a healthcare provider to ensure it's safe to include pomegranate juice in your diet.

Incorporating pomegranate juice into your daily routine can offer a delicious and natural way to boost antioxidant intake and support men's health, alongside a balanced diet and healthy lifestyle.

Tribulus Terrestris and Zinc Tonic for Male Vitality.

The combination of Tribulus Terrestris extract and zinc creates a potent tonic for enhancing male vitality and overall health. Tribulus Terrestris, a herb used in traditional medicine across various cultures, is reputed for its ability to increase libido, improve sexual function, and support healthy testosterone levels. Zinc, an essential mineral, plays a critical role in hormone production, immune function, and cellular metabolism, making it vital for male reproductive health and general well-being.

Ingredients:

- Tribulus Terrestris extract (dosage as per product recommendation)
- Zinc supplement (as per recommended dietary allowance, or RDA, which is 11 mg for adult men) or zinc-rich foods (such as pumpkin seeds, beef, lentils, or chickpeas)

Instructions:

- If using a zinc supplement, take the recommended dose of Tribulus Terrestris extract alongside the zinc supplement with water. Follow the dosage instructions on the product labels carefully.
- Alternatively, you can incorporate zinc-rich foods into your diet and supplement with Tribulus Terrestris extract according to the product's dosage recommendation. For example, adding pumpkin seeds to your breakfast cereal or including beef or lentils in your meals can boost your zinc intake.
- For best absorption and efficacy, consider taking the Tribulus Terrestris extract and zinc with a meal.

What to Expect:

Regular consumption of the Tribulus Terrestris and Zinc Tonic can lead to improved male vitality, enhanced libido, and possibly better sexual performance. The tonic may also contribute to increased energy levels,

improved mood, and enhanced overall health due to the synergistic effects of Tribulus Terrestris and zinc on hormone balance and cellular function.
While this tonic is beneficial for supporting male vitality, it's essential to consult with a healthcare provider before starting any new supplement regimen, especially for individuals with underlying health conditions or those taking medications, to ensure the combination is safe and appropriate for your specific health needs.
Incorporating the Tribulus Terrestris and Zinc Tonic into your routine can offer a natural and effective way to support male reproductive health and vitality, but it should be part of a comprehensive approach to wellness that includes a balanced diet, regular exercise, and adequate rest.

FENUGREEK SEED TEA FOR MEN'S HEALTH.

Fenugreek Seed Tea is a natural remedy known for its benefits in supporting men's health, particularly in enhancing testosterone levels. Fenugreek seeds contain compounds that are believed to increase libido, support healthy testosterone levels, and improve overall vitality in men. Additionally, fenugreek has been shown to have positive effects on energy, muscle strength, and body composition.
Ingredients:

- 1-2 teaspoons of fenugreek seeds
- 1 cup of boiling water

Instructions:

- Crush the fenugreek seeds slightly to release their active compounds. You can use a mortar and pestle or the back of a spoon.
- Place the crushed fenugreek seeds in a tea infuser or directly in a heat-resistant cup.
- Pour 1 cup of boiling water over the seeds, ensuring they are fully submerged.
- Cover and allow the tea to steep for about 10-15 minutes. Covering the cup during steeping helps to preserve the volatile oils and flavors.
- After steeping, remove the tea infuser or strain the tea to remove the seeds.
- Optional: Fenugreek seed tea has a somewhat bitter, maple-syrup-like flavor. You can add honey or lemon to enhance its taste, though many prefer it plain to enjoy its full benefits.

What to Expect:
Drinking Fenugreek Seed Tea regularly can contribute to improved men's health, including supporting healthy testosterone levels and enhancing libido. Many men report increased energy and improved performance in physical activities, as well as better overall vitality.

While fenugreek seed tea is beneficial for many, it's important to start with a small amount to assess your body's reaction, as some individuals may experience mild gastrointestinal upset. Additionally, because fenugreek can affect hormone levels, it's crucial to consult with a healthcare provider before beginning any new supplement regimen, especially for those with hormone-sensitive conditions or those taking medications.
Incorporating Fenugreek Seed Tea into your daily routine can be a simple and natural way to support men's health, but it should complement a balanced diet and healthy lifestyle for optimal results.

GINSENG TEA FOR VITALITY.

Ginseng Tea, made from the root of the ginseng plant, is renowned for its remarkable benefits in boosting vitality and energy levels. Ginseng is one of the most popular herbal remedies worldwide, valued for its adaptogenic properties, which help the body withstand stress and enhance overall well-being. There are several types of ginseng, including Asian (Panax) ginseng and American ginseng, both known for their ability to improve energy, mental performance, and immune function.
Ingredients:

- 1-2 grams of ginseng root (fresh or dried)
- 1 cup of boiling water

Instructions:

- Thinly slice the ginseng root. If using dried ginseng, break it into small pieces to increase the surface area for infusion.
- Place the sliced or dried ginseng root in a tea infuser or directly in a heat-resistant cup.
- Pour 1 cup of boiling water over the ginseng, ensuring it's fully submerged.
- Cover and allow the tea to steep for about 5-10 minutes. The steeping time can be adjusted according to taste preference and the desired strength of the tea.
- After steeping, remove the tea infuser or strain the tea to remove the ginseng pieces.
- Optional: Ginseng tea has a distinct, somewhat earthy flavor. You can add honey, lemon, or a small amount of sweetener to enhance its taste.

What to Expect:
Drinking Ginseng Tea can lead to an increase in energy and vitality, making it a great choice for those looking to naturally boost their stamina and mental alertness. Regular consumption of ginseng tea may also support immune health, improve cognitive function, and aid in stress management.

While ginseng is generally safe for most people, it's important to be mindful of potential side effects, such as headaches, sleep disturbances, or digestive upset, especially with high doses or long-term use. Additionally, ginseng may interact with certain medications, including blood thinners and insulin, so consulting with a healthcare provider before starting any new herbal remedy is advisable.

Incorporating Ginseng Tea into your daily routine can be an effective way to enhance overall vitality and well-being. However, it's best to use ginseng as part of a balanced lifestyle that includes a nutritious diet, regular exercise, and adequate rest for optimal health benefits.

Zinc-rich Herbal Mix for Male Health.

This Zinc-rich Herbal Mix combines pumpkin seeds, watermelon seeds, and sunflower seeds, all of which are natural sources of zinc, an essential mineral crucial for male health. Zinc plays a vital role in testosterone production, fertility, and prostate health. Regular consumption of these seeds can help maintain optimal zinc levels, supporting overall male reproductive health and immune function.

Ingredients:

- ¼ cup pumpkin seeds
- ¼ cup watermelon seeds
- ¼ cup sunflower seeds

Instructions:

- Mix equal parts of pumpkin seeds, watermelon seeds, and sunflower seeds in a bowl. Ensure that the seeds are raw and unsalted to maximize their nutritional benefits.
- Once mixed, store the seed blend in an airtight container to keep them fresh.
- Consume a handful of this mix daily, either on its own as a snack or sprinkled over salads, yogurt, or smoothies.

What to Expect:

Integrating this Zinc-rich Herbal Mix into your diet can contribute to improved male health, including:

- Enhanced testosterone levels: Zinc is a key mineral in testosterone production, which is essential for libido, muscle growth, and overall vitality.
- Improved fertility: Zinc contributes to sperm quality and motility, playing a critical role in male fertility.
- Prostate health: Adequate zinc intake is associated with a lower risk of prostate issues.

Pumpkin seeds, watermelon seeds, and sunflower seeds also provide other vital nutrients such as magnesium, selenium, and healthy fats, contributing to heart health, immune support, and overall well-being.
While this herbal mix is beneficial for boosting zinc intake naturally, it's important to maintain a balanced and varied diet to ensure you're getting a wide range of nutrients essential for health. For those with specific health conditions or dietary needs, consulting with a healthcare provider or a nutritionist is advisable to tailor dietary choices to individual health requirements.
Incorporating this Zinc-rich Herbal Mix into your daily routine can be a simple and tasty way to support male health and ensure adequate zinc intake, alongside other healthful lifestyle practices.

CHAPTER 7: EXTERNAL BODY HEALTH AND CARE.

HERBAL REMEDIES FOR SKIN HEALTH AND CARE.

CALENDULA SALVE FOR ECZEMA.

Calendula Salve is a gentle, natural remedy for soothing eczema and other skin irritations. Calendula, known for its anti-inflammatory and healing properties, can help reduce itching, redness, and dryness associated with eczema. When infused in olive oil and combined with beeswax, it creates a protective salve that nourishes and repairs the skin.

Ingredients:

- 1 cup dried calendula petals
- 1 cup olive oil
- 1/4 cup beeswax pellets

Instructions:

- Infuse Calendula in Olive Oil:
    - Place the dried calendula petals in a clean, dry jar.
    - Pour the olive oil over the petals, ensuring they are completely submerged.
    - Seal the jar and place it in a warm, sunny spot for 2 weeks, shaking it gently every day to distribute the petals.
    - After 2 weeks, strain the oil through a cheesecloth or fine mesh strainer to remove the petals. The resulting oil should have a rich, golden color.
- Prepare the Salve:
    - In a double boiler, gently heat the strained calendula-infused oil.
    - Add the beeswax pellets to the oil, stirring continuously until the beeswax is completely melted and the mixture is well combined.
    - Remove from heat and let it cool slightly.
- Pour and Set:
    - Carefully pour the warm salve mixture into clean, dry containers.
    - Allow the salve to cool and solidify at room temperature. This may take a few hours.
- Label and Store:
    - Label your salve jars with the contents and date of production.
    - Store the salve in a cool, dark place. The salve should be good for up to a year.

Usage:

- Apply a small amount of the Calendula Salve to the affected areas of the skin as needed for relief. The salve is gentle and can be used several times a day.

What to Expect:

Using Calendula Salve can provide soothing relief from the symptoms of eczema, such as itching, inflammation, and dryness. With regular application, you may notice a reduction in skin irritation and an improvement in skin hydration and healing.

While Calendula Salve is generally safe and well-tolerated, it's always a good idea to patch test any new product on a small area of skin before widespread use, especially if you have sensitive skin or allergies. If irritation occurs, discontinue use.

Creating your own Calendula Salve is a rewarding process that results in a natural, effective remedy for managing eczema and promoting healthy skin.

Aloe Vera Gel for Sunburn.

Aloe Vera Gel is renowned for its cooling, soothing, and healing properties, making it an excellent natural remedy for sunburn. The gel extracted from the aloe vera plant contains compounds that provide pain relief, reduce inflammation, and promote skin healing. Applying aloe vera gel directly to sunburnt skin can help alleviate discomfort and accelerate the healing process.

Instructions:

- Extract Aloe Vera Gel:
    - Choose a healthy, mature aloe vera leaf from the plant. A larger leaf is preferable as it contains more gel.
    - Use a sharp knife to slice off the leaf from the base of the plant.
    - Stand the leaf upright in a cup or bowl for a few minutes to allow the yellow sap (aloin, which can be irritating) to drain out.
    - After the sap has drained, lay the leaf flat on a cutting board. Slice off the serrated edges of the leaf.
    - Carefully slice the leaf open lengthwise to expose the clear gel inside.
    - Use a spoon or knife to scrape out the gel. Be gentle to avoid including any parts of the green leaf skin, which might contain aloin.
- Apply Aloe Vera Gel:
    - Apply the freshly extracted aloe vera gel directly to the sunburnt skin using clean fingers or a soft cotton pad.

- Gently spread the gel over the affected area, allowing it to form a thin layer.
- Let the gel air dry on your skin for maximum absorption and relief.
- Reapply as needed, especially after bathing or when the skin feels dry.

What to Expect:
Upon application, you should feel an immediate cooling and soothing sensation on the sunburnt areas. Aloe vera gel helps to moisturize the skin, prevent peeling, and accelerate healing. With regular application, you can expect a reduction in redness and discomfort associated with sunburn.
For severe sunburns, or if symptoms persist, it's important to seek medical advice, as additional treatment may be necessary.
Storage:
If you have extra aloe vera gel, it can be stored in a clean, airtight container in the refrigerator for up to one week. For longer storage, freeze the gel in ice cube trays and transfer the frozen cubes to a freezer bag. This method not only preserves the gel but also provides an extra cooling effect when applied to sunburnt skin.
Using Aloe Vera Gel is a simple, effective way to provide relief for sunburn, leveraging the natural healing power of the aloe vera plant to soothe and repair damaged skin.

TEA TREE OIL BLEND FOR ACNE.

Tea Tree Oil Blend is a natural and effective remedy for treating acne due to its potent antibacterial and anti-inflammatory properties. Diluting tea tree oil with water minimizes the risk of skin irritation while maintaining its effectiveness in targeting acne-causing bacteria and reducing inflammation.
Ingredients:

- 1 part tea tree oil
- 9 parts water

Instructions:

- Prepare the Blend:
    - In a clean container, mix 1 part tea tree oil with 9 parts water. For example, you could use 1 teaspoon of tea tree oil and 9 teaspoons of water.
    - Shake or stir the mixture well to ensure the tea tree oil is evenly distributed in the water.
- Application:
    - Dip a clean cotton ball or a cotton swab into the diluted tea tree oil blend.

- Gently apply the mixture to the acne spots or affected areas of the skin. Avoid applying it to the entire face if not necessary, as tea tree oil is potent and best used as a spot treatment.
    - Allow the mixture to dry naturally on the skin. There is no need to rinse it off unless you experience irritation.
- Storage:
    - Store any leftover blend in a clean, airtight container in a cool, dark place. Consider refrigerating the blend to preserve its potency, especially if you've made a large batch.

What to Expect:
With regular application, you can expect a reduction in acne severity and inflammation. Tea tree oil's antibacterial action helps to clear acne-causing bacteria, while its anti-inflammatory properties reduce redness and swelling.
Important Notes:

- Always perform a patch test before using tea tree oil on your face, especially if you have sensitive skin. Apply a small amount of the diluted blend to your forearm and wait 24 hours to see if any irritation occurs.
- If you experience dryness, irritation, or an allergic reaction, discontinue use immediately and rinse the area with water.
- Tea tree oil should never be applied undiluted to the skin, as it can cause severe irritation and allergic reactions in some individuals.

Tea Tree Oil Blend for Acne offers a simple, natural alternative for managing acne, helping to clear and soothe the skin without the harsh effects of chemical treatments.

Plantain Leaf Poultice for Skin Irritations.

Plantain Leaf Poultice is a traditional remedy used for centuries to soothe various skin irritations, including bites, stings, burns, and rashes. Plantain leaves, from the Plantago major or Plantago lanceolata species, contain natural anti-inflammatory and antimicrobial properties, making them effective in promoting healing and reducing discomfort on the skin.
Instructions:

- Collect Fresh Plantain Leaves: Choose fresh, green plantain leaves. Ensure they are clean and free from pesticides - wild, unsprayed leaves are ideal.
- Crush the Leaves: Use a mortar and pestle to crush the leaves thoroughly until they release their juice. If you don’t have a mortar and pestle, you can chop the leaves finely and then crush them using the back of a spoon or by simply using your hands.

- Apply the Poultice: Once the leaves are crushed and juicy, apply them directly to the affected area of the skin. If the area is large or if you prefer a cleaner application, you can spread the crushed leaves on a clean cloth or gauze and then place it on the skin.
- Secure the Poultice: Use a bandage or medical tape to hold the poultice (or cloth/gauze with the poultice) in place. Ensure it's secure but not too tight.
- Leave on for 1-2 hours: For best results, leave the poultice on for at least 1-2 hours, or even longer if possible. For ongoing issues, you can apply a fresh poultice several times a day.

What to Expect:
Applying a Plantain Leaf Poultice can quickly soothe skin irritations by reducing inflammation, itching, and discomfort. The natural healing properties of plantain may also expedite the healing process of minor wounds or skin abrasions. Users often report a cooling sensation upon application, followed by a gradual relief from irritation.
While Plantain Leaf Poultice is generally safe and effective for topical use, it's always wise to perform a patch test on a small area of skin first to ensure there's no allergic reaction. Additionally, if the skin irritation is severe, persistent, or if there's an underlying condition, consulting with a healthcare professional is advisable.
Incorporating Plantain Leaf Poultice into your natural first aid kit can offer a readily available and effective remedy for treating minor skin irritations and promoting skin health with the power of nature.

YARROW COMPRESS FOR WOUND HEALING.

Yarrow Compress is a traditional remedy valued for its potent wound-healing properties. Yarrow, scientifically known as Achillea millefolium, has been used for centuries in herbal medicine for its ability to stop bleeding, reduce inflammation, and promote the healing of cuts, scrapes, and bruises. The herb contains active compounds such as flavonoids and alkaloids that contribute to its therapeutic effects.
Instructions:

- Prepare Yarrow Tea:
  - Take 1-2 tablespoons of dried yarrow.
  - Pour 1 cup of boiling water over the dried yarrow in a heat-resistant bowl.
  - Cover and allow the yarrow to steep for about 15 minutes. This creates a strong infusion that will be used for the compress.
- Soak the Cloth:

- After the yarrow has steeped, strain the liquid to remove the plant material.
    - Soak a clean cloth or gauze in the yarrow infusion until it is fully saturated.
- Apply the Compress:
    - Gently wring out the cloth or gauze to remove excess liquid without making it too dry.
    - Apply the soaked cloth directly to the wound or affected area. If the wound is open or sensitive, you can place the compress on the surrounding skin rather than directly on the wound.
    - Secure the cloth in place with a bandage or medical tape if necessary, ensuring it's not too tight.
- Leave on for up to 1 hour:
    - Allow the compress to sit on the affected area for up to 1 hour, refreshing with more yarrow infusion if it dries out.
    - You can apply a fresh yarrow compress 2-3 times a day as needed for continued relief and healing.

What to Expect:
Using a Yarrow Compress can accelerate the healing process of wounds by reducing inflammation, promoting clotting, and preventing infection due to yarrow's antimicrobial properties. Many people report a decrease in pain and swelling after application, along with quicker wound closure and healing.
While Yarrow is generally safe for topical use, it's important to ensure that the wound is clean before applying the compress. Also, individuals with allergies to plants in the Asteraceae family should use caution. For deep, puncture, or severe wounds, or if there is any sign of infection, seek medical attention promptly.
Incorporating a Yarrow Compress into your first aid practices can be an effective natural remedy for managing minor wounds and supporting the body's healing process.

BURDOCK ROOT INFUSION FOR ACNE.

Burdock Root Infusion is a traditional herbal remedy known for its detoxifying and blood-purifying properties, making it particularly effective in treating acne from within. Burdock root, scientifically known as Arctium lappa, contains powerful antioxidants, anti-inflammatory, and antimicrobial compounds that help to cleanse the blood, improve liver function, and reduce skin inflammation. By addressing the internal imbalances that can lead to acne, burdock root infusion offers a holistic approach to skin health.
Ingredients:

- 1 tablespoon dried burdock root
- 4 cups of water

Instructions:

- Add 1 tablespoon of dried burdock root to 4 cups of water in a medium-sized pot.
- Bring the water to a boil, then reduce the heat and simmer the burdock root for about 30 minutes. This long simmering process extracts the active compounds from the burdock root, creating a potent infusion.
- After simmering, remove the pot from the heat and allow it to cool slightly.
- Strain the infusion to remove the burdock root pieces, leaving you with the clear liquid.
- The infusion can be consumed warm or cooled. It has a mildly sweet and earthy flavor that can be enhanced with a teaspoon of honey or lemon juice if desired.

What to Expect:

Drinking Burdock Root Infusion can lead to gradual improvements in skin health, including a reduction in acne outbreaks, clearer skin, and an overall decrease in inflammation. It works from the inside out, cleansing the blood and supporting liver detoxification, which are essential for healthy skin.

It's important to consume the infusion consistently for several weeks to observe significant results, as natural remedies often require time to take effect. A daily serving of the burdock root infusion can be a beneficial addition to your skincare regimen.

While Burdock Root Infusion is safe for most individuals, it's advisable to start with a small amount to ensure tolerance. Pregnant or breastfeeding women, individuals with chronic health conditions, or those on medication should consult with a healthcare provider before incorporating burdock root into their diet.

Incorporating Burdock Root Infusion into your daily routine can offer a natural and effective solution for managing acne, promoting not only clearer skin but also overall health and well-being.

Calendula Infused Oil for Skin Irritations.

Calendula Infused Oil harnesses the healing properties of calendula flowers, known for their anti-inflammatory, antimicrobial, and skin-regenerative qualities. This natural remedy is excellent for soothing skin irritations, rashes, and minor wounds, promoting healing and reducing inflammation. The infusion process extracts the beneficial compounds from the calendula flowers into the carrier oil, making it an ideal topical treatment for a variety of skin conditions.

Ingredients:

- Dried calendula flowers
- Carrier oil (such as olive oil, almond oil, or coconut oil)

Instructions:

- Prepare the Calendula and Oil Mixture:
    - Fill a clean, dry jar about half full with dried calendula flowers.
    - Pour your choice of carrier oil over the flowers until the jar is nearly full, ensuring the flowers are completely submerged in the oil.
- Infuse the Oil:
    - Seal the jar tightly with a lid.
    - Place the jar in a warm, sunny spot for 4-6 weeks to allow the flowers to infuse into the oil. A windowsill that receives plenty of sunlight is ideal. Shake the jar gently every few days to mix the contents.
- Strain the Infused Oil:
    - After the infusion period, strain the oil through a fine mesh sieve or cheesecloth into a clean container to remove the calendula flowers. For a clearer oil, strain a second time.
- Store the Calendula Oil:
    - Transfer the strained oil into a clean, dry bottle or jar. Label the container with the date and contents. Store the oil in a cool, dark place.

How to Use:

- Apply the calendula infused oil directly to the affected area of the skin. Gently massage a small amount of the oil into the skin until absorbed.
- Use as needed for skin irritations, rashes, dry skin, or as a general moisturizer for sensitive skin.

What to Expect:

With regular application, you can expect a soothing effect on irritated skin, reduced redness and inflammation, and accelerated healing of minor wounds or rashes. Calendula oil is gentle and suitable for most skin types, including sensitive skin.

While calendula infused oil is generally safe for topical use, it's always advisable to perform a patch test on a small area of skin first to ensure there's no allergic reaction. If you're pregnant or nursing, or if you have any major health concerns, consult with a healthcare provider before using calendula oil.

Incorporating Calendula Infused Oil into your skincare routine can provide a gentle, natural solution for managing skin irritations and enhancing skin health.

TEA TREE OIL SPOT TREATMENT FOR ACNE.

Tea Tree Oil Spot Treatment is a natural and effective remedy for targeting acne spots. Tea tree oil, derived from the leaves of the Melaleuca alternifolia tree, is known for its potent antimicrobial and anti-inflammatory properties, making it ideal for reducing acne lesions and preventing new breakouts. It's important to dilute tea tree oil before application to minimize skin irritation.
Ingredients:

- 2-3 drops of tea tree oil
- 1 teaspoon of water or carrier oil (such as jojoba oil, coconut oil, or almond oil)

Instructions:

- Dilute the Tea Tree Oil:
  - In a small bowl, mix 2-3 drops of tea tree oil with 1 teaspoon of water or a carrier oil of your choice. Carrier oils can provide additional moisturizing benefits and help prevent irritation, making them a preferred option for sensitive skin.
- Application:
  - Dip a clean cotton swab into the diluted tea tree oil mixture.
  - Gently dab the mixture directly onto the acne spots. Avoid rubbing the area to prevent irritation.
  - Let the treatment dry naturally. There's no need to rinse it off unless you experience discomfort.
- Frequency of Use:
  - You can apply the tea tree oil spot treatment 1-2 times daily, depending on your skin's sensitivity. Starting with once daily application is advisable to assess skin tolerance.

What to Expect:
With regular use, you can expect a reduction in the severity and frequency of acne spots. Tea tree oil's antimicrobial action helps to kill acne-causing bacteria, while its anti-inflammatory properties reduce redness and swelling, promoting healing. However, results may vary, and it may take several weeks to see significant improvements.
While tea tree oil is effective for many people, those with sensitive skin should proceed with caution. It's always recommended to perform a patch test on a small area of skin before using a new product broadly, especially on the face. If irritation or an allergic reaction occurs, discontinue use immediately and consult a healthcare provider if necessary.

Incorporating Tea Tree Oil Spot Treatment into your skincare routine can be a powerful way to combat acne naturally, complementing other skincare practices for clear and healthy skin.

OATMEAL AND CHAMOMILE BATH FOR ECZEMA.

An Oatmeal and Chamomile Bath is a natural remedy designed to soothe eczema and irritated skin. Oatmeal has anti-inflammatory and moisturizing properties that help to relieve itching and reduce redness, while chamomile is known for its calming and healing effects on the skin, making this combination ideal for sensitive or eczema-prone skin.

Ingredients:

- 1 cup colloidal oatmeal (finely ground oatmeal)
- 1/2 cup dried chamomile flowers

Instructions:

- Blend 1 cup of colloidal oatmeal with 1/2 cup of dried chamomile flowers until you achieve a fine powder. A coffee grinder or food processor works well for this.
- Draw a warm bath to a comfortable temperature. Avoid hot water, as it can further irritate eczema.
- While the tub is filling, add the oatmeal and chamomile blend directly to the bathwater, stirring well to ensure it disperses evenly.
- Once the bath is ready, soak in the oatmeal and chamomile-infused water for 15-20 minutes. Use your hands to gently scoop up some of the water and pour it over areas of your skin that are not submerged.
- After soaking, pat your skin dry with a towel. Avoid rubbing the skin, as this can cause irritation.
- Follow up with a gentle, fragrance-free moisturizer to lock in hydration.

What to Expect:

Taking an Oatmeal and Chamomile Bath can provide immediate relief from the discomfort associated with eczema, such as itching, redness, and dryness. The anti-inflammatory properties of both oatmeal and chamomile work together to soothe and heal the skin, reducing flare-ups and promoting recovery.

For best results, consider incorporating this bath into your skincare routine 1-2 times a week or as needed during eczema flare-ups. It's also important to maintain a regular moisturizing regimen and avoid known irritants that may trigger eczema symptoms.

While this natural remedy is gentle and effective for many, it's always a good idea to perform a patch test with both oatmeal and chamomile before fully immersing yourself in the bath, especially if you have highly sensitive skin or allergies to these ingredients. If you experience any adverse reactions, discontinue use and consult with a healthcare provider.

WITCH HAZEL AND LAVENDER SKIN TONER.

The combination of witch hazel extract and lavender essential oil creates a gentle, natural skin toner that is effective for managing acne and reducing inflammation. Witch hazel is known for its astringent properties, which help to tighten pores and refine skin texture, while lavender essential oil offers soothing, anti-inflammatory benefits, making this toner ideal for calming irritated skin and promoting a clear complexion.

Ingredients:

- 1 cup witch hazel extract
- 5-10 drops lavender essential oil

Instructions:

- In a clean, sterilized bottle or jar, pour 1 cup of witch hazel extract.
- Add 5-10 drops of lavender essential oil to the witch hazel. The amount of lavender oil can be adjusted based on personal preference and skin sensitivity. Start with fewer drops and increase as desired, keeping in mind that essential oils are potent.
- Cap the bottle or jar and shake well to mix the ingredients thoroughly.
- To use, soak a cotton pad with the witch hazel and lavender toner and gently apply it to cleansed skin, focusing on areas prone to acne and inflammation. Avoid the eye area.
- Allow the toner to dry naturally on the skin before applying moisturizer.

What to Expect:

Using this Witch Hazel and Lavender Skin Toner as part of your daily skincare routine can help reduce acne breakouts, minimize pores, and calm skin inflammation. Witch hazel's astringent properties work to cleanse and tighten the skin, while lavender's calming effect helps to soothe redness and irritation.

This toner is suitable for most skin types, including oily and acne-prone skin. However, it's always a good idea to perform a patch test before using new skincare products, especially those containing essential oils, to ensure they do not cause irritation or allergic reactions.

For optimal results, use the toner twice daily after cleansing and before moisturizing. Consistent use can help maintain balanced, clear, and calm skin.

Remember, while this natural toner can be an effective addition to your skincare regimen, maintaining a healthy lifestyle, staying hydrated, and following a balanced diet also contribute significantly to skin health.

COMFREY SALVE FOR WOUND HEALING.

Comfrey Salve is a potent herbal remedy renowned for its remarkable healing properties. Comfrey, scientifically known as Symphytum officinale, contains allantoin, a compound that promotes cell regeneration and speeds up the healing process of wounds, bruises, and skin irritations. When combined with beeswax, the infused oil transforms into a protective salve that can be directly applied to the skin to aid healing.

Ingredients:

- 1 cup comfrey leaves, dried and finely chopped
- 1 cup carrier oil (such as olive oil, coconut oil, or almond oil)
- 1/4 cup beeswax pellets

Instructions:

- Infuse Comfrey Leaves in Oil:
    - Place the dried comfrey leaves in a glass jar and cover them with the carrier oil of your choice.
    - Seal the jar and place it in a warm, sunny spot for 4-6 weeks, shaking it every few days to ensure even infusion. For a quicker method, you can gently heat the oil and comfrey leaves in a double boiler for about 2-3 hours on low heat, making sure not to overheat or boil the oil.
    - After infusion, strain the oil through a cheesecloth or fine mesh sieve to remove the comfrey leaves, retaining the infused oil.
- Making the Comfrey Salve:
    - In a double boiler, gently heat the infused comfrey oil. Once warm, add the beeswax pellets.
    - Stir the mixture until the beeswax is completely melted and well incorporated into the oil.
    - Remove from heat and allow the mixture to cool slightly before pouring it into sterilized tins or jars.
    - Let the salve cool and solidify completely before sealing with a lid.

Usage:

- Apply a small amount of the Comfrey Salve to clean wounds, bruises, or skin irritations. Gently massage it into the area and allow it to absorb.
- Use the salve 2-3 times daily until the wound or bruise has healed.

What to Expect:

The Comfrey Salve works by promoting faster cell regeneration and reducing inflammation, which can significantly speed up the healing process of the skin. Its natural, protective barrier also helps keep the wound moist and safe from external irritants.

While comfrey is highly effective in wound healing, it should be used with caution. Avoid applying the salve to deep, open wounds or ingesting it, as comfrey contains compounds that can be harmful if absorbed internally in large amounts. It's best suited for superficial skin issues.
Always consult with a healthcare provider before using herbal remedies, especially on serious wounds or if you have underlying health conditions. Comfrey Salve is a wonderful addition to your natural first aid kit, offering a gentle yet powerful solution for skin healing and care.

CHICKWEED OINTMENT FOR ITCHY SKIN.

Chickweed Ointment is an effective natural remedy for soothing itchy and irritated skin. Chickweed (Stellaria media) has cooling and anti-inflammatory properties, making it ideal for treating skin conditions like eczema, psoriasis, rashes, and minor burns. When infused in oil and combined with beeswax, chickweed creates a soothing ointment that can be applied directly to affected areas to relieve discomfort.
Ingredients:

- 1 cup chickweed, finely chopped (fresh or dried)
- 1 cup carrier oil (such as olive oil, coconut oil, or sweet almond oil)
- 1/4 cup beeswax pellets

Instructions:

- Infuse Chickweed in Oil:
    - Place the chickweed in a glass jar and cover it with the carrier oil of your choice.
    - Seal the jar tightly and place it in a warm, sunny location for 4-6 weeks, shaking it every few days to ensure the chickweed is fully infused into the oil. For a quicker infusion, you can gently heat the oil and chickweed in a double boiler on low heat for 2-3 hours, being careful not to boil the oil.
    - After the infusion period, strain the oil through a cheesecloth or fine mesh strainer to remove the chickweed. Retain the infused oil for the ointment.
- Making the Chickweed Ointment:
    - In a double boiler, gently heat the infused chickweed oil. Once warm, add the beeswax pellets.
    - Stir continuously until the beeswax is completely melted and combined with the oil.
    - Remove from heat and let the mixture cool slightly. Before it solidifies, pour it into clean, sterilized tins or jars.
    - Allow the ointment to cool and solidify at room temperature before securing the lids.

Usage:

- Apply a small amount of Chickweed Ointment to the affected itchy or irritated skin areas. Massage gently until absorbed.
- Use the ointment 2-3 times a day or as needed to relieve symptoms.

What to Expect:
Chickweed Ointment can provide immediate relief from itching and discomfort caused by dry skin, eczema, psoriasis, and other skin irritations. Its natural cooling effect helps soothe the skin, while its anti-inflammatory properties reduce redness and swelling.
As with any topical remedy, it's advisable to do a patch test before widespread use, especially if you have sensitive skin or allergies. Apply a small amount of the ointment to a discreet area and wait 24 hours to ensure there's no adverse reaction.
While Chickweed Ointment is a gentle and effective remedy for itchy and irritated skin, severe or persistent skin conditions should be evaluated by a healthcare professional. Incorporating this ointment into your skin care regimen can offer natural, soothing relief for minor skin irritations.

Burdock Root Tea for Skin Detoxification.

Burdock Root Tea is a traditional herbal remedy known for its powerful detoxifying properties, particularly beneficial for the skin. Made from the root of the burdock plant (Arctium lappa), this tea aids in purifying the blood and removing toxins that can lead to skin issues like acne, eczema, and psoriasis. Its diuretic effect also supports kidney function, further promoting the elimination of toxins from the body and resulting in clearer, healthier skin.
Ingredients:

- 1-2 teaspoons dried burdock root
- 2 cups water

Instructions:

- Add 1-2 teaspoons of dried burdock root to 2 cups of water in a saucepan.
- Bring the mixture to a boil, then reduce the heat and simmer for about 15-20 minutes. This allows the active compounds in the burdock root to be extracted into the water.
- After simmering, strain the tea to remove the burdock root pieces.
- Allow the tea to cool to a comfortable drinking temperature.

Serving Suggestion:

- The tea can be consumed warm or chilled, depending on personal preference. It has a slightly earthy and sweet flavor that can be enhanced with a teaspoon of honey or a slice of lemon if desired.
- For skin detoxification, drink 1-2 cups of Burdock Root Tea daily.

What to Expect:
Regular consumption of Burdock Root Tea can lead to visible improvements in skin health and complexion. Its detoxifying effects help to cleanse the blood and reduce the occurrence of skin blemishes and irritations. Additionally, burdock root's anti-inflammatory properties may soothe skin conditions and promote a more even skin tone.
While Burdock Root Tea is beneficial for detoxifying the skin and improving complexion, it's essential to use it as part of a balanced diet and healthy lifestyle. Also, individuals with certain medical conditions, particularly those related to the kidneys or liver, should consult with a healthcare provider before incorporating burdock root into their regimen.
Incorporating Burdock Root Tea into your daily routine can be a simple and natural way to support skin health from the inside out, leveraging the purifying benefits of this traditional herbal remedy.

Chickweed Infused Oil for Itchy Skin.

Chickweed Infused Oil is a natural remedy highly regarded for its soothing properties on itchy and irritated skin. Chickweed (Stellaria media) is known for its anti-inflammatory and mild antiseptic effects, making it an excellent choice for treating various skin conditions such as eczema, rashes, and minor burns. When infused in a carrier oil, chickweed imparts its healing properties, creating a versatile and gentle solution for skin discomfort.
Ingredients:

- 1 cup dried chickweed
- 1-2 cups carrier oil (such as olive oil, coconut oil, or jojoba oil)

Instructions:

- Prepare the Chickweed:
    - Ensure the chickweed is completely dried to prevent moisture from causing the oil to spoil.
    - Roughly chop or crush the dried chickweed to increase its surface area.
- Infuse Chickweed in Oil:
    - Place the dried chickweed in a clean, dry jar.
    - Pour the carrier oil over the chickweed, making sure it is completely submerged. Use enough oil to cover the chickweed by at least an inch to allow for expansion.
    - Seal the jar tightly and place it in a warm, sunny spot for 4-6 weeks to allow the chickweed to infuse into the oil. Shake the jar daily to mix the contents.

    - For a quicker infusion, you can gently heat the oil and chickweed in a double boiler on low heat for 2-3 hours, being careful not to overheat or cook the herb.
- Strain the Infused Oil:
    - After the infusion period, strain the oil through a cheesecloth or fine mesh strainer to remove the chickweed. Squeeze or press the herb to extract as much oil as possible.
    - Pour the strained oil into clean, dry bottles or jars.

Usage:

- Apply the chickweed infused oil directly to itchy, irritated skin areas as needed. Massage gently until the oil is absorbed.
- The oil can be used several times a day, depending on the severity of the itchiness or irritation.

What to Expect:

Chickweed infused oil provides immediate soothing relief for itchy and irritated skin. Its anti-inflammatory properties help to calm the skin, reduce redness, and promote healing. With regular application, you may notice an improvement in skin condition and a reduction in discomfort.

This remedy is gentle and suitable for most skin types. However, as with any new topical application, it's a good idea to perform a patch test on a small area of skin first to ensure there's no adverse reaction.

Chickweed infused oil is a simple, effective way to harness the soothing properties of chickweed for skin relief. It can be a valuable addition to your natural skincare regimen, offering a gentle alternative to commercial itch-relief products.

WITCH HAZEL AND ALOE VERA GEL FOR SKIN IRRITATIONS.

The combination of witch hazel extract and aloe vera gel creates a powerful, natural remedy for soothing skin irritations. Witch hazel is known for its astringent and anti-inflammatory properties, making it excellent for reducing inflammation, calming irritation, and tightening pores. Aloe vera, on the other hand, is renowned for its healing, moisturizing, and soothing effects, particularly on burns, cuts, and other skin irritations. Together, they form a gentle yet effective treatment for a variety of skin concerns.

Ingredients:

- 1/4 cup witch hazel extract
- 1/4 cup aloe vera gel

Instructions:

- In a clean bowl, combine 1/4 cup of witch hazel extract with 1/4 cup of aloe vera gel. Use pure aloe vera gel for the best results, free from added colors, fragrances, or alcohol.

- Stir the mixture thoroughly until the witch hazel and aloe vera gel are well blended.
- Transfer the mixture to a clean, airtight container for storage. A pump bottle or a jar with a lid works well.
- To use, apply a small amount of the mixture to the affected area of the skin. Gently massage it in until fully absorbed. You can use this remedy 2-3 times a day or as needed to soothe irritation.

What to Expect:

Applying the Witch Hazel and Aloe Vera Gel to skin irritations can provide immediate relief from discomfort, reduce redness and swelling, and promote faster healing. The astringent properties of witch hazel help to cleanse the skin and minimize pores, while aloe vera's hydrating nature ensures that the skin remains moisturized and heals without leaving dry patches.

This combination is suitable for all skin types, including sensitive skin, and can be used to treat sunburns, razor burns, insect bites, and minor cuts or abrasions. It's also effective as a calming after-sun treatment or to soothe irritation after shaving.

While this mixture is generally safe and beneficial for most people, it's always a good idea to perform a patch test on a small area of skin first, especially if you have sensitive skin or allergies. If you experience any adverse reaction, discontinue use immediately.

The Witch Hazel and Aloe Vera Gel is a versatile, easy-to-make remedy that harnesses the natural healing powers of both ingredients, offering a gentle solution for managing skin irritations and promoting healthy, calm skin.

Neem Leaf Paste for Acne and Eczema.

Neem leaf paste is a traditional remedy revered for its potent antiseptic, anti-inflammatory, and antimicrobial properties, making it highly effective in treating skin conditions like acne and eczema. Neem, derived from the Azadirachta indica tree, contains compounds that not only soothe irritated skin but also help in reducing redness, swelling, and infection associated with acne breakouts and eczema flare-ups.

Ingredients:

- 2 tablespoons neem leaf powder
- Enough water to form a paste

Instructions:

- In a small bowl, mix 2 tablespoons of neem leaf powder with water. Add the water gradually until you achieve a thick, but spreadable, paste consistency.
- Before application, cleanse the skin with a gentle, non-drying cleanser to remove impurities and excess oil.

- Apply the neem leaf paste directly to the affected areas of the skin using clean fingers or a spatula. If you have sensitive skin, you may want to do a patch test on a small area first to ensure there is no adverse reaction.
- Leave the paste on the skin for about 10-20 minutes or until it dries.
- Rinse off the paste with lukewarm water and gently pat the skin dry with a clean towel. Follow up with a gentle, non-comedogenic moisturizer to keep the skin hydrated.
- For best results, use the neem leaf paste 2-3 times a week.

What to Expect:

The application of neem leaf paste can significantly improve acne and eczema symptoms. Its antibacterial properties help to kill the bacteria that cause acne, while its anti-inflammatory effects reduce redness and swelling. In cases of eczema, neem can provide relief from itching and irritation and help to heal the damaged skin barrier.

Regular use of neem leaf paste may lead to clearer, healthier skin. However, as with any natural remedy, results can vary from person to person. While neem is generally safe for topical use, it's important to observe your skin's reaction, especially if you have sensitive skin, and discontinue use if any irritation occurs.

Neem leaf paste offers a natural, chemical-free alternative for managing skin conditions, harnessing the healing power of nature to support skin health.

Witch Hazel and Calendula Acne Treatment.

Combining witch hazel extract with calendula-infused oil creates an effective, natural treatment for acne-prone skin. Witch hazel is renowned for its astringent and anti-inflammatory properties, making it excellent for reducing acne inflammation and minimizing pores without over-drying the skin. Calendula, known for its soothing and healing capabilities, helps to calm irritated skin, reduce redness, and promote skin regeneration. This synergistic blend is gentle yet potent, offering a holistic approach to managing acne.

Ingredients:

- 1/2 cup witch hazel extract
- 1/4 cup calendula-infused oil

Instructions:

- Prepare calendula-infused oil in advance by steeping dried calendula petals in a carrier oil (such as olive oil or almond oil) for several weeks or gently heating the mixture for a few hours. Strain the oil to remove the petals.
- In a clean bottle or container, mix 1/2 cup of witch hazel extract with 1/4 cup of calendula-infused oil. Shake well to combine.

- To use, apply a small amount of the mixture to a cotton ball or pad and gently dab onto acne-prone areas after cleansing. Avoid rinsing, allowing the treatment to penetrate and act on the skin.
- Apply this treatment 1-2 times daily, especially after washing your face in the morning and at night.

What to Expect:
The Witch Hazel and Calendula Acne Treatment can significantly reduce the appearance of acne and soothe irritated skin. With regular use, you can expect a decrease in inflammation, redness, and acne breakouts, as well as an overall improvement in skin texture and tone.
This natural remedy is suitable for all skin types, including sensitive skin. However, as with any topical treatment, it's wise to perform a patch test on a small area of skin first to ensure no adverse reaction occurs.
By incorporating this Witch Hazel and Calendula Acne Treatment into your skincare routine, you can harness the natural healing properties of both witch hazel and calendula, providing a gentle yet effective solution for managing acne and promoting healthy, clear skin.

Plantain Leaf and Yarrow Wound Salve.

This Plantain Leaf and Yarrow Wound Salve is a powerful, natural remedy designed to promote the healing of cuts and wounds. Plantain leaf (Plantago major) is renowned for its antibacterial and anti-inflammatory properties, making it ideal for wound care. Yarrow (Achillea millefolium), on the other hand, is celebrated for its ability to stop bleeding and heal skin tissue. Combined in a salve with beeswax, these herbs offer a protective barrier that nurtures the skin and accelerates healing.
Ingredients:

- 1/2 cup plantain leaves, finely chopped or crushed
- 1/2 cup yarrow, finely chopped or crushed
- 1 cup carrier oil (such as olive oil, coconut oil, or almond oil)
- 1/4 cup beeswax pellets

Instructions:

- Infuse the Herbs in Oil:
    - Combine the chopped plantain leaves and yarrow with the carrier oil in a double boiler. If you don’t have a double boiler, you can use a glass or metal bowl set over a pot of simmering water.
    - Gently heat the mixture for 2-3 hours on low heat, ensuring it does not boil. This process infuses the oil with the medicinal properties of the herbs.

    - After infusion, strain the oil through a cheesecloth or fine mesh strainer to remove the herb particles, retaining the infused oil.
- Making the Salve:
    - Return the infused oil to the cleaned double boiler and gently heat.
    - Add the beeswax pellets to the infused oil and stir until completely melted and combined.
    - Remove from heat and allow to cool slightly before pouring into small tins or jars.
    - Let the salve cool and solidify before sealing with lids.

Usage:

- Clean the cut or wound thoroughly before application.
- Apply a small amount of the Plantain Leaf and Yarrow Wound Salve directly to the affected area.
- Cover with a bandage if necessary.
- Reapply 2-3 times daily until the wound is healed.

What to Expect:

Using this salve can significantly reduce healing time for cuts and wounds. Plantain and yarrow work together to reduce inflammation, prevent infection, and promote the regeneration of skin cells. The beeswax forms a protective layer that moisturizes the skin and keeps out irritants.

This natural wound salve is gentle and suitable for all skin types. However, as with any topical treatment, it's advisable to do a patch test first, especially if you have sensitive skin or plant allergies.

Incorporating this Plantain Leaf and Yarrow Wound Salve into your first-aid kit ensures you have a natural, effective remedy for skin injuries at hand, harnessing the healing power of these remarkable herbs.

CALENDULA AND HONEY HEALING OINTMENT.

The Calendula and Honey Healing Ointment is a natural, potent remedy designed to promote healing and soothe skin irritations. Calendula, known for its anti-inflammatory and antimicrobial properties, aids in wound healing and skin regeneration. Honey, with its natural antibacterial qualities and ability to draw moisture into the skin, enhances the ointment's healing capabilities. Combined with beeswax, this ointment creates a protective barrier on the skin while providing moisture and reducing inflammation.

Ingredients:

- 1 cup calendula-infused oil (Prepare by infusing dried calendula petals in a carrier oil like olive or almond oil for 4-6 weeks or gently heat for a few hours to speed up the process)
- 1/4 cup beeswax pellets

- 2 tablespoons honey, preferably raw and organic

Instructions:

- Prepare the Calendula-Infused Oil: If not already prepared, infuse dried calendula petals in your choice of carrier oil. After infusion, strain the oil to remove the petals.
- Making the Ointment:
    - In a double boiler, gently heat the calendula-infused oil. Once warm, add the beeswax pellets.
    - Stir until the beeswax is completely melted and well incorporated into the oil.
    - Remove from heat and allow the mixture to cool slightly before adding the honey. Stir thoroughly to ensure the honey is evenly distributed throughout the mixture.
    - Before the mixture solidifies, pour it into clean, sterilized jars or tins.
    - Allow the ointment to cool and set completely before sealing with lids.

Usage:

- Clean the affected area of the skin before application.
- Apply a small amount of the Calendula and Honey Healing Ointment to cuts, scrapes, burns, or any skin irritations.
- Use the ointment 2-3 times daily or as needed to promote healing and soothe the skin.

What to Expect:

The Calendula and Honey Healing Ointment provides a natural and effective way to support skin healing. Users can expect reduced inflammation, minimized risk of infection, and accelerated healing of wounds. The ointment also moisturizes the skin, making it feel soft and supple.

This healing ointment is suitable for all skin types, including sensitive skin. However, individuals with allergies to pollen or bee products should proceed with caution and consider a patch test before widespread use.

Incorporating this Calendula and Honey Healing Ointment into your skincare regimen or first-aid kit offers a gentle yet powerful solution for managing skin injuries and irritations, leveraging the natural healing properties of its ingredients.

Tea Tree and Witch Hazel Acne Solution.

The Tea Tree and Witch Hazel Acne Solution harnesses the potent antimicrobial and anti-inflammatory properties of tea tree oil combined with the astringent benefits of witch hazel. This natural remedy is effective for treating acne-prone skin, helping to reduce inflammation, kill bacteria, and minimize the appearance of pores without over-drying the skin.

Ingredients:

- 10 drops tea tree oil
- 1/4 cup witch hazel extract

Instructions:

- In a clean, sterilized container, add 1/4 cup of witch hazel extract.
- Add 10 drops of tea tree oil to the witch hazel. This dilution is strong enough to be effective yet gentle on the skin. If you have sensitive skin, you may start with fewer drops and adjust according to your skin's tolerance.
- Cap the container and shake well to ensure the tea tree oil is thoroughly mixed with the witch hazel.
- To use, apply a small amount of the solution to a cotton ball or pad and gently dab onto acne-prone areas after cleansing. Avoid the eye area.
- Use the solution 1-2 times daily, particularly in the evening after washing your face, to treat and prevent acne.

What to Expect:

Incorporating the Tea Tree and Witch Hazel Acne Solution into your skincare routine can lead to a noticeable improvement in acne and skin clarity. Tea tree oil's antimicrobial properties help to combat acne-causing bacteria, while witch hazel's astringent qualities reduce inflammation and tighten pores, resulting in clearer, healthier-looking skin.

While this solution is suitable for acne-prone skin, it's essential to observe how your skin reacts to tea tree oil, especially if you have sensitive skin. Always perform a patch test on a small area of skin before widespread use. If irritation occurs, dilute the solution further or discontinue use.

By using the Tea Tree and Witch Hazel Acne Solution regularly, you can achieve a balanced and clearer complexion naturally. Remember, consistency is key in skincare, and it's important to complement this treatment with a healthy lifestyle and proper skin hygiene for the best results.

Comfrey and Plantain Leaf Healing Balm.

This Comfrey and Plantain Leaf Healing Balm harnesses the natural healing properties of comfrey and plantain leaves, making it an excellent remedy for minor cuts, skin irritations, and abrasions. Comfrey, known scientifically as Symphytum officinale, contains allantoin, which promotes cell regeneration and speeds up wound healing. Plantain leaves (Plantago major) are renowned for their anti-inflammatory and antiseptic properties, providing relief from skin irritations and promoting healing. Combined with beeswax, this balm creates a protective barrier that moisturizes, soothes, and heals the skin.

Ingredients:

- 1/2 cup dried comfrey leaves
- 1/2 cup dried plantain leaves
- 1 cup carrier oil (such as olive oil, coconut oil, or almond oil)
- 1/4 cup beeswax pellets

Instructions:

- Infuse Comfrey and Plantain Leaves in Oil:
    - Combine the dried comfrey and plantain leaves with the carrier oil in a double boiler. If a double boiler is not available, you can use a glass bowl over a pot of simmering water.
    - Gently heat the mixture on low for 2-3 hours to allow the oil to infuse with the medicinal properties of the herbs. Avoid boiling.
    - Strain the infused oil through a cheesecloth or fine mesh sieve to remove the herb particles, capturing the infused oil in a clean container.
- Making the Healing Balm:
    - Return the infused oil to the double boiler and add the beeswax pellets.
    - Heat gently, stirring until the beeswax is completely melted and combined with the oil.
    - Once fully blended, carefully pour the mixture into small tins or jars.
    - Allow the balm to cool and solidify before sealing with lids.

Usage:

- Clean the affected area thoroughly before applying the balm.
- Apply a small amount of the Comfrey and Plantain Leaf Healing Balm directly to minor cuts, scrapes, or skin irritations.
- Use as needed, 2-3 times daily, until the area is healed.

What to Expect:

The application of this healing balm can significantly accelerate the healing process for minor wounds and skin irritations. Its natural anti-inflammatory and antiseptic properties help to prevent infection while soothing the skin and promoting cell regeneration. The beeswax in the balm forms a protective layer that locks in moisture, supporting the skin's natural healing process.

While this balm is designed to be gentle and effective for most skin types, it's always advisable to perform a patch test before widespread use, especially if you have sensitive skin or are prone to allergies.

Incorporating the Comfrey and Plantain Leaf Healing Balm into your skincare routine or first aid kit provides a natural, effective solution for skin healing, leveraging the powerful medicinal properties of these healing herbs.

Borage Seed Oil for Dermatitis and Eczema.

Borage Seed Oil is a potent natural remedy for skin conditions such as dermatitis and eczema, thanks to its high gamma-linolenic acid (GLA) content. GLA is an omega-6 fatty acid that plays a crucial role in maintaining skin health, reducing inflammation, and restoring the skin's moisture barrier. Borage seed oil's unique properties make it an excellent choice for soothing irritated skin and promoting healing.

Usage:

- Apply a small amount of borage seed oil directly to the affected areas of the skin.
- Gently massage the oil into the skin until it is fully absorbed.
- For best results, use the oil twice daily, in the morning and at night, after cleansing the skin.

What to Expect:

Regular topical application of borage seed oil can lead to noticeable improvements in the condition of the skin affected by dermatitis or eczema. You may observe a reduction in redness, itching, and inflammation, as well as an overall improvement in skin hydration and texture. The high GLA content in borage seed oil helps to repair the skin's natural barrier, preventing further moisture loss and protecting against irritants.

Borage seed oil is generally well-tolerated, but as with any topical treatment, it's wise to perform a patch test on a small area of skin first, especially if you have sensitive skin or allergies. Discontinue use if any adverse reactions occur.

While borage seed oil offers a natural and effective solution for managing dermatitis and eczema, it's important to remember that skin conditions can be complex and may require a multifaceted approach to treatment. Incorporating borage seed oil into your skincare routine should complement other recommended treatments and lifestyle adjustments advised by a healthcare provider.

By integrating borage seed oil into your care regimen, you're leveraging a powerful, natural source of GLA to support skin healing and comfort, offering relief from the symptoms of dermatitis and eczema.

Calendula and Chamomile Skin Soothing Lotion.

Combining the healing properties of calendula and chamomile with the soothing effect of aloe vera gel, this skin lotion is a perfect remedy for calming irritated, sensitive, or dry skin. Calendula, known for its anti-inflammatory and wound-healing properties, works well with chamomile, which offers calming and anti-irritant benefits. Aloe vera gel adds moisture and enhances the skin's healing process, making this lotion ideal for a variety of skin concerns.

Ingredients:

- 1/2 cup calendula flowers (dried)
- 1/2 cup chamomile flowers (dried)
- 1 cup carrier oil (such as almond oil, coconut oil, or olive oil)
- 1/4 cup aloe vera gel
- 1-2 tablespoons beeswax (adjust for desired thickness)

Instructions:

- Infuse Calendula and Chamomile in Oil:
  - Combine the dried calendula and chamomile flowers with the carrier oil in a double boiler.
  - Gently heat the mixture on low for 2-3 hours, allowing the herbs to infuse into the oil. Alternatively, place the herbs and oil in a jar and let them infuse in a sunny spot for 4-6 weeks.
  - Strain the oil through cheesecloth or a fine mesh strainer to remove the herb particles, retaining the infused oil.
- Prepare the Lotion:
  - Return the infused oil to the double boiler and add beeswax. Heat gently until the beeswax is fully melted, stirring well.
  - Remove from heat and let the mixture cool slightly. Before it begins to harden, whisk in the aloe vera gel until the mixture is smooth and homogeneous.
  - If the lotion is too thick, add more aloe vera gel. If it's too thin, you can return it to heat and add a bit more beeswax.
- Bottle the Lotion:
  - Once the lotion reaches your desired consistency, pour it into clean, sterilized jars or bottles.
  - Allow the lotion to cool completely before sealing with lids.

Usage:

- Apply the Calendula and Chamomile Skin Soothing Lotion to clean skin, focusing on areas that are dry, irritated, or inflamed.
- The lotion can be used daily, both morning and night.

What to Expect:

With regular application, you can expect to see a reduction in skin irritation, inflammation, and dryness. The combination of calendula, chamomile, and aloe vera works to soothe the skin, promote healing, and provide a barrier of moisture that protects against environmental stressors.

This natural lotion is suitable for all skin types, including sensitive skin. However, always do a patch test before using any new skincare product extensively, especially if you have allergies or sensitive skin.

This Calendula and Chamomile Skin Soothing Lotion offers a gentle, effective way to care for your skin, utilizing the powerful healing properties of natural ingredients to maintain healthy, soothed, and hydrated skin.

GREEN TEA AND HONEY FACIAL TONIC FOR ACNE.

The Green Tea and Honey Facial Tonic is a natural, antioxidant-rich remedy ideal for acne-prone skin. Green tea is celebrated for its anti-inflammatory and antimicrobial properties, which can help reduce acne breakouts and soothe irritated skin. Honey, known for its natural antibacterial and healing properties, aids in preventing acne while moisturizing and healing the skin. Together, they create a potent tonic that not only targets acne but also enhances skin health.

Ingredients:

- 1 cup water
- 1-2 green tea bags (or 1-2 teaspoons of loose-leaf green tea)
- 1 tablespoon raw honey

Instructions:

- Boil 1 cup of water and pour it over the green tea bag or loose-leaf green tea. Allow it to steep for 3-5 minutes for a strong infusion. If using loose-leaf tea, strain the leaves after steeping.
- Let the green tea cool to room temperature. Cooling is essential to avoid degrading the beneficial properties of honey when it's added.
- Once the tea is cool, remove the tea bag or strain the leaves, and mix in 1 tablespoon of raw honey until fully dissolved.
- Transfer the tonic to a clean, airtight container. A glass bottle with a spray nozzle or a simple jar works well.

Usage:

- To apply, soak a cotton pad with the Green Tea and Honey Facial Tonic and gently pat it onto cleansed skin, focusing on acne-prone areas. Alternatively, you can use a spray bottle to mist the tonic directly onto your face, then pat it in with clean hands.
- Allow the tonic to dry naturally on your skin before applying any other products.
- Use this tonic in the morning and evening after cleansing for the best results.

What to Expect:

With regular application, the Green Tea and Honey Facial Tonic can help reduce the severity and frequency of acne breakouts, soothe skin inflammation, and promote a clearer, more radiant complexion. The tonic's gentle formula makes it suitable for daily use and all skin types, including sensitive skin.

As with all skincare products, especially homemade ones, it's wise to conduct a patch test on a small skin area before full application to ensure no allergic reaction occurs.
Incorporating this natural tonic into your skincare routine can offer a simple, effective way to leverage the acne-fighting and skin-healing benefits of green tea and honey, leaving your skin healthy and glowing.

ALOE VERA AND CALENDULA GEL FOR SUNBURN.

The combination of aloe vera gel and calendula-infused oil creates a powerful, soothing gel ideal for treating sunburnt skin. Aloe vera is widely known for its cooling, healing, and anti-inflammatory properties, making it a go-to remedy for sunburn relief. Calendula, with its natural anti-inflammatory and skin-healing abilities, enhances the soothing effects of aloe vera, promoting faster skin recovery and reducing the risk of peeling.
Ingredients:

- 1/2 cup pure aloe vera gel
- 2 tablespoons calendula-infused oil

Instructions:

- Prepare Calendula-Infused Oil: (If you don't have pre-made calendula oil, you can create it by steeping dried calendula petals in a carrier oil like olive or almond oil for several weeks or gently heating for a few hours, then straining.)
- In a clean bowl, combine 1/2 cup of pure aloe vera gel with 2 tablespoons of calendula-infused oil. Ensure the aloe vera gel is as pure as possible, without added fragrances or alcohol, which can irritate sunburnt skin.
- Mix the aloe vera gel and calendula oil thoroughly until you achieve a smooth, homogeneous consistency.
- Transfer the mixture to a clean, airtight container for storage. A glass jar or a bottle with a pump dispenser works well.

Usage:

- Gently apply a generous amount of the Aloe Vera and Calendula Gel to the sunburnt areas of your skin. Reapply several times a day, as needed, to keep the skin hydrated and to soothe discomfort.
- For an extra cooling effect, you can refrigerate the gel before applying it to the skin.

What to Expect:
Using the Aloe Vera and Calendula Gel on sunburnt skin can provide immediate soothing relief, significantly reduce redness and inflammation, and help accelerate the healing process. The gel's moisturizing properties also help to prevent peeling and maintain skin hydration.

This natural remedy is gentle and suitable for all skin types. However, it's always a good idea to patch test a small amount of the gel on your skin before widespread use, especially if you have sensitive skin or allergies to plants. Incorporating this Aloe Vera and Calendula Gel into your after-sun care routine can effectively soothe and heal sunburnt skin, leveraging the natural healing powers of both aloe vera and calendula for faster recovery and relief.

YARROW AND WITCH HAZEL SKIN TONER.

The Yarrow and Witch Hazel Skin Toner is a natural and effective remedy, combining the astringent and healing properties of both yarrow and witch hazel. Yarrow, known for its ability to soothe and heal the skin, works alongside witch hazel, which tightens pores, reduces inflammation, and helps heal skin irritations. This toner is particularly beneficial for acne-prone and oily skin types, providing a gentle yet powerful solution for maintaining clear and healthy skin.

Ingredients:

- 1/2 cup dried yarrow flowers
- 1/2 cup witch hazel bark
- 2 cups distilled water

Instructions:

- Prepare the Infusion:
  - Combine the dried yarrow flowers and witch hazel bark in a saucepan.
  - Add 2 cups of distilled water to the saucepan and bring the mixture to a boil.
  - Once boiling, reduce the heat and allow the mixture to simmer gently for about 20-30 minutes. This process extracts the beneficial compounds from the yarrow and witch hazel.
  - After simmering, remove the saucepan from the heat and let the infusion cool to room temperature.
- Strain the Toner:
  - Use a fine mesh sieve or cheesecloth to strain the infusion, removing the solid parts. Ensure you capture the liquid, which is now your skin toner.
  - Transfer the strained toner into a clean, sterilized bottle. A bottle with a spray nozzle can be particularly convenient for application, but any airtight container will work.
- Application:
  - To use, apply the Yarrow and Witch Hazel Skin Toner to a clean cotton pad or ball.
  - Gently swipe across the face, focusing on areas prone to oiliness and acne. Avoid the delicate eye area.

- Allow the toner to dry naturally on your skin before applying moisturizer or other skincare products.

What to Expect:

Using the Yarrow and Witch Hazel Skin Toner regularly can lead to a noticeable improvement in skin tone and texture. Its astringent properties help reduce pore size and control excess oil, while its healing effects soothe redness and skin irritations, promoting a balanced and clear complexion.

This toner is gentle enough for daily use and can be incorporated into both morning and evening skincare routines. For those with sensitive skin, it's advisable to perform a patch test before widespread use to ensure compatibility.

With its natural ingredients and healing benefits, the Yarrow and Witch Hazel Skin Toner is an excellent addition to any skincare regimen, offering a simple and effective way to maintain healthy, vibrant skin.

BORAGE AND FLAXSEED OIL ECZEMA RELIEF BLEND.

Combining borage oil with flaxseed oil creates a powerful Eczema Relief Blend, leveraging the natural healing properties of both oils to soothe eczema and improve skin health. Borage oil, rich in gamma-linolenic acid (GLA), helps to reduce inflammation and moisturize the skin. Flaxseed oil, abundant in omega-3 fatty acids, further supports skin healing and reduces inflammation. Together, these oils offer a synergistic effect that can alleviate the discomfort associated with eczema and promote healthier skin.

Ingredients:

- 1 part borage oil
- 1 part flaxseed oil

Instructions:

- In a clean container, mix equal parts of borage oil and flaxseed oil. For example, combine 1 tablespoon of borage oil with 1 tablespoon of flaxseed oil.
- Shake or stir the mixture thoroughly to ensure the oils are well blended.
- Store the Eczema Relief Blend in a cool, dark place to preserve its potency.

Usage:

- Apply a small amount of the Borage and Flaxseed Oil Eczema Relief Blend to the affected areas of the skin. Gently massage it in until it is absorbed.
- Use the blend 2-3 times daily, especially after bathing while the skin is still damp, to lock in moisture.

- Consistent application over time is key to seeing improvements in skin condition and relief from eczema symptoms.

What to Expect:

With regular use, you may notice a reduction in the dryness, itching, and overall discomfort associated with eczema. The blend's moisturizing properties can help restore the skin's barrier, preventing further moisture loss and protecting against irritants.

While this natural remedy can be highly effective for many individuals, it's always a good idea to perform a patch test before widespread use, especially if you have sensitive skin or allergies. Additionally, consulting with a healthcare provider or dermatologist is advisable before starting any new topical treatment for eczema, particularly if you are currently using prescription medications or have severe eczema.

The Borage and Flaxseed Oil Eczema Relief Blend offers a gentle, natural option for managing eczema and supporting skin health, making it a valuable addition to your skincare routine.

SEA BUCKTHORN BERRY JUICE FOR SKIN AND OVERALL HEALTH.

Sea Buckthorn Berry Juice is a nutrient-packed beverage derived from the berries of the sea buckthorn plant. It's celebrated for its high content of vitamins, minerals, antioxidants, and omega fatty acids, which collectively support skin health and promote overall vitality.

Ingredients:

- Pure sea buckthorn berry juice (ready-to-drink or concentrate)

Instructions:

- If using sea buckthorn berry concentrate, dilute it according to the product's instructions, typically mixing with water or another juice for a palatable taste.
- Consume the prepared juice directly if you have the ready-to-drink variety.

What to Expect:

Regular consumption of Sea Buckthorn Berry Juice can significantly enhance skin health, thanks to its rich vitamin C and E content, which aid in collagen production and provide antioxidant protection. The omega-7 fatty acids present are particularly beneficial for maintaining skin hydration and elasticity. This juice supports immune function, reduces inflammation, and promotes healing, contributing to a state of well-being and enhanced energy levels.

COMFREY AND HONEY WOUND HEALING OINTMENT.

The Comfrey and Honey Wound Healing Ointment is a natural and effective remedy for treating minor wounds, cuts, and abrasions. Comfrey, known scientifically as Symphytum officinale, has been used historically for its rapid cell regeneration properties, making it excellent for healing. Honey adds antibacterial and anti-inflammatory benefits, further promoting the healing process. When combined with beeswax, these ingredients create a protective barrier that moisturizes, soothes, and accelerates the healing of the skin.

Ingredients:

- 1/2 cup comfrey leaf-infused oil (Prepare by infusing dried comfrey leaves in a carrier oil, such as olive or coconut oil, for several weeks or gently warming the leaves in oil over low heat for a few hours, then straining)
- 2 tablespoons beeswax pellets
- 1 tablespoon raw honey

Instructions:

- Prepare the Comfrey Leaf-Infused Oil: If not already prepared, infuse dried comfrey leaves in your choice of carrier oil, strain, and set aside 1/2 cup for this recipe.
- Melt the Beeswax: In a double boiler, gently melt 2 tablespoons of beeswax pellets. If you don't have a double boiler, you can use a heat-proof bowl over a pot of simmering water.
- Combine Ingredients: Once the beeswax is melted, add the 1/2 cup of comfrey leaf-infused oil to the double boiler and mix well. Remove from heat and quickly stir in 1 tablespoon of raw honey until fully incorporated.
- Pour Into Containers: While the mixture is still liquid, carefully pour it into clean, dry containers. Small tins, jars, or lip balm tubes work well, depending on your preference.
- Let it Solidify: Allow the ointment to cool and solidify at room temperature. This may take a few hours. Once solid, cap the containers.
- Label and Date: Label your containers with the contents and date made for future reference.

Usage:

- Clean the wound or cut thoroughly before application.
- Apply a small amount of the Comfrey and Honey Wound Healing Ointment to the affected area.
- Cover with a bandage if necessary.
- Reapply 2-3 times daily until the wound heals.

What to Expect:

You should notice accelerated healing of minor wounds and cuts, reduced inflammation, and minimized scarring thanks to the regenerative properties of comfrey and the antibacterial benefits of honey. The ointment also provides a moisture barrier, protecting the wound from further irritation.
Cautions:

- Comfrey should not be used on deep wounds or broken skin, as it can heal the top layer of skin too quickly, trapping bacteria.
- Always patch test before using a new topical product, especially if you have sensitive skin.
- Consult with a healthcare professional before using herbal remedies, particularly on children, pregnant or nursing women, or if you have existing health conditions.

This Comfrey and Honey Wound Healing Ointment is a valuable addition to your home first aid kit, offering a natural alternative for minor wound care.

Herbal Remedies for Hair and Scalp Health.

Rosemary and Nettle Hair Rinse for Hair Growth.

The Rosemary and Nettle Hair Rinse is a natural, herbal solution aimed at promoting hair growth and enhancing scalp health. Rosemary is widely recognized for its ability to stimulate blood circulation to the scalp, which encourages hair growth and strengthens hair roots. Nettle, rich in vitamins A and C, iron, and other minerals, nourishes the hair follicles and can help in reducing hair loss. Together, these herbs create a potent rinse that revitalizes the scalp and supports healthy hair growth.
Ingredients:

- 2 tablespoons dried rosemary leaves
- 2 tablespoons dried nettle leaves
- 1 liter (about 4 cups) boiling water

Instructions:

- Combine the dried rosemary and nettle leaves in a large heat-resistant bowl or pitcher.
- Pour the boiling water over the herbs, ensuring they are fully submerged.
- Cover and allow the mixture to steep for at least 30 minutes to an hour. This long steeping time allows for the maximum extraction of the beneficial compounds from the herbs.
- After steeping, strain the liquid to remove the herb particles, transferring the hair rinse into a clean container.
- Once cooled to a comfortable temperature, the rinse is ready for use.

Usage:

- After shampooing and conditioning your hair as usual, pour the Rosemary and Nettle Hair Rinse slowly over your scalp and hair as a final rinse. Massage the scalp gently to ensure the rinse is evenly distributed.
- You can choose to leave the rinse in your hair without rinsing it out for maximum benefits, or lightly rinse with cool water after a few minutes.
- Use this herbal rinse 1-2 times a week to support hair growth and scalp health.

What to Expect:

With regular use, you may notice an improvement in hair texture, a reduction in scalp issues such as dandruff, and an increase in hair growth over time. The natural properties of rosemary and nettle work together to stimulate the scalp, improve blood circulation, and provide essential nutrients to the hair follicles.

This herbal hair rinse is suitable for all hair types and is particularly beneficial for those experiencing thinning hair or looking to enhance their hair growth naturally. As it is made from natural ingredients, it is gentle on the scalp and unlikely to cause irritation.

Incorporating the Rosemary and Nettle Hair Rinse into your hair care routine is a simple and effective way to leverage the power of nature in promoting healthy, strong, and vibrant hair.

HORSETAIL SILICA RINSE FOR HAIR STRENGTHENING.

Horsetail Silica Rinse leverages the power of horsetail (Equisetum arvense), a plant known for its high silica content, to strengthen hair and improve its texture and shine. Silica is a vital mineral that contributes to the health and elasticity of hair, promoting stronger strands and reducing breakage. This natural rinse can be an excellent addition to your hair care routine if you're looking for ways to enhance hair vitality and resilience.

Ingredients:

- 1/4 cup dried horsetail herb
- 1 liter (about 4 cups) boiling water

Instructions:

- Place the dried horsetail herb in a large heat-resistant bowl or pot.
- Pour the boiling water over the horsetail, ensuring it's fully submerged.
- Cover the bowl or pot and let the horsetail infuse in the hot water for at least 1 hour, allowing all the silica and other beneficial compounds to be extracted.

- After steeping, strain the infusion to remove the horsetail herb, transferring the liquid to a clean container. Allow it to cool to room temperature or slightly warm, which is comfortable for application.

Usage:

- After shampooing (and conditioning, if that's part of your routine), pour the Horsetail Silica Rinse slowly over your scalp and hair as a final rinse. For ease of application, you might want to use a spray bottle or a cup.
- Massage the scalp gently and ensure that the rinse has been evenly distributed throughout your hair.
- You can choose to leave the rinse in your hair to dry naturally, maximizing the benefits of the silica and other nutrients absorbed by your hair and scalp.

What to Expect:

With regular use of the Horsetail Silica Rinse, you should notice an improvement in your hair's strength and elasticity. The high silica content in the horsetail helps fortify the hair strands from the inside out, promoting a reduction in hair breakage and split ends. Additionally, your hair may appear shinier and feel smoother due to the overall health boost provided by the rinse.

This rinse is suitable for all hair types and is especially beneficial for individuals experiencing brittle hair or those looking to enhance hair growth and health naturally. It's a gentle, chemical-free way to support hair health, making it a safe choice for regular use.

Incorporating the Horsetail Silica Rinse into your hair care regimen is a simple, effective way to harness the benefits of nature's own hair strengthening solution, promoting healthier, more resilient hair.

Herbal Remedies for Eye Health.

Bilberry Extract for Vision Support.

Bilberry Extract is derived from the fruit of the bilberry plant (Vaccinium myrtillus), closely related to blueberries and known for its high content of anthocyanins and antioxidants. These compounds are highly beneficial for eye health, particularly in supporting vision, improving night vision, and protecting against eye conditions related to oxidative stress and inflammation. Taking bilberry extract is a convenient way to supplement your diet with these potent antioxidants for enhanced vision support.

Usage:

- Follow the dosage instructions provided on the packaging of the commercially prepared bilberry extract. The recommended dosage can vary depending on the concentration of the extract.
- Bilberry supplements are often available in capsule or liquid form. Choose the form that best suits your preference and follow the manufacturer's instructions for use.

What to Expect:
Regular intake of Bilberry Extract can offer several benefits for eye health, including:

- Enhanced night vision and improved adaptation to darkness.
- Support for retinal health, which is crucial for maintaining sharp vision.
- Potential reduction in eye fatigue, especially for those who spend long hours in front of computer screens or engaged in activities that strain the eyes.
- Antioxidant protection against oxidative stress, which can contribute to the development of age-related eye diseases.

While Bilberry Extract is considered safe for most individuals, it's always a good idea to consult with a healthcare provider before starting any new supplement, especially if you have existing health conditions or are taking other medications. This is to ensure that the supplement won't interact with your medications or conditions.
Incorporating Bilberry Extract into your routine can be a simple and effective way to support overall eye health and maintain good vision. However, it's also important to follow a healthy lifestyle that includes a balanced diet rich in fruits and vegetables, regular eye check-ups, and proper eye care practices to support eye health comprehensively.

EYEBRIGHT TEA FOR EYE STRAIN.

Eyebright Tea, made from the dried herb Euphrasia officinalis, has been traditionally used for centuries to relieve eye strain and irritation. Eyebright contains natural compounds that are thought to have anti-inflammatory and astringent properties, making it beneficial for reducing redness, swelling, and discomfort associated with eye strain, as well as improving overall eye health.
Ingredients:

- 1-2 teaspoons dried eyebright herb
- 1 cup boiling water

Instructions for Drinking:

- Place 1-2 teaspoons of dried eyebright herb in a tea infuser or directly in a cup.
- Pour 1 cup of boiling water over the herb.

- Cover and allow it to steep for about 10-15 minutes. Covering the cup helps to retain the essential oils and medicinal properties of the herb.
- Strain the tea to remove the herb particles.
- You can drink eyebright tea 1-2 times daily to help relieve eye strain and support eye health.

Instructions for Eyewash:

- Follow the same steps as above to prepare the eyebright tea.
- Let the tea cool down to room temperature and ensure it is strained thoroughly to remove all herb particles to avoid any irritation when using it as an eyewash.
- To use the tea as an eyewash, you can use an eye cup or add a few drops to a clean cloth and gently apply it to the eyes.
- Ensure that any instrument used for the eyewash is sterilized to prevent infection.

What to Expect:

Using Eyebright Tea can provide relief from eye strain, particularly for those who spend long hours in front of computer screens or engaged in detailed work that tires the eyes. Drinking the tea can offer internal support for eye health, while using it as an eyewash can directly soothe and reduce external eye irritation and discomfort.

It's important to note that while Eyebright is generally considered safe, it's essential to ensure the highest quality of herb to avoid contamination. Additionally, if you have pre-existing eye conditions, allergies, or are pregnant or nursing, consult with a healthcare provider before using eyebright internally or externally.

Incorporating Eyebright Tea into your routine can be a natural and effective way to alleviate eye strain and support healthy vision. However, if symptoms persist or you experience significant eye discomfort, seeking advice from a healthcare professional or an eye care specialist is recommended.

EYEBRIGHT AND CHAMOMILE EYE WASH FOR EYE STRAIN.

Combining Eyebright and Chamomile into an eye wash creates a soothing, anti-inflammatory remedy that is ideal for relieving eye strain and irritation. Both herbs are renowned for their calming and healing properties. Eyebright (Euphrasia officinalis) has been traditionally used for eye-related issues, while Chamomile (Matricaria chamomilla) offers gentle relief for inflammation and discomfort, making this blend particularly effective for tired, strained, or irritated eyes.

Ingredients:

- 1 teaspoon dried Eyebright herb
- 1 teaspoon dried Chamomile flowers

- 1 cup boiled water

Instructions:

- Combine 1 teaspoon of dried Eyebright herb and 1 teaspoon of dried Chamomile flowers in a heat-resistant bowl or jar.
- Pour 1 cup of freshly boiled water over the herbs, ensuring they are fully submerged.
- Cover and allow the mixture to steep for about 10-15 minutes. This steeping time allows the therapeutic properties of the herbs to infuse into the water.
- After steeping, strain the mixture thoroughly using a fine mesh strainer or cheesecloth to remove all herb particles. It's crucial to ensure the liquid is completely free of any debris to avoid irritating the eyes.
- Allow the solution to cool to room temperature before using it as an eye wash.

Usage:

- To use the eye wash, you can use an eye cup or add a few drops to a clean cloth and gently apply it to the closed eyelids. Alternatively, you can dip a clean cloth in the solution and place it over your eyes as a compress.
- Ensure the solution is at a comfortable temperature before applying it to your eyes.
- Use the eye wash 1-2 times a day, especially after prolonged reading, computer work, or when experiencing eye discomfort.

What to Expect:

The Eyebright and Chamomile Eye Wash can provide immediate soothing relief for eye strain and irritation. With regular use, you may notice reduced redness, discomfort, and a refreshing feeling for tired eyes. This natural remedy supports healthy vision and can help alleviate symptoms associated with prolonged eye use, such as dryness and strain.

While this eye wash is gentle and safe for most people, it's always advisable to perform a patch test or consult with a healthcare provider before using new herbal remedies, especially if you have sensitive eyes or pre-existing eye conditions.

Incorporating this Eyebright and Chamomile Eye Wash into your eye care routine can offer a natural and effective way to maintain eye health and comfort, leveraging the soothing properties of these traditional herbs.

BILBERRY AND GOJI BERRY TEA FOR VISION SUPPORT.

Bilberry and Goji Berry Tea combines the powerful vision-supporting properties of bilberries with the nutrient-rich goji berries to create a potent herbal tea for eye health. Bilberries are well-known for their high content of anthocyanins, which can improve night vision and protect against eye conditions related to oxidative stress. Goji berries are packed with antioxidants, including zeaxanthin and lutein, which are crucial for protecting the eyes from damage caused by free radicals and enhancing visual acuity. Together, these berries offer a synergistic effect to support and maintain healthy vision.

Ingredients:

- 1 tablespoon dried bilberries
- 1 tablespoon dried goji berries
- 1 liter (about 4 cups) boiling water

Instructions:

- Combine the dried bilberries and goji berries in a large teapot or heat-resistant pitcher.
- Pour the boiling water over the berries, ensuring they are fully submerged.
- Cover and let the mixture steep for 10-15 minutes. The longer steeping time allows for a more potent extraction of the beneficial compounds from the berries.
- After steeping, strain the tea to remove the berry solids. The resulting liquid should have a deep, rich color, indicative of the nutrients and antioxidants leached from the berries.
- Serve the tea warm, or let it cool and enjoy it chilled. You can add a natural sweetener like honey or a slice of lemon for added flavor, if desired.

What to Expect:

Drinking Bilberry and Goji Berry Tea regularly can contribute to improved eye health and vision support. You may notice enhanced night vision, reduced eye strain, and overall improved visual acuity with consistent consumption. The antioxidants in the tea can also help protect the eyes from age-related conditions and damage from exposure to screens and environmental factors.

This herbal tea is a delightful and beneficial addition to your diet, especially if you are looking for natural ways to support your eye health. However, it's important to remember that while herbal teas can provide nutritional support, they should not replace medical treatments or regular eye examinations by a healthcare professional.

Integrating Bilberry and Goji Berry Tea into your daily routine can be a delicious and natural way to nourish your eyes and support your vision, alongside maintaining a balanced diet and healthy lifestyle for overall well-being.

Herbal Remedies for Oral Health.

Clove and Myrrh Mouthwash for Oral Hygiene.

Clove and Myrrh Mouthwash harnesses the natural antiseptic and analgesic properties of clove alongside the soothing, antibacterial effects of myrrh to create a potent herbal mouthwash. This combination is particularly effective in maintaining oral health, alleviating toothache, and preventing gum disease. Clove oil contains eugenol, a compound known for its pain-relieving properties, while myrrh has been used for centuries to treat mouth ulcers and inflamed gums.

Ingredients:

- 1 teaspoon ground cloves or 5-10 whole cloves
- 1 teaspoon myrrh resin or powder
- 1 cup water

Instructions:

- Prepare the Infusion:
    - In a small saucepan, combine 1 teaspoon of ground cloves (or 5-10 whole cloves) and 1 teaspoon of myrrh resin or powder with 1 cup of water.
    - Bring the mixture to a boil, then reduce the heat and simmer gently for 10-15 minutes, allowing the herbs to infuse the water.
    - Remove from heat and let the mixture cool to room temperature.
- Strain the Mouthwash:
    - Once cooled, strain the mouthwash through a fine mesh sieve or cheesecloth to remove the clove pieces and myrrh resin. Ensure all solid particles are removed to avoid irritation when using the mouthwash.
- Store the Mouthwash:
    - Transfer the strained mouthwash to a clean, airtight container. A glass bottle or jar is preferred to preserve the mouthwash's potency. Store it in a cool, dark place or in your refrigerator to extend its shelf life.

Usage:

- Use the Clove and Myrrh Mouthwash by swishing a small amount (about 1-2 tablespoons) in your mouth for 30 seconds to 1 minute, then spit it out. Do not swallow the mouthwash.
- For best results, use at least once or twice daily, especially after brushing your teeth or whenever you need relief from oral discomfort.

What to Expect:
Regular use of Clove and Myrrh Mouthwash can lead to improved oral hygiene, reduced gum inflammation, and alleviation of toothaches. The antiseptic properties of the ingredients help to kill harmful bacteria in the mouth, preventing plaque buildup, cavities, and gum disease.
While this homemade mouthwash is effective for oral health maintenance and natural pain relief, it's not a substitute for professional dental care. Continue with regular dental check-ups and consult with your dentist if you experience ongoing oral health issues.
This natural mouthwash offers a simple, effective way to support your oral hygiene routine with the healing power of herbs, providing a chemical-free alternative to commercial mouthwashes.

SAGE AND SEA SALT GARGLE FOR SORE THROATS.

The Sage and Sea Salt Gargle combines the antibacterial and anti-inflammatory properties of sage with the healing effects of sea salt to create a powerful remedy for soothing sore throats and oral inflammations. Sage has been traditionally used for its medicinal properties, including reducing inflammation and treating throat infections, while sea salt helps to reduce swelling, cleanse the throat, and accelerate healing.
Ingredients:

- 1 tablespoon dried sage leaves
- 1 cup boiling water
- 1 teaspoon sea salt

Instructions:

- Prepare the Sage Infusion:
    - Place 1 tablespoon of dried sage leaves in a heat-resistant bowl or cup.
    - Pour 1 cup of boiling water over the sage leaves.
    - Cover and allow the sage to steep for about 10-15 minutes to create a strong infusion.
    - Strain the sage infusion to remove the leaves, collecting the liquid in a clean container.
- Add Sea Salt:
    - While the sage infusion is still warm, add 1 teaspoon of sea salt.
    - Stir until the sea salt is completely dissolved in the sage infusion.
- Using the Gargle:
    - Allow the sage and sea salt mixture to cool to a comfortable temperature for gargling.

- Take a small sip of the mixture, tilt your head back, and gargle for 30 seconds to 1 minute, then spit it out.
- Repeat several times a day as needed, especially after meals and before bed, to soothe the sore throat and reduce inflammation.

What to Expect:

Using the Sage and Sea Salt Gargle can provide immediate relief from sore throat discomfort. The sage works to reduce inflammation and kill bacteria that can cause throat infections, while the sea salt helps to draw out infections, reduce swelling, and soothe irritated throat tissues.

This natural remedy is a simple and effective way to relieve sore throat symptoms and can be used in conjunction with other treatments to speed up the healing process. However, if your sore throat persists for more than a few days or is accompanied by other symptoms such as fever, it's important to seek medical advice.

Adding the Sage and Sea Salt Gargle into your self-care routine during times of throat discomfort offers a natural and holistic approach to health, utilizing the healing properties of simple kitchen ingredients to provide relief and support recovery.

CONCLUSION AND LAST WORD.

As we conclude "Over 350 Barbara O'Neill Inspired Herbal Healing Home Remedies & Natural Medicine: Volume 2," I extend my deepest gratitude and congratulations to you, the reader. Your dedication to exploring the depth of natural healing and integrating these remedies into your life is truly commendable. This volume, rich with over 300 detailed recipes and remedies, was crafted to serve not merely as a reference but as a constant companion on your journey toward holistic wellness. It stands as a testament to the belief that understanding and working with nature's gifts can profoundly impact our health and well-being.

This book was born out of the recognition that the wealth of knowledge stemming from Barbara O'Neill's teachings and the vast array of herbal remedies could not be confined to a single volume. By diving deeper into each remedy, we've provided a structured and comprehensive guide that ensures clarity and ease of use. It's designed for you to come back to time and again, whether to address a specific health concern or to find inspiration for maintaining overall wellness.

Your feedback is a cornerstone of this journey. It not only helps us refine and enhance the content but also joins us in a collaborative effort to share and spread this invaluable knowledge. We warmly invite you to share your experiences, insights, and suggestions, whether through a review on Amazon or direct communication via email. Each piece of feedback is a precious opportunity for growth, enabling us to incorporate your suggestions and enhance the content with each iteration.

As you continue to navigate through the world of herbal healing, remember that this book, and the knowledge it contains, is a resource meant to empower you. It encourages a personalized approach to health, reminding you to listen to your body and adapt remedies to fit your unique needs. This personalized journey is not just about physical health; it's about nurturing a deep and meaningful connection with the natural world, aligning with its rhythms for a more balanced and fulfilling life.

Thank you for allowing this volume to be a part of your journey. May it inspire you, guide you, and support you as you explore the rich landscape of herbal medicine. Here's to your health, wellness, and the continued exploration of the healing power of nature.

With heartfelt wishes for your journey ahead,

Margaret Willowbrook

INDEX

REFERENCES

1. **"The Herbal Apothecary: 100 Medicinal Herbs and How to Use Them"** by JJ Pursell (2015)

2. **"The Herbal Medicine-Maker's Handbook: A Home Manual"** by James Green (2000)

3. **"Making Plant Medicine"** by Richo Cech (2000)

4. **"The Complete Herbal Tutor"** by Anne McIntyre (2010)

5. **"Rosemary Gladstar's Medicinal Herbs: A Beginner's Guide"** by Rosemary Gladstar (2012)

6. **"Back To Eden"** by Jethro Kloss (1939)

7. **"Common Herbs for Natural Health"** by Juliette de Bairacli Levy (1974)

8. **"Complete Earth Medicine Handbook"** by Susanne Fischer-Rizzi (1996)

9. **"Herbal: 100 Herbs from the World's Healing Traditions"** by Mimi Prunella Hernandez (2021)

10. **"The Way of Herbs"** by Michael Tierra (1998)

11. **"Alchemy of Herbs"** by Rosalee de la Forêt (2017)

12. **"Herbal Recipes for Vibrant Health"** by Rosemary Gladstar (2008)

13. **Books and lectures** from Barbara O'Neill.

Bonus Page: Video Short Tutorials by Barbara O'Neill

Thank you for joining us on this journey through the world of herbal healing and natural medicine. To enrich your learning experience, we're thrilled to offer you exclusive access to a collection of video short tutorials featuring Barbara O'Neil. These tutorials, extracted directly from her lectures, provide practical, visual guidance on implementing the natural health practices discussed in this book.

By subscribing, you'll not only gain instant access to our current video library but also be updated with new videos as we continue to add to our collection. This is a fantastic way to stay connected with the latest in herbal healing and natural medicine, ensuring you're always equipped with the knowledge to support your wellness journey.

How to Access:

Simply scan the QR code below or follow the provided link to subscribe and unlock your access. This is our way of saying thank you and enhancing your journey toward holistic health with the invaluable wisdom of Barbara O'Neill.

@INFINITEWELLNESSWAVE

https://www.instagram.com/infinitewellnesswave

As new tutorials become available, you'll be the first to know, allowing you to continuously expand your understanding and application of natural health principles.

We hope these video tutorials serve as a valuable resource in your quest for wellness, bringing the teachings of Barbara O'Neill to life in a new and engaging way. Your feedback and suggestions are always welcome as we grow this library together.

A MESSAGE FROM THE PUBLISHER:

Are you enjoying the book? We would love to hear your thoughts!

Many readers do not know how hard reviews are to come by and how much they help a publisher. We would be incredibly grateful if you could take just a few seconds to write a brief review on Amazon, even if it's just a few sentences!

Please be aware that this is an ongoing project, and we are continuously improving the book's content thanks to your feedback. While it may not be perfect yet, your support greatly helps us!

Please go here to leave a quick review:

https://amazon.com/review/create-review?&asin=B0CSDCGZFK

We would greatly appreciate it if you could take the time to post your review of the book and share your thoughts with the community. If you have enjoyed the book, please let us know what you loved the most about it and if you would recommend it to others. Your feedback is valuable to us, and it helps us to improve our services and continue to offer high-quality literature to our readers.

Made in the USA
Columbia, SC
22 August 2024

78fedf9d-a885-4dc6-b36a-47d04eeba8adR01